NURSING PHOTOBOOK™

Helping Geriatric Patients

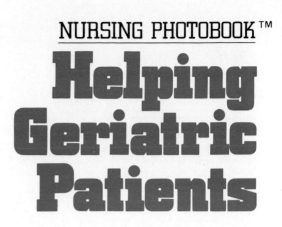

NURSING85 BOOKS™
SPRINGHOUSE CORPORATION
SPRINGHOUSE, PENNSYLVANIA

NURSING85 BOOKS™

NURSING PHOTOBOOK™ SERIES
Providing Respiratory Care
Managing I.V. Therapy
Dealing with Emergencies
Giving Medications
Assessing Your Patients
Using Monitors
Providing Early Mobility
Giving Cardiac Care
Performing GI Procedures
Implementing Urologic Procedures
Controlling Infection
Ensuring Intensive Care
Coping with Neurologic Disorders
Caring for Surgical Patients
Working with Orthopedic Patients
Nursing Pediatric Patients
Helping Geriatric Patients
Attending Ob/Gyn Patients
Aiding Ambulatory Patients
Carrying Out Special Procedures

NEW NURSING SKILLBOOK™ SERIES
Giving Emergency Care Competently
Monitoring Fluid and Electrolytes Precisely
Assessing Vital Functions Accurately
Coping with Neurologic Problems Proficiently
Reading EKGs Correctly
Combatting Cardiovascular Diseases Skillfully
Nursing Critically Ill Patients Confidently
Dealing with Death and Dying
Managing Diabetics Properly
Giving Cardiovascular Drugs Safely

NURSE'S REFERENCE LIBRARY®
Diseases
Diagnostics
Drugs
Assessment
Procedures
Definitions
Practices
Emergencies

NURSING NOW™ SERIES
Shock
Hypertension
Drug Interactions
Cardiac Crises
Respiratory Emergencies
Pain

NURSE'S CLINICAL LIBRARY™
Cardiovascular Disorders
Respiratory Disorders
Endocrine Disorders
Neurologic Disorders
Renal and Urologic Disorders
Gastrointestinal Disorders
Neoplastic Disorders
Immune Disorders
Infectious Disorders

Nursing85 **DRUG HANDBOOK™**

NURSING PHOTOBOOK™ Series

PROGRAM DIRECTOR
Jean Robinson

CLINICAL DIRECTOR
Barbara McVan, RN

ART DIRECTOR
Lisa A. Gilde

**Springhouse Corporation
Book Division**

CHAIRMAN
Eugene W. Jackson

PRESIDENT
Daniel L. Cheney

VICE-PRESIDENT AND DIRECTOR
Timothy B. King

VICE-PRESIDENT, BOOK OPERATIONS
Thomas A. Temple

VICE-PRESIDENT, PRODUCTION AND
PURCHASING
Bacil Guiley

Staff for this volume

BOOK EDITOR
Patricia K. Lawson

SENIOR CLINICAL EDITOR
Paulette J. Strauch, RN

CLINICAL EDITOR
Carol H. Best, RN, CNRN

ASSOCIATE EDITOR
Paul Vigna, Jr.

SPECIAL ASSIGNMENTS EDITORS
Katherine W. Carey
Patricia R. Urosevich

PHOTOGRAPHER
Paul A. Cohen

ASSOCIATE DESIGNERS
Linda Jovinelly Franklin
Scott M. Stephens
Carol Stickles

ASSISTANT PHOTOGRAPHER
Thom Staudenmayer

EDITORIAL/GRAPHIC COORDINATOR
Doreen K. Stowers

CLINICAL/GRAPHIC COORDINATOR
Evelyn M. James

COPY EDITOR
Sharyl D. Wolf

EDITORIAL STAFF ASSISTANT
Cynthia A. O'Connell

PHOTOGRAPHY ASSISTANT
Frank Margeson

ART PRODUCTION MANAGER
Robert Perry

ARTISTS
Lorraine Carbo
Virginia Crawford
Marsha Drummond
Donald G. Knauss
Robert H. Renn
George Retseck
Craig Siman
Sandra Simms
Louise Stamper
Joan Walsh
Robert Walsh
Ron Yablon

RESEARCHER
Vonda Heller

TYPOGRAPHY MANAGER
David C. Kosten

TYPOGRAPHY ASSISTANTS
Janice Haber
Ethel Halle
Diane Paluba
Nancy Wirs

PRODUCTION MANAGERS
Wilbur D. Davidson
Robert L. Dean, Jr.

PRODUCTION ASSISTANT
Terry Gallagher

ILLUSTRATORS
Michael Adams
ArtPeople
Dimitrios Bastas
John Dougherty
Ralph Giguere
Tom Herbert
Robert Jackson
Bob Jones
Eileen Rudisill
Bud Yingling

SERIES GRAPHIC DESIGNER
John C. Isely

COVER PHOTO
Photographic Illustrations

**Clinical consultants
for this volume**

Linda Blocker, RN, BSN, BA
Assistant Director of Nursing Service
Germantown Hospital and Medical Center
Philadelphia

Marion B. Dolan, RN
Executive Director
Newfound Area Nursing Association
Bristol, N.H.

Amended reprint, 1985
© 1982 by Springhouse Corporation,
1111 Bethlehem Pike, Springhouse, Pa. 19477
All rights reserved. Reproduction in whole or part by any means whatsoever without written permission of the publisher is prohibited by law.
Printed in the United States of America.

PB-040185

Library of Congress Cataloging in Publication Data

Main entry under title:

Helping geriatric patients.

(Nursing photobook)
"Nursing82 books."
Bibliography: p.
Includes index.
1. Geriatric nursing. I. Series.
RC954.H4   1982   610.73'65   82-11959
ISBN 0-916730-46-8

Contents

Contributors

At the time of original publication, these contributors held the following positions.

Susan P. Belding is a nursing supervisor with the Visiting Nurse Association of Eastern Montgomery County in Abington, Pennsylvania. She holds a BSN degree from Temple University in Philadelphia.

Linda Blocker, an advisor for this PHOTOBOOK, is assistant director of Nursing Service at Germantown Hospital and Medical Center in Philadelphia. She earned a BSN degree at Gwynedd-Mercy College, Gwynedd Valley, Pennsylvania, and a BA degree at Gordon College, Wenham, Massachusetts. Ms. Blocker is an MSN degree candidate specializing in adult health and aging at Pennsylvania State University in University Park, Pennsylvania.

Marion B. Dolan, an advisor for this PHOTOBOOK, is executive director of the Newfound Area Nursing Association in Bristol, New Hampshire. A diploma graduate of St. Mary's Hospital School of Nursing, she is studying health administration and planning at the University of New Hampshire in Durham. Ms. Dolan is a member of Hospice Affiliates of New Hampshire and the National League for Nursing. She is president-elect of the New Hampshire National League for Nursing.

Mary P. Farmer is an assistant professor in the Hahnemann Medical College and Hospital A.D. nursing program in Philadelphia. She holds a nursing diploma from Fitzgerald-Mercy Hospital School of Nursing in Darby, Pennsylvania, and a BSN degree from Villanova (Pa.) University. In addition, she earned an MAEd degree at St. Joseph University in Philadelphia. Ms. Farmer is a member of the American Nurses' Association and the Gerontological Society.

Sharyn Q. Figgins, an oncology nurse at Mercy Hospital in Cedar Rapids, Missouri, is a BSN degree graduate of the University of Maryland, Baltimore. Ms. Figgins holds memberships in the Oncology Nursing Society, the American Nurses' Association, and the Iowa Nurses' Association.

Sister Angela Fox, SSJ, is an aide at the adult day care center of St. Joseph's Villa in Flourtown, Pennsylvania. She earned a BSEd degree at Villanova (Pa.) University.

Marilyn D. Harris is executive director of the Visiting Nurse Association of Eastern Montgomery County, Abington, Pennsylvania. A diploma graduate of Abington (Pa.) Memorial Hospital School of Nursing, Ms. Harris earned both BSN and MSN degrees at the University of Pennsylvania, Philadelphia.

Kay C. Heiss is employed as a staff RN and visiting nurse by the Visiting Nurse Association of Eastern Montgomery County in Abington, Pennsylvania. She earned a nursing diploma at Philadelphia's Lankenau Hospital School of Nursing and a BS degree at Southern Connecticut State College in New Haven, Connecticut.

Sister Rose Josepha is the nurse coordinator of the adult day care center at St. Joseph's Villa in Flourtown, Pennsylvania. She is a diploma graduate of St. Joseph's Hospital School of Nursing in Philadelphia.

Sister Leona Killian works as a licensed physical therapist at St. Joseph's Villa in Flourtown, Pennsylvania. She holds a certificate degree in physical therapy from Hahnemann Medical College and Hospital in Philadelphia, as well as a BS degree in biology from Chestnut Hill College, also in Philadelphia. Sister Leona is a member of the American Physical Therapy Association's section on geriatrics.

Sister Rose Michele, SSJ, is director of the inservice program for orienting nurses and training new aides at St. Joseph's Villa, Flourtown, Pennsylvania, and is also head nurse of residents there. Sister Rose earned a BSN degree at Our Lady of the Angels College in Aston, Pennsylvania.

Theresa M. Rager is a nursing supervisor with the Visiting Nurse Association of Eastern Montgomery County in Abington, Pennsylvania, and a BSN degree graduate of Pennsylvania State University in University Park.

Sister St. Gregory directs the adult day care program of St. Joseph's Villa in Flourtown, Pennsylvania. She holds a BS degree in education from Chestnut Hill College in Philadelphia and completed a certificate program in gerontology at College Misericordia in Dallas, Pennsylvania. She is a member of the Gerontological Society of America and the National Council on the Aging. She is also a member of Alzheimer's Disease and Related Disorders Association.

Mary Beth Tittle, an adult advanced registered nurse practitioner, is an instructor at the University of Florida's College of Nursing, Gainesville. She holds an MSN degree and a certificate in gerontology from the University of Florida. Ms. Tittle holds memberships in both Sigma Theta Tau and Phi Kappa Phi.

Introduction

What does geriatric nursing mean to you? If you haven't worked with many geriatric patients, you may have a number of misconceptions about them. And you may not fully understand the kind of nursing care they'll require—both in terms of general approach and specific procedures. If so, this PHOTOBOOK is just the preparation you need.

Our first section focuses on the patient. It describes the aging process in detail—and shows you the most positive way to guide your patient through it. In addition, it gives you specifics on physical aging changes, to help you distinguish normal changes from disease processes.

Now, consider the care your patient's body systems require *because* of aging. We devote the book's next four sections to procedures commonly performed in geriatric nursing. Note the accent on preventive procedures, so you can use your skills to help avoid problems stemming from aging changes. In addition, we emphasize self-care, to help your patient stay active and independent. You'll find page after page of patient-teaching information, as well as home care aids.

In the second section, we cover such basics as daily hygiene and skin care. And we give special attention to joint problems, because so many older people have them. In the third section we give guidelines for oxygen administration in the home and introduce you to the latest equipment. In addition, we describe step-by-step rehabilitative care for a patient who's had a stroke. Declining appetite and changing lifestyle can lead your patient to neglect nutrition—the foundation of good health. Read the fourth section to learn how to give a thorough nutritional assessment and correct any problems. You'll also find simple—yet effective—measures to promote good bowel and urinary function. In the fifth section you'll learn about cataract surgery as well as contact lenses for geriatric patients. We'll also describe different hearing aid models and give detailed maintenance and trouble-shooting instructions.

Feel like you have a good grasp of the basic nursing care involved? Then, round out your knowledge by reading the sixth section. Here, we discuss ways to help your patient maintain an independent lifestyle. For example, you can teach him how to adapt his home for his safety and comfort and how to make use of services available in the community. However, living in a nursing home may eventually become necessary for your patient. We tell you how to help him and his family make the wisest possible choice. Finally, if you're caring for a dying geriatric patient, you'll find the information on hospice care helpful in coping sensitively with this life phase.

But don't stop here. This brief summary must have sparked a dozen questions in your mind about each topic we've discussed. If so, look for the answers in the text, illustrations, photos, and charts in the pages of this book.

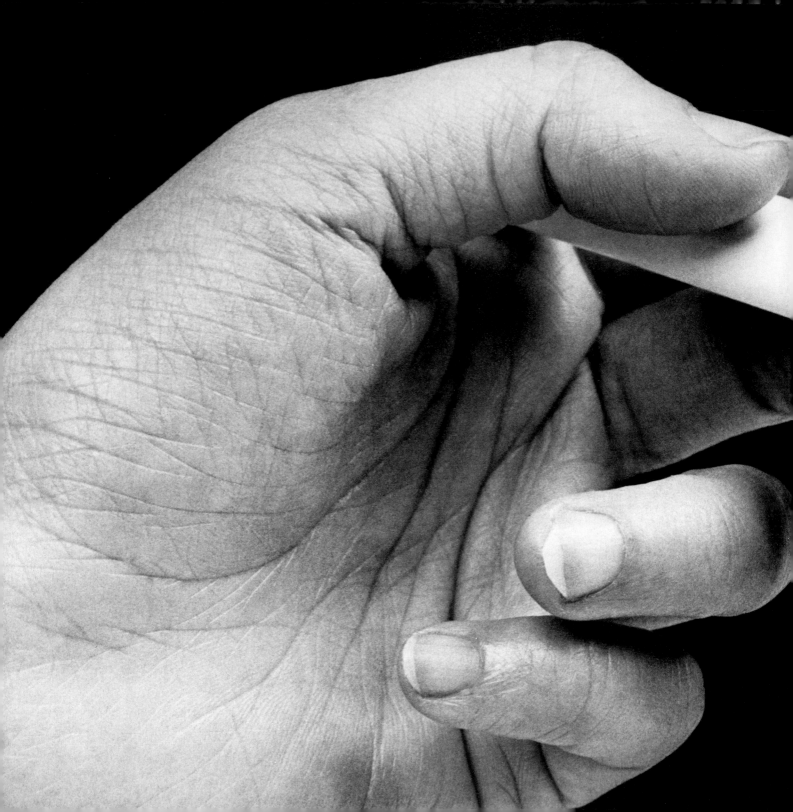

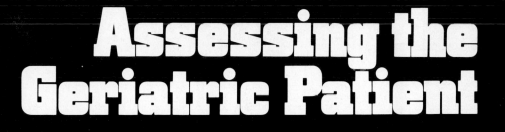

Assessing the Geriatric Patient

Aging considerations

Assessment

Aging considerations

Who is the geriatric patient? In the next few pages, we'll introduce you to him. He is, after all, a very special patient who requires all the dedicated personal attention you can give. Why? Because he's in a phase of his life cycle where his body functions are slowing—and perhaps declining—so he needs both preventive health care and conscientious nursing care when he's ill.

Read the following pages to learn more about your geriatric patient, how society views him, and how he views himself. Find out why he benefits from a strong positive approach. Then, study the general guidelines we give you for conducting your day-to-day patient care.

Aging considerations

How well do you understand the aging process? Did you realize that aging isn't simply a set of physiologic changes? Rather, it's the *total* physical, intellectual, and developmental experience that adults live out until death. Aging occurs at a different rate in each individual, but almost all people eventually experience certain changes. The physical component of aging includes changes in general appearance (such as wrinkling, stooping posture, and graying hair); diminished sensory function (such as hearing and vision loss); decreased body system function (for example, lowered respiratory capacity); and vulnerability to diseases (such as arthritis, diabetes, and cardiovascular disease).

Intellectual changes may include decreased reaction time, or impaired short-term memory. *Social or developmental* changes may include retirement and adjustment to a new set of daily activities; loss of spouse, friends, or family; change in lifestyle or environment; and preparation for death.

Perhaps most of the aging changes mentioned sound negative. However, a number of positive changes occur as well, such as having more free time to pursue personal interests. The text on page 10 refutes some common misconceptions about aging. Also, you can help your patient prevent or control negative changes through diet, exercise, and social activity.

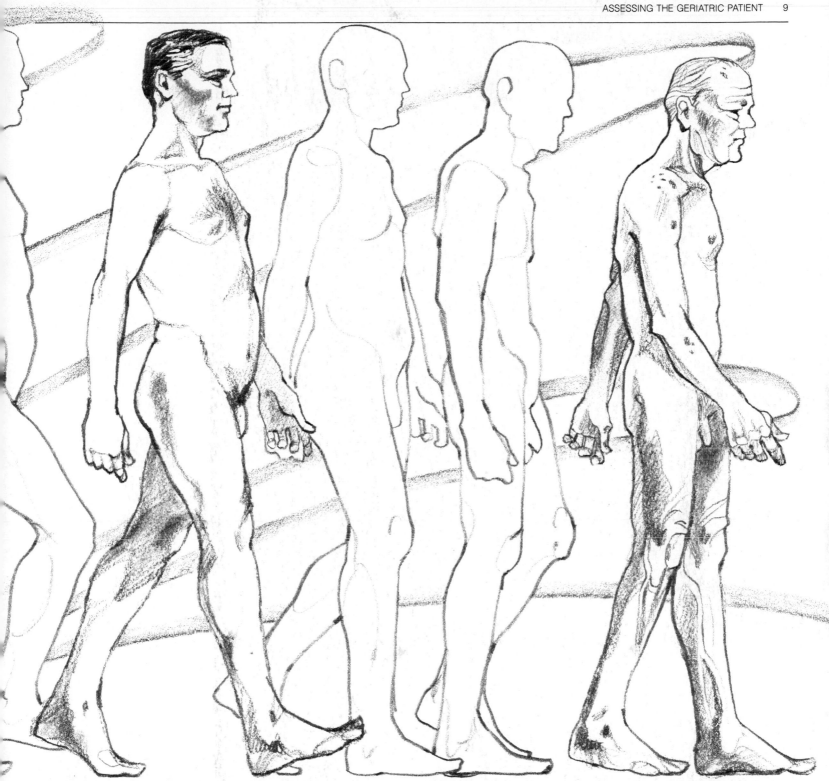

At what age is your patient considered a geriatric patient? Most health-care professionals agree on age 65. But remember, you're caring for an individual patient, not an age-group. Chronologic age (age in years) and physiologic age (age which reflects biologic changes in cells and tissues) can be two very different things. A 65-year-old may have relatively smooth skin and erect posture, while a 50-year-old may be wrinkled and stooped. Of course, your patient's birth date gives you his chronologic age. However, you'll evaluate his physiologic age by checking such factors as appearance, visual and hearing keenness, basal metabolism, and lung function. Because your patient's physiologic age determines his health, life span, and ability to tolerate stresses such as surgery or disease, your care plan should be based on it.

Perhaps you're wondering *why* your geriatric patient ages. A number of theories attempt to explain aging in terms of evolution, genetics, or stress, to name a few approaches. Evolutionary theory proposes that the human life span is keyed to allow optimum reproduction of the species. Genetic theory proposes that genes are programmed for a given life span. Stress theories maintain that repeated use over a lifetime exhausts cells and tissues. Other biological theories focus on cell waste accumulation, DNA linkages, limits to cell reproduction, and autoimmune responses.

Aging considerations

Common misconceptions about aging

Contemporary society tends to view aging negatively. Young people may find older people strange or unappealing. Middle-aged people may fear their own aging, which they see manifested in the elderly. Even older people may share mistaken notions about aging.

You'll probably confront such attitudes in your patient's family and friends, other staff members, your patient, and perhaps even yourself. Maybe you know a staff member on your unit who avoids geriatric patients or gives them only hasty, impersonal care.

If you're caring for a geriatric patient, you'll have to resist this stereotyping. You must teach everyone who comes in contact with him that he needs a positive approach for optimum well-being.

Remember: Social conditioning can cause many psychological aging symptoms. If you *expect* erratic or impaired behavior from a patient, he'll be much more likely to exhibit it.

Here are some common misconceptions concerning the elderly:
• *Most older adults suffer extreme unhappiness.* Actually, how happy or sad older people feel generally reflects their temperament during youth.
• *Most older adults are senile or psychotic.* Actually, researchers estimate that only about 5% are psychotic or have severe intellectual impairment. About 20% have measurable memory impairment. About 20% have some sort of psychological disorder (ranging from mild neurosis to psychosis).
• *Older adults are incompetent.* Although older people may have slowed reaction time and take longer to perform certain tasks requiring psychomotor skills, older workers have more consistent output, less job turnover, fewer accidents, and less absenteeism.
• *Most older adults need help with everyday activities because of poor health.* Although certain degenerative changes and diseases afflict older people, about 80% can maintain a functional lifestyle. Only about 5% are institutionalized, and only about 15% have a handicapping chronic health problem.
• *Older adults isolate themselves socially.* Actually, most maintain close relationships with relatives or friends and stay active in community life. The majority live within one-half hour travel time of one of their children. However, many researchers feel that loneliness *is* the major mental health problem of the elderly.

Though no one would deny that older adults face many difficulties, they also have some distinct advantages. Instead of resenting retirement, most can appreciate relief from workday pressures and anxieties, while still receiving some form of income (although their income may be fixed). Instead of regretting loss of a job, they can appreciate new freedom to pursue long-neglected personal interests. Instead of feeling behind the times, they can rest secure in stable value systems developed from real-life experience. Instead of lapsing into helplessness, they can use the good judgment developed from long experience to pursue constructive lives. These more positive attitudes allow them to view old age as another phase of the life cycle, with its own opportunities for growth and happiness, *not* as an unfortunate decline.

General guidelines for geriatric patient care

You may be caring for a geriatric patient in a variety of settings: the hospital, his home, a boarding home, a day-care center, or a nursing home. Because your elderly patient functions better both mentally and physically in familiar surroundings, try to arrange medical care for him in the home or community, rather than in an institutional setting. Of course, some acute problems require patient hospitalization.

How can you provide constructive geriatric patient care? Educate the health team that cares for your patient to view him as an *individual* rather than labeling him as a geriatric patient with stereotypical problems. Also, to help prevent mental and physical pathology, foster a *wellness* approach. People who stay healthy into their eighties usually remain active physically, intellectually, and socially.

Your patient requires special attention in the following areas.

Adequate nutrition allows optimum physical and mental function (see fourth section). Older adults may neglect nutrition from ignorance of its importance, worry over expense, lack of appetite, poor dental health, cultural factors, or aversion to eating alone.

Rest and relaxation includes adequate sleep as well as relaxing activities, such as hobbies, meditation, and biofeedback. Sleep should fulfill the person's individual requirements rather than a rigid 8-hours-per-night schedule (see page 14).

Exercise improves circulation, increases oxygenation, and reduces muscle pain. Morning exercise helps correct joint stiffness, and evening exercise relaxes a person to promote restful sleep (see page 58).

Preventive medical care, such as regular blood pressure screenings, Pap smears, eye tests, and general check-ups, helps avoid the escalation of small problems into life-threatening ones and facilitates early treatment of serious conditions.

Dental care and good oral hygiene help the patient retain his teeth and avoid the reduced self-esteem and discomfort associated with losing them (see pages 31 and 32).

Positive mental attitudes help retard the aging process. They stem from:
• *Personal independence.* Encourage self-care in dressing, feeding, and bathing.
• *Control over environment.* If possible, encourage living at home rather than in an institution.
• *Social interaction.* Encourage letters, phone calls, and visits. Older people need to foster social skills for establishing contact with other people, exercise empathy to deepen relationships, and experience physical touch through handshaking, hugging, kissing, and dancing. They need to strengthen social bonds by sharing experiences and possessions. Understand that your geriatric patient may participate less actively in social situations. He may tend to sit and observe rather than dominate a conversation. But, this level of involvement can fulfill his needs.
• *Accentuating the positive.* Encourage him to express enjoyment and recall happy occasions. Allow your patient to relive past accomplishments. It will help him view himself positively and help you learn more about him.
• *Mental stimulation.* Encourage continuing education and development of new talents. Senior citizen group activities and travel can help him maintain interest in life. Remind older patients that forgetting happens to younger as well as older people, and intelligence doesn't necessarily decline with age.

Pleasant, considerate daily contact helps preserve your patient's self-esteem. Observe the following guidelines:
• Maintain a primary care relationship with your patient.
• Reduce anxiety by explaining procedures thoroughly. Provide

constant reassurance.
- When you leave your patient, let him know when you'll return.
- Use touch to establish rapport, unless your patient objects to it.
- When you talk to your patient, face him so he can see your lips and eyes. (See the positions recommended for communication below.)
- Pay special attention to nonverbal communication.
- Don't exceed your patient's attention span or physical limitations.
- Involve family members in patient care as much as possible.
- Respect your patient's privacy.

For your patient in bed: Position her comfortably with the head of the bed elevated. Make sure she can see your lips and eyes.

For your hard-of-hearing, vision-impaired, or sensorily deprived patient in bed: Position her comfortably, so she's facing you. Bring your face very close to hers. Use touch as appropriate.

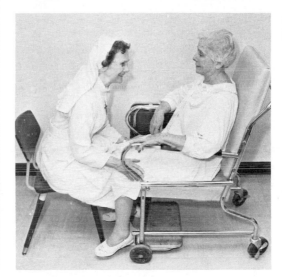

For your hard-of-hearing, vision-impaired, or sensorily deprived patient in a chair: Move very close to her. Face her frontally and put your knees between her knees to establish physical contact. Use touch as appropriate.

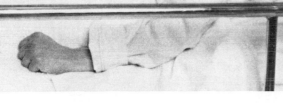

For your patient in a wheelchair: Position yourself to one side rather than directly in front of her, to bring you closer.

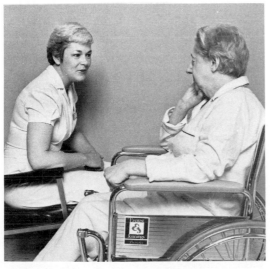

For your patient who's withdrawn: Sit on a footstool in front of your patient, to bring your head below or to the same level as his. He'll probably find this position less threatening. Be cautious about touching him; he may object to it.

Assessment

Are you ready to assess your geriatric patient? Of course, your first step is to take a comprehensive nursing history. To assist you, we'll give you special interviewing techniques to use with your geriatric patient which will help elicit the greatest amount of information.

You probably already know what a general history should include. But, we'll show you how to slant your questions to detect an *older* person's problems. For example, you must question your patient closely about his nutrition and sleep habits. Also, you should pay particular attention to the psychological component of your history, to determine whether your patient needs help coping with life crises.

Finally, to help you perform an accurate physical assessment, we've provided an illustrated chart of the typical aging changes you can expect to see, as well as some problems your aging patient might develop.

Taking a history

Victoria Redburn, a 65-year-old laboratory worker, has been admitted to the hospital for hypertension. Taking a history from an older adult requires special sensitivity. These guidelines should help you approach your patient properly.

• Create a comfortable environment, whether you perform the assessment at a community center, at the hospital, or at home. Consider using increased illumination (without glare) to help compensate if your patient has poor vision. Also, provide privacy for your patient. If she's uncomfortable with family members present, you may need to have them leave the room. (But remember, you may need to ask them questions your patient can't answer, so make sure they stay close by.)

• Begin your history by making general observations from the first moment you see your patient. Is she heavy, thin, or of average weight? Does she appear healthy and energetic, or ill and fatigued? Is her breathing labored? Does she seem to be in pain? Does she seem comfortable or ill-at-ease? Note her skin color, posture, gait, grooming, and any significant odors. As you shake hands, note her skin temperature and her strength.

• Address your patient in respectful terms. She may prefer that you call her Mrs. Redburn rather than Victoria. Be sure to ask her preference.

• Position your patient comfortably so she's facing you. Now, begin your assessment, using the format we outline at right under *Assessment areas.*

• Phrase your questions simply, addressing only one point at a time. Your patient may have hearing loss, so face her directly, letting her see your lips and eyes clearly. (See suggested communication positions on page 11.) Enunciate carefully to help her lip-read. For severe hearing loss, you may need to use electronic amplifying equipment. *Important: Never* shout at your patient. Doing so ob-

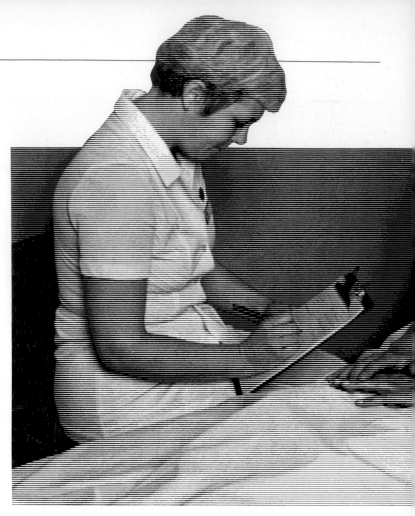

scures consonants and amplifies only the vowels, so it won't help your patient understand you. If necessary, communicate in writing. If you do, remember to make sure your patient can read, and that she's wearing glasses, if she uses them.

• Allow your patient plenty of time to respond. Her reaction time may be slower than a younger person's. Try to adapt to her pace. If you need more time to conduct a thorough interview, consider scheduling a second session. *Remember:* You need to cover *all* areas mentioned here, but not necessarily in one session. Also, keep in mind that assessment is an ongoing process.

• As you talk to your patient, observe her facial expressions, mood, speech, and orientation level. Don't underestimate her intelligence; chances are, it hasn't declined at all. Verbal function doesn't show any significant decrease with age, although short-term memory may decline. However, if you *do* perceive memory or learning disorders, be sure to repeat questions, instructions, and

explanations, if needed.

To assess orientation, use the guidelines on page 14. If your patient's extremely confused, obtain a history from a relative or somebody who knows her well. Presence of a family member or friend during the physical assessment may have a calming effect on the patient. Also, explicitly describe each action *just before* and *as* you perform it. If your patient shows signs of hunger, give her a snack. If she needs to go to the bathroom, don't make her wait. Remember, because of her confusion, she may have very little control over her needs and impulses.

Important: Keep in mind that you could mistake confusion, disorientation, memory loss, slowed reaction time, or anxiety from alcohol or drugs for physiological mental dysfunction.

• Try to establish rapport with your patient. Remember, your older patient may hesitate to give her history, because she doesn't want her fears of poor health confirmed. Also, she may feel that your questions about lifestyle and family are intrusive.

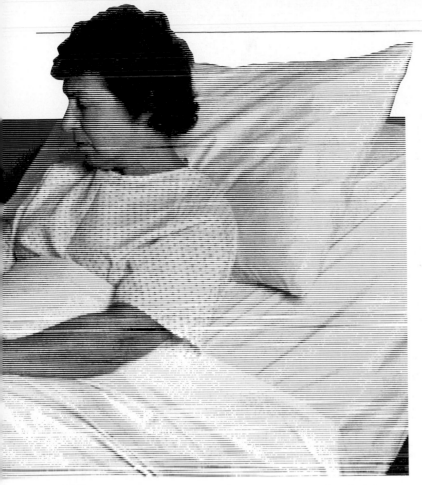

Assessment areas

Now you understand the special approach your geriatric patient requires. But what specific information should you obtain from her? Be sure to cover these basics:

• *Reason for visit.* Ask your patient why she's in the hospital. Have her describe any signs and symptoms and give the approximate date of occurrence, what she was doing at the time, whether the onset was gradual or sudden, and how long the sign or symptom lasted. Be aware that older people often have *multiple* health problems, rather than just one.

• *Family history.* Find out the health history of her immediate family; for example, her father, mother, siblings, children, and grandparents. Identify any diseases they have, and ask about causes of death. This information may reveal tendencies toward diabetes mellitus or cardiovascular disease, for example. Also, a family history will provide information about your patient's support system.

• *Personal history.* Obtain some basic statistics about your patient, such as her height, weight, date of her birth, and education. Tactfully inquire about her economic resources and financial management. Ask about her living environment. Does she live with her family or alone? Has she lived at her present residence long? In what kind of neighborhood and housing does she live? For example, does she live in a house or in a high-rise?

Also, ask about her daily routine. When does she usually get up, and how does she spend a typical day? Does she do her own housework? Her own shopping? Does she participate in any group or community activities? Does she get regular exercise? When does she usually go to bed? (To find out about her sleeping habits, use the assessment tool on page 14.)

Certain areas of your patient's personal history deserve special attention. She may have psychological problems, problems with alcohol, or sexual concerns. If your patient seems withdrawn or depressed, make a special effort to detect suicidal tendencies. (For detailed information on assessing these areas, see pages 14 to 17.)

• *Medication history.* Find out what medications your patient's taking. For each drug, ask its name, dose, route of administration, how often she is to take it, who administers it, and what your patient knows about the medication. If she doesn't know the name of the medication, ask her to describe its color, shape, and purpose. Find out if she takes her medication as often as prescribed.

Because your older patient metabolizes medication differently (from slowed metabolism and decreased liver and kidney function) she may be more vulnerable to drug reactions. Also, since she may take a number of different drugs, she has a greater chance of adverse interactions.

Be sure to ask about any *unprescribed* medication your patient's taking, including vitamins, cough syrups, or tonics. Frequently misused medications include laxatives and enemas (which may lead to potassium deficiency or malnourishment), tranquilizers, and sleeping medications. If your patient has alcohol problems, alcohol-based medication, such as some liquid cold medications, may compound her problem.

Finally, don't forget to ask about medication the doctor ordered, but the patient has stopped taking without the doctor knowing or which she refuses to take.

• *Nutritional status.* Ask your patient to describe her eating habits in detail. Does she eat three meals each day? What does she eat for each meal? How much liquid does she drink each day? In what form (coffee, tea, soda, water, or liquid or soft foods)? Does she have any culturally based food preferences? Is she on a special diet; for example, a low-cholesterol, low-sodium diet? Does she normally eat only soft food, because of chewing problems?

Does she take supplemental vitamins or minerals? Does she shop for herself, or does someone shop for her? Who prepares her meals? With whom does she eat?

• *Bowel habits.* Does she have regular bowel movements, or is she frequently constipated? What time of day does she have a bowel movement? What is the color and consistency of the stool? Does she use laxatives, suppositories, or enemas? Has she had any recent change in bowel habits? What was the date, time, and appearance of her most recent bowel movement?

• *Urinary patterns.* When she urinates, does she feel as though she's completely emptied her bladder, or as though she still needs to go? Does she have any burning, pain, or bleeding when urinating? Does she have urinary frequency? Does she get up at night to urinate? Has she ever had a urinary tract infection?

• *Past medical history.* Ask your patient about any diseases (including childhood illnesses), previous hospitalizations, diagnostic tests, and immunizations. Your patient may not remember every medical problem she's had in her life, but she'll probably remember the most important ones.

• *Body systems review.* Finally, review each body system listed in the physical assessment chart on pages 18 to 27. Ask your patient about any signs and symptoms or changes she's noted. For each one, ask for the date and circumstances of occurrence. Have your patient locate the sign or symptom anatomically. If she has pain, ask her to describe pain type and intensity. (Remember, however, that an older patient may have diminished deep-pain sensation.) Also, be sure to ask if she's had previous treatment for this problem.

Document *all* the data your patient provides; you can sift through it later to determine whether it's relevant.

Assessment

Assessing your patient's orientation level

If you suspect your patient's confused or disoriented, perform the following reality check. Keep in mind that his confusion has a number of possible causes, such as drug reactions, alcohol, malnutrition, or mental dysfunction from organic brain syndrome. So, don't jump to any conclusions. Instead, try to gather enough information in your overall history and physical assessment to help determine the cause. Also, be sure to take into consideration any hearing or vision problems, aphasia, dysarthria, or language barrier.

To test orientation, ask your patient:
• What's your name?
• Do you know who I am?
• Where are you now?
• What day of the week is it? (If necessary, ask, "Is it Monday? Is it Tuesday?")
• What's the date? (Again, you may suggest dates.)
• What year is it?

To test your patient's memory, ask him the following questions:
• *(For distant memory)* Where were you born? In what year?
• *(For recent memory)* What did you have for breakfast today? Where were you yesterday?
• *(For immediate memory)* Remember the numbers 3, 5, and 9. I'll ask you to repeat them to me in a few minutes. (A few minutes later)—What numbers did I ask you?

Note: You must obtain the correct answers to the questions assessing distant and recent memory, either from your patient's history or by asking other staff members.

Other questions that will help reveal mental function include:
• *(For arithmetic)* How much is 100 minus 50? Can you count from 1 to 10?
• *(For judgment)* If you're alone at night, how can you get help?
• *(For emotions)* Do you ever cry? How often? Would you describe yourself as a happy person? Do you ever see or hear anything out of the ordinary?

If your patient answers a number of these questions incorrectly or inappropriately, notify the doctor. (Also, see the fifth section for guidelines on orienting techniques.)

Understanding sleep requirements

As a person ages, his sleep patterns change and his sleep requirements diminish. As you can see from the chart at right, an older person will get less deep, stage 4 sleep and more stage 2 and 3 sleep. And, he'll probably get less REM (rapid-eye-movement) sleep, the type necessary for mental well-being. (REM sleep is indicated in black on chart.) An older person usually sleeps fitfully and awakens very easily from leg cramps, nightmares, the need to urinate, or noises.

Always include a sleep assessment in your nursing history. Ask your patient:
• What time do you go to bed at night? Do you nap during the day?
• What bedtime rituals, such as reading, snacking, or watching TV, do you have?
• What medication do you take at bedtime? Do you take any sleep medications?
• What's your most comfortable position in bed?
• In what room temperature, ventilation, and lighting do you like to sleep?
• How well do you sleep?
• How often do you wake up at night?
• What time do you get up in the morning?
• How much do you exercise?

Although sleep patterns change and sleep requirements diminish with aging, your geriatric patient needs a certain amount of uninterrupted sleep. But, don't automatically obtain an order for sedatives for the patient who sleeps poorly. Medication may interfere with the REM stages of sleep, even though your patient appears to be sleeping soundly. Instead, try to recreate his optimum sleeping conditions. Sometimes, simple observance of bedtime rituals can help him sleep well. If your patient does wake up before morning, encourage him to perform some restful activity until he feels tired, rather than lying awake worrying about his inability to sleep. Or, as an alternative to sleeping all night long, your patient may develop a napping pattern that gives him adequate rest.

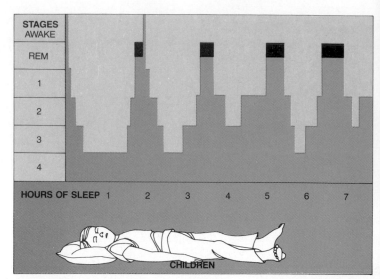

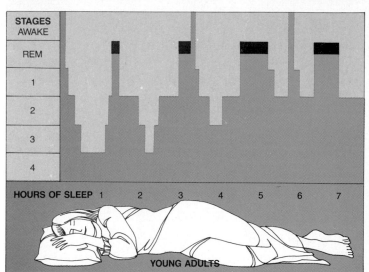

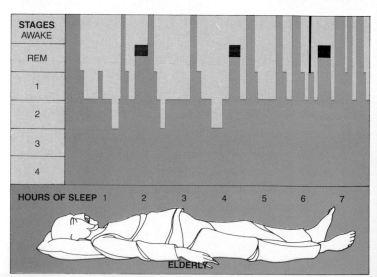

Reprinted by permission from Kales, A., and J.D. Kales. *Sleep Disorders*, NEW ENGLAND JOURNAL OF MEDICINE, 290:487, 1974.

Understanding your patient's sexual needs

Perhaps you're reluctant to consider your geriatric patient's sexuality. Many people feel that age makes a person physiologically incapable of performing sexual intercourse, or that sexual activity could physically harm him. But, these concerns have little basis in fact. True, with increasing age, male testosterone levels gradually decline. And after menopause, women may experience vaginal changes. Also, each phase of the sex act takes longer for an older adult to perform. Although these physical changes can affect sexual function or enjoyment to some extent, they don't rule out satisfying sexual activity.

In many cases, older people maintain a level of sexual activity that correlates with their activity in young adulthood (ages 20 to 40). If they were sexually active when young, they'll probably remain sexually active as they age. Often, women show more interest in sex than before, because they no longer fear pregnancy. Men may only experience decreased libido after testosterone level reduction, which may not happen until very late in life, if at all. Most male impotence at this time probably arises from lack of self-confidence, because men have been led to *expect* to perform poorly. If their partner adopts an understanding attitude, the problem should quickly be resolved.

Rather than being harmful, sexual intercourse keeps the sexual organs healthy and responsive. And, it doesn't require excessive energy. Actually, prolonged sexual frustration can consume just as much energy. So, a person need only curtail sexual activity if he has a severe physical impairment and the doctor orders him to.

Besides physiological considerations, other factors inhibiting sexual activity include cultural taboos, rigid moral principles, negative self-image, and physical problems such as fatigue, illness, and medication side effects.

Your first step in helping your geriatric patient overcome handicapping attitudes is a thorough assessment. But, remember, if your patient shows displeasure or hostility when you ask him about sexual matters, stop your questioning and resume it later, after you've established a closer relationship. Consider asking these questions:
• Do you have sexual intercourse regularly? How often?
• If you don't, what's your reason? Do you feel you shouldn't because you're older? Do you think you won't enjoy sexual activity as much or that you can't perform as well as you used to? Do you have any physical limitations that interfere with sexual intercourse? Perhaps you don't have a sexual partner?
• Do you ever express your sexuality in some manner other than through sexual intercourse, such as masturbation?
• In what other physical ways do you express and receive affection?

Discuss your patient's fears as objectively as possible. Make sure he understands that age hasn't physically impaired him. If your female patient experiences vaginal dryness during coitus, suggest that she apply water-soluble lubricating jelly liberally. For a male who's having problems with erection, suggest a special penile sheath.

Remind your patient that sexual expression can take other forms than just coitus. Oral or manual genital stimulation can provide satisfactory substitutes. And, of course, kissing, hugging, and hand-holding all help fulfill the need for sexual contact.

Your patient shouldn't limit affectionate physical contact to a sexual partner. Relatives, friends, and children can also help fill this need. *Remember:* Older people have a special need for love and affection, to help them cope with the losses and crises in their lives.

Finally, if your patient has severely inhibiting attitudes, he may need sexual counseling. If he has a physically incapacitating problem, he may need medical treatment as well.

Learning about psychological problems

The far-reaching aging changes we've described will probably have some psychological effects. Consider the life crises elderly people may face: retirement, with accompanying loss of status and independence; loss of spouse; sensory loss; and possibly, disease, pain, surgery, and institutionalization. Depending on the strength of the person's coping mechanisms, any one of these could precipitate psychological problems. The cumulative effect can overwhelm even an emotionally strong, healthy person.

Psychological disorders

Researchers estimate that 15% to 20% of people over age 65 have some psychological problem. The most common psychological disorders affecting the elderly are *functional* disorders (those assumed to have an emotional basis), such as depression, neurosis, paranoia, and schizophrenia. Older adults probably experience depression more frequently than any other problem. Major signs and symptoms include profound sadness, insomnia with early morning waking, anorexia and weight loss, helplessness, slowed thinking, poor self-esteem, self-reproach, decreased activity level, and hypochondria. Keep in mind that emotional difficulties may cause psychosomatic physical symptoms.

Most often, however, rather than causing a specific mental problem, old age only intensifies an inherent personality weakness or deficit.

Assessment

To assess your patient's emotional status, ask him the following questions:
• How would you describe yourself and your attitude toward life?
• What do you like best about yourself? Least?
• Do you like to be alone or with others?
• How well do you relate to strangers?
• What are your current goals? Have you met your previous goals?
• What makes you feel guilty?
• Who do you feel closest to?
• Do you feel dependent on your family and friends, or do you feel that you function independently?
• Do you feel you have control over your life?
• Do you usually feel happy? What situations or persons make you feel that way?
• What makes you feel upset? Do you ever cry? How often?
• What do you do to relieve tension or stress? Do you suppress your feelings or give vent to them? Do you distract yourself with another activity? Take a tranquilizer or a drink?

If you feel your patient's depressed or has some other emotional problem, notify his doctor and social worker, who may refer him for counseling.

Document your assessment in your nurses' notes.

Is your patient suicidal?

You may be surprised to learn that older adults make up 16% to 25% of the suicides in this country. They have a suicide rate 40% to 60% higher than the rest of the population. White males over age 65 have the highest suicide rate of any population group, perhaps because they feel that life accomplishments determine personal self-worth. This may make the dependency and decreased activity of old age harder to accept.

A sense of helplessness and uselessness seem to correlate most highly with suicide. An older person may feel that through suicide, he can once again exercise complete control over his life. Isolation may also play a part. Any major change in lifestyle, environment, or territory can provoke suicidal thoughts or feelings. Events that commonly precipitate suicide include death of a spouse and admission to a nursing home.

Many older suicide victims plan their deaths successfully and carry them out without confiding in anyone. They rarely threaten suicide.

Important: Keep in mind that a person may attempt passive suicide by alcohol or drug abuse or starvation.

However, about 75% of the older people who commit suicide do see a health-care professional within a month before death. That's why your accurate assessment can be important. Always assess elderly white male patients (as well as any patient who seems depressed) for suicidal tendencies.

In your assessment, note such clues as a depressed appetite and insomnia lasting more than a year. The following behavior changes are also very significant. Ask your patient's family if he's been:
- visiting relatives not seen for years
- making a will
- giving away precious personal items
- acting unusually animated
- indulging in uncharacteristic behavior, such as suddenly buying a gun.

Also take enough time to look for the following characteristics in your patient:
- loss of the will to live
- loss of independence
- loss of income, employment, and status
- loss of self-confidence and self-esteem
- loss of a spouse, close friend, or sibling
- major changes in physical appearance from surgery
- loss of hair, teeth, or mobility
- addiction to drugs or alcohol
- psychological problems
- multiple physical problems
- admission to a nursing home
- pathologic family relationships.

To assess your patient's suicide potential, ask him the following direct questions:
- If you could think of one word to describe your past life, what would it be? Your future life?
- How do you feel most of the time?
- Do you ever think of dying? Under what circumstances?
- Have you ever thought of taking your own life? How would you do it? When?

If your assessment indicates your patient may be suicidal, notify the doctor, social worker, and his family. If he practices a religion, contact his clergyman.

Understanding alcohol abuse

Older people don't have as high a rate of alcohol abuse as younger people. In general, they tend to drink less. But, a number of older people (perhaps as many as 7.5% of people over age 55) *do* have an alcohol problem. Of these, some may be long-term alcoholics. Others may have begun to drink only with age, to ease mental anguish, reduce anxiety, or forget their loneliness. Loneliness and isolation seem to correlate more highly with alcohol abuse than do any other factors.

Alcohol abuse negatively affects an elderly person's life in various ways; for example, he may experience nutrient depletion, self-neglect, confusion, and physical injury.

If he combines alcohol with drugs, he'll have special problems. Most drugs older people take don't mix well with alcohol (see chart at right). Reactions include a wide range of signs and symptoms, such as hypotension, vomiting, and central nervous system depression. A severe reaction could cause death.

Assessment

You probably won't find assessing your patient for alcohol abuse an easy task. For one thing, you may confuse the signs and symptoms of alcoholism with those of a chronic illness such as diabetes or organic brain syndrome, or with malnutrition. Also, if your patient has a serious problem, he may deny it (and his family may cover for him as well).

Try asking the following questions:
- How much alcohol do you drink each day?
- What do you drink? Beer? Wine? Hard liquor?
- Do you have a drink at a definite time each day?
- Do you want one first thing in the morning?
- How does drinking affect you?
- Have you always drunk the amount you drink now? Does it seem to affect you in the same way?
- Why do you drink? Does it help you feel less shy with people? Do you drink to escape worries or troubles? Does a drink help you get to sleep?
- Do you drink alone?
- Does drinking interfere with your daily activities?
- Does drinking strain relations with other people?
- Have you ever had memory loss or a blackout after drinking?
- Have you ever had medical treatment for drinking?

Note: Moderate alcohol use may benefit your patient by relaxing him and improving circulation and appetite. So don't overreact if your patient has a daily glass of wine or beer.

When you assess your patient, look for such signs and symptoms as impaired sensation in hands and feet, poor coordination, confusion, facial edema, alcohol on breath, liver enlargement, jaundice, and ascites. Your patient may have a seizure either from alcohol abuse or withdrawal from alcohol. Other withdrawal signs and symptoms may include trembling or fidgeting.

If you suspect your patient has an alcohol problem, refer him for counseling. Geriatric patients usually respond quickly to a program of antidepressant medication and group social activities, administered through an outpatient center.

Nurses' guide to alcohol and drug interactions

The following chart shows how the types of drugs older people commonly take may interact with alcohol. For each medication class mentioned, we've listed a few examples of drugs that are frequently prescribed. But remember, if your older patient is taking *any* medication, make sure he checks with his doctor about alcohol use.

Class	Generic names	Interaction with alcohol					
		No known interaction	Potentiating	Antagonistic	Potentiating toward an adverse reaction	Unpredictable	Adverse, life-threatening
Nonnarcotic analgesics	Aspirin, acetaminophen					●	
Antiarrhythmics	All except phenytoin sodium	●					
Antihypertensives	Guanethidine sulfate, hydralazine hydrochloride, methyldopa, peripheral vasodilators, reserpine		●				
Antidiabetics/ hypoglycemics	Acetohexamide, chlorpropamide, tolazamide, tolbutamide				●		●
Antidepressants	Tricyclics (amitriptyline hydrochloride, desipramine hydrochloride)		●	●			
Corticosteroids	Hydrocortisone, prednisone	●					
Antihistamines	Diphenhydramine hydrochloride		●				
Major tranquilizers	Phenothiazines (chlorpromazine hydrochloride, thioridazine hydrochloride)				●		●
Minor tranquilizers	Benzodiazepines, meprobamate					●	

Assessment

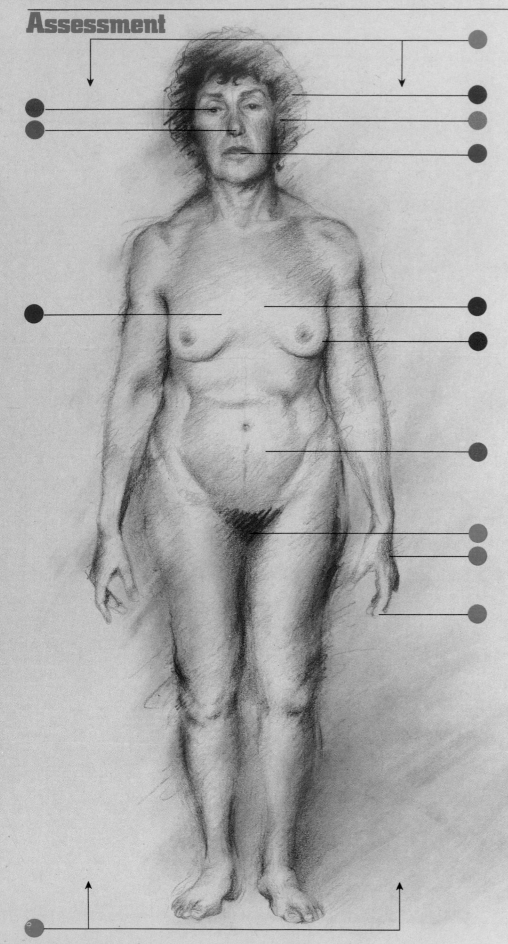

Performing a physical assessment

You've obtained a thorough history from Mrs. Redburn. Now, you're ready to perform a physical assessment. The chart on the following pages shows you what to do. The first part tells you how to examine your patient. The second part shows you what to look for. Your primary concern in assessing an older patient is to distinguish natural aging changes from pathologic changes. To help you do so, we've grouped common aging changes under the heading *Typical changes*. (We've included here a few changes that *are* pathologic, but only if a majority of older people experience them.) Under the heading *Possible problems*, we list those pathologic conditions or diseases that you'll see *more frequently* in older patients than in younger patients, but not inevitably. Study both sets of information carefully.

Remember, assessment is an ongoing process. After doing several assessments, you'll know your patient's condition well enough to distinguish normal aging changes from any new signs of problems.

How to examine

● Skin and nails

- Make sure you have adequate lighting.
- Perform a general inspection. Then, follow up with a closer examination, using a magnifying glass where necessary (see photo), to pick up more detail.
- Observe for scars. If your patient has any, find out if they're from surgery (including cosmetic surgery).
- Inspect fingernails and toenails thoroughly.

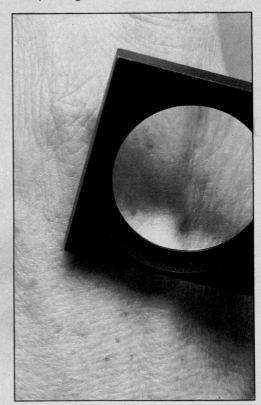

Hair

- Check body and scalp for hair distribution, amount, texture, and signs of a hair transplant.

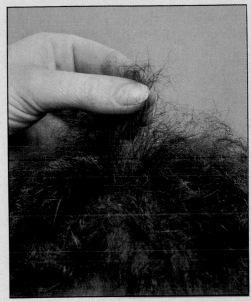

Eyes

- Place light source *behind* patient since geriatric patients usually have decreased glare tolerance. (However, darken room for pupil check and ophthalmoscope exam.)
- Examine lens with ophthalmoscope.
- Check visual acuity with and without corrective lenses, using a Snellen chart and a newspaper or book.
- Test peripheral vision by holding an object 18″ (45.7 cm) to the side of her head behind her range of vision and bringing it slowly forward until she can see it (see photo).

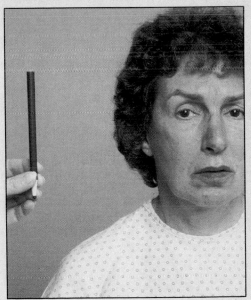

Ears

- Use an otoscope to check internal auditory canal and eardrum. If cerumen buildup obscures your view of her eardrum, you may need to soften the cerumen with drops and irrigate her ear before proceeding further. *Important:* If you have difficulty seeing ear landmarks, don't ask your patient to hold her nose and swallow, as you would a younger adult. Doing this could affect her equilibrium.
- Test hearing *after* the otoscope exam. Perform Weber's test by holding a tuning fork by its stem and striking it on your hand. Then, press the stem firmly against the patient's skull in the center top of her head (see photo). If she hears sounds *better* in one ear, she may have hearing problems in *that* ear.
- Perform the Rinne test by striking the tuning fork on your hand and placing it on your patient's mastoid bone. When your patient says she no longer hears sound, place the fork near her external auditory meatus. She should hear sound again. For normal results, she should hear sounds conducted by air longer than sounds conducted by bone.

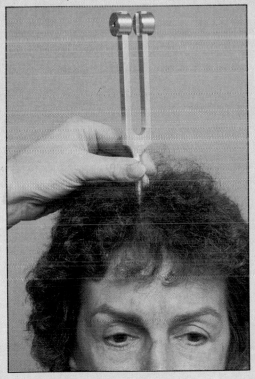

Nose

- Perform visual inspection for symmetry.
- Palpate nose for change in structure.
- Use an otoscope to visualize internal nose, including the nasal mucosa. Also, observe for nasal septum deviation.
- Check patency of nostrils by occluding one nostril and asking the patient to inhale through the other with her mouth closed (see photo). Repeat for the other nostril.

- To test olfactory nerve function, ask patient to identify distinct smells such as coffee or garlic.
- Palpate paranasal sinuses for tenderness.

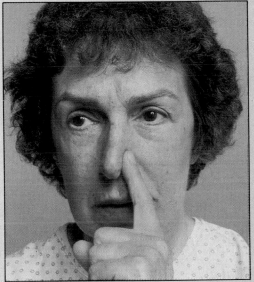

Mouth

- Examine mouth, using penlight or other light source and tongue depressor (see photo). Observe color and condition of mucosa.
- Note presence and condition of teeth. Check patient's gum line for irritation or recession.
- Check dental occlusion (bite) visually.
- Palpate entire oral cavity with a finger cot or glove, checking for ulcerations or lesions.
- Withdraw tongue with gauze sponge and inspect all surfaces.
- Note quantity, appearance, and odor of saliva.
- Remove dentures, if any, and inspect gums carefully. Evaluate the dentures for proper fit.

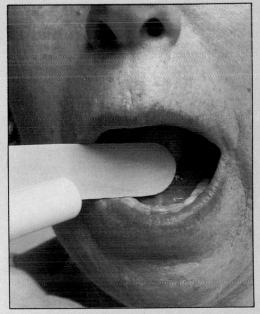

Assessment

Performing a physical assessment continued

● Respiratory

• Observe respiratory rate, depth, and changes in chest configuration. Note patient's use of accessory muscles during respiration, which may indicate chronic obstructive pulmonary disease (COPD).
• Palpate for proper tracheal alignment.
• Palpate for tenderness along ribs.
• Percuss for chest tones (see photo).
• Auscultate for breath sounds.
• Since respiratory and cardiac systems are closely related, assess cardiovascular system especially carefully in the presence of respiratory changes.

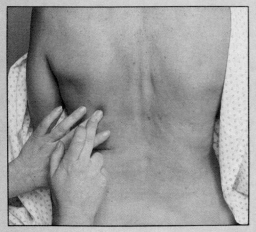

● Cardiovascular system

• Observe chest and abdomen for pulsation and rib retraction.
• Observe and palpate the jugular vein for distention or filling defect.
• Palpate all pulses and apex of heart, as well as the abdominal aorta.
• Auscultate for heart sounds and blood pressure.
• Percuss heart for enlargement.
• Take blood pressure in both arms with the patient lying, sitting, and standing.
• Check legs for skin temperature, skin color, and varicosities (see photo).

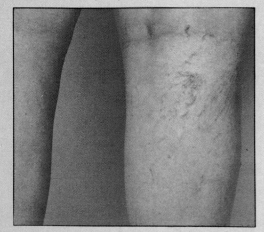

● Breasts

• Examine female patient in both supine position and sitting with her arms extended over her head, unless degenerative joint disease or cardiac or respiratory problems make this impossible.
• If kyphosis or respiratory problems are present, they may cause a forward thrust of her chest wall. You'll find palpating her breasts easier if you have your patient bend forward so her breasts hang away from the chest wall (see photo).
• Inspect breasts for symmetry, in both the supine and sitting positions.
• Palpate breasts and underarms for masses or lesions (with patient in supine position, if possible). Use flat part of hand to feel for masses and tissue thickening. Note any tender areas.
• Compress nipple between thumb and forefinger. Note color, amount, and odor of any discharge.
• Teach female how to examine her own breasts. Instruct her to examine them at least once every month.
• If you suspect a mass in the breast of a male patient with gynecomastia (breast enlargement), use a pocket flashlight to transilluminate it. Light won't pass through the tissue mass, which will appear darker than normal tissue.

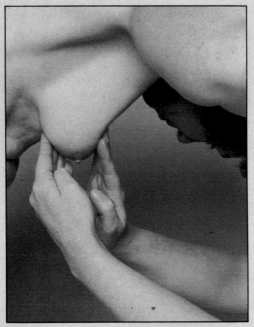

● Gastrointestinal system

• Observe abdomen for symmetry and presence of masses.
• Inspect abdominal skin for scars, striae, rashes, dilated veins, lesions, and other changes.
• Auscultate for bowel sounds.
• Percuss for liver, spleen, and stomach size and location.
• Palpate lightly for tenderness and muscle guarding (see photo); palpate deeply for rebound tenderness; perform ballottement to detect masses.

• Palpate the anal sphincter. (Or, you may do this during the genitourinary exam.)

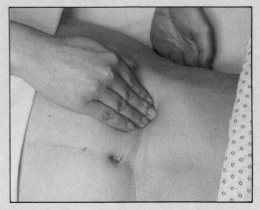

● Genitourinary system
(FEMALE)

• Have your patient urinate first; then position her in the lithotomy position. However, if this causes discomfort, try the side-lying or some other comfortable position.
• Wear examining gloves.
• Inspect and palpate external genitalia for changes (see photo). If you observe discharge, culture it.
• Perform internal exam, if appropriate. Lubricate insertion finger. Check vaginal outlet to determine necessary speculum size. If patient isn't sexually active, you may need to use a small speculum.
• Change gloves for rectal exam. Lubricate insertion finger. Evaluate the anus and lower segment of the rectum. Note sphincter tone; palpate for any tenderness, irregularities or nodes. When withdrawing your finger from the anal area, observe the glove for any signs of bleeding.
• Percuss for a distended bladder.

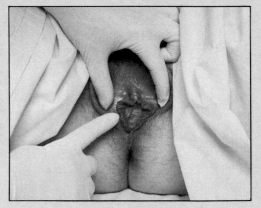

● Genitourinary system
(MALE)

• Let your patient urinate first; then place him in Sims' position.
• Inspect the scrotal sac and penis. Retract the foreskin in an uncircumsized patient.
• Palpate scrotal sac.
• Palpate prostate through rectum, using a gloved finger. Lubricate insertion finger. You'll

feel the prostate anteriorly as a two-lobed structure with a groove between the two lobes. Evaluate the anus and rectum as for a female.
• Percuss bladder for distention.

Musculoskeletal system

• Inspect and palpate all joints. Note presence of crepitus.
• Note patient's gait, posture, and how she sits, positions herself, and uses her hands.
• Test muscle strength by having patient grasp your index and third fingers with her hands and squeeze firmly (see photo).
• For more details, see the NURSING PHOTOBOOK WORKING WITH ORTHOPEDIC PATIENTS.

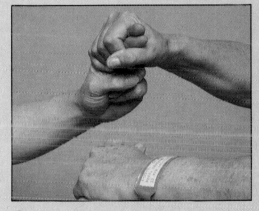

Neurologic system

• Evaluate behavior and consciousness level.
• Observe for tremors, clumsiness, involuntary movements, and a tendency to use only one side of body.
• Have patient walk heel-to-toe.
• Palpate for muscle laxity, tenderness, fasciculations, or rigidity.
• Test deep-tendon reflexes (see photo). To do so, you may need to use reinforcement techniques such as having patient clench her fists or the back of a chair while you try to elicit the reflex. *Note:* If patient has joint disease, be careful not to cause her unnecessary pain. You may need to *palpate* for reflexes rather than using a hammer.
• For more details, see the NURSING PHOTOBOOK WORKING WITH NEUROLOGIC PATIENTS.

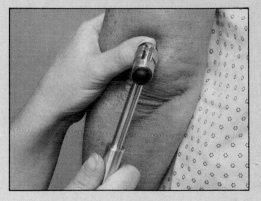

Aging changes

Skin and nails

Typical changes
• Decreased sebaceous and sweat gland activity
• Dry skin
• Decreased subcutaneous fat
• Increased thinning of skin, especially on backs of hands and forearms
• Skin creasing and wrinkling. Patient may have frown lines on forehead, crow's-feet at outer corners of eyes, and comma-shaped lines on either side of mouth.
• Loss of elasticity
• Skin drooping. Look for ptosis of eyelids, double chin, or jowls. *Note:* When evaluating skin turgor, pinched fold of skin will take longer to return to normal. (This would be a sign of dehydration in a younger patient.)
• Changes in skin pigmentation, causing decreased overall pigmentation in face and neck, but increased clusters of brownish, pigmented flat spots (liver spots, lentigines, or senile lentigo). Liver spots may be benign or precancerous.
• Seborrheic keratosis (see illustration below), a benign, raised, wartlike lesion with fingerlike projections. May be dark and greasy or yellowish and dry. Varies from pinhead size to 1″ (2.54 cm) in diameter. Usually appears on hairline, neck, upper chest, or back.

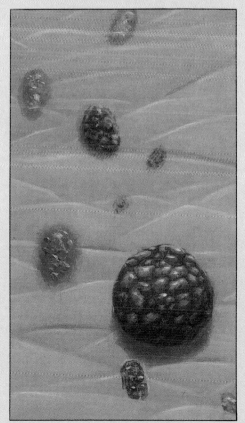

• Cherry angioma (see illustration below), a benign, red-to-purple overgrowth of dilated blood vessels, which is a form of senile angioma. Varies in size from 1 to 5 mm in diameter. Usually appears on chest, trunk, or extremities.

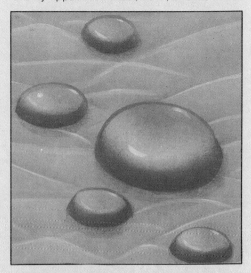

• Venous lake, a papular, bluish-black vascular discoloration occurring singly or in groups, which is a form of senile angioma. Indicates increasing blood pressure in superficial veins and usually appears on face, neck and ears.
• Acrochordon (skin tag), a benign, soft, stalklike, flesh-colored growth which usually appears on neck, underarms, and upper chest (see illustration below).

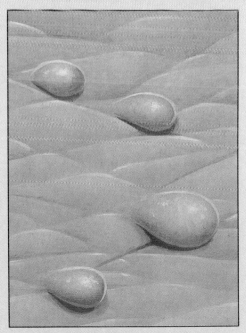

• Diminished body odors
• Slower-growing and thicker nails, which become brittle and more likely to crack, split, or peel

Assessment

Performing a physical assessment continued

Possible problems
- Pruritus (indicated by scratch marks)
- Severe dry skin, causing burning, stinging, or itching
- Ichthyosis (fish-scale appearance; see illustration below)

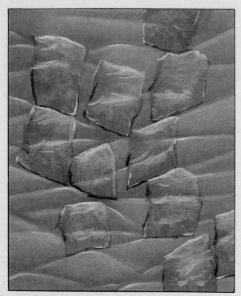

- Pressure sores
- Skin lesions. Be sure to ask your patient about changes in size of birthmarks, moles, or warts, development of new moles or warts, or bleeding from lesions.
- Increased vulnerability to hypothermia and hyperthermia
- Irritant or contact dermatitis
- Increased bruising
- Actinic or senile keratosis (see illustration below), a precancerous, papular, brown lesion that may involve keratin buildup and lead to development of cutaneous horn. Usually appears on face, ears, neck, hands, and arms.

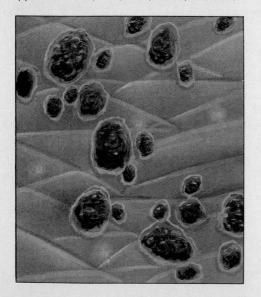

- Squamous cell carcinoma (see illustration below), a cancerous lesion with a high incidence of metastasis. Lesion resembles actinic keratosis. Begins as a flesh-colored nodule; then becomes red and scaly; finally becomes hard and wartlike with a gray top, or ulcerated with raised borders. Usually appears on face, neck, ears, and hands (body areas most exposed to the sun).

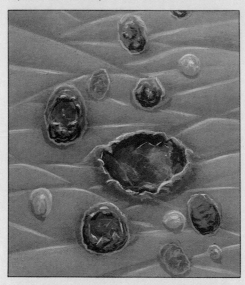

- Basal cell carcinoma (see illustration below), a cancerous lesion with a low incidence of metastasis. Appears as a raised lesion with a pearly border; may be pigmented. Usually appears on forehead, eyelids, cheeks, nose, and lips.

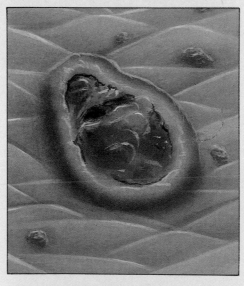

- Fingernail problems such as hangnails
- Thickened toenails, leading to onychogryphosis (Ram's Horn deformity) or ingrown toenails
- Fungal nail infection, causing discolored and deteriorated nails

Hair

Typical changes
- Thinning and pigmentation loss of scalp hair. Males tend to bald or develop a receding hairline (see illustration below)
- Coarsening and straightening of hair texture
- Possible increased thickness and amount of facial hair in women
- Loss of body hair, beginning with extremities; decreased underarm and pubic hair

Possible problems
- Increased vulnerability to hypothermia or hyperthermia

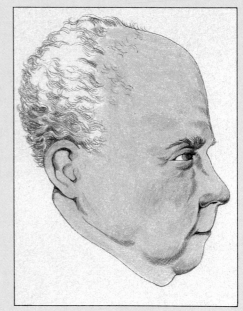

Eyes

Typical changes
- Darkening of skin around eye orbits
- Atrophy of lid muscles and loss of skin elasticity, causing drooping lids (ptosis)
- Pouches under eyes
- Appearance of crow's-feet at peripheral border of eyelids
- Pale conjunctivae
- Xanthelasmas (see illustration below), thin, yellowish lipid deposits on inner portion of upper and lower eyelid

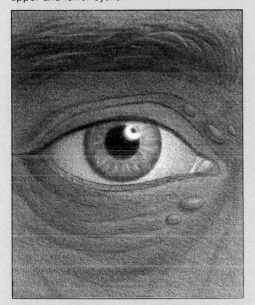

- Pingueculas (see illustration below), fat pads at either the inner or outer conjunctivae

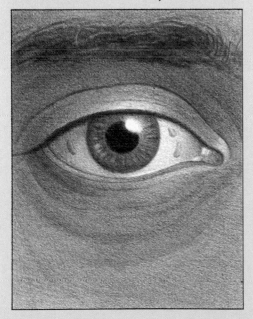

- Arcus senilis (see illustration), an opaque, grayish, or greenish-yellow lipid ring deposited around cornea

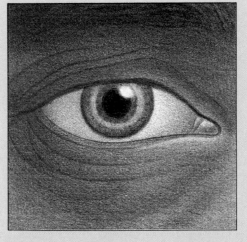

- Pale iris with degenerative changes; for example, normal pigment is replaced with brown areas
- Reduced pupil size and irregular pupil shape. Reaction may occur with less briskness, and accommodation to light may take longer, but both eyes should show same reaction time.
- Pale retina and disc, with arteries and veins appearing similar in size. Arteries may have a thin, wirelike appearance, while retinal vessels may show increased tortuosity.
- Presbyopia (farsightedness)
- Decreased quantity and quality of tears
- Decreased peripheral vision and decreased adaptation to darkness

Possible problems
- Entropion (inverted lid) or ectropion (everted lid). (See illustrations below.) Eyelashes irritate conjunctiva and may lacerate cornea.

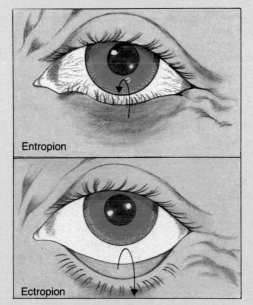

Entropion

Ectropion

- Blepharochalasis (extreme drooping of upper eyelid skin over eye)
- Intraocular pressure greater than 25 to 30 mm Hg, indicating glaucoma. (The doctor performs a test to determine intraocular pressure.)
- Cataract formation, indicated by lens opacity or cloudy areas on lens
- Keratitis sicca (burning, dry, or irritated eyes)
- Ulcerated cornea
- Manifestations of glaucoma, hypertension, and diabetes in internal eye vessels (see illustrations below)

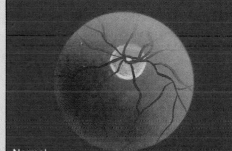

Normal

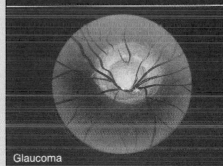

Glaucoma

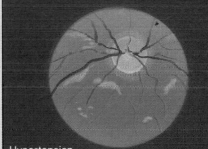

Hypertension

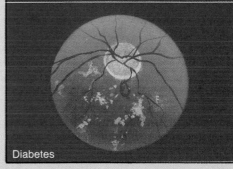

Diabetes

Assessment

Performing a physical assessment continued

 ### Ears

Typical changes
- Presbycusis (loss of auditory acuity) from auditory nerve degeneration
- Increase in lobe length from continuous cartilage deposition. Also, cartilage changes may distort the shape of the auditory canal.
- Dry skin on external ear
- Increased hair growth in ear
- Thickened eardrum; decreased cone of light is seen through otoscope
- Coarsening and stiffening of internal ear cilia
- Buildup of cerumen in ear, which may interfere with patient's hearing. Ask your patient about use of cotton swabs or wax softeners to clean ears. These may only aggravate cerumen problems.

Possible problems
- Yeast or fungal infection in the ear canal; possible scarring of eardrum from repeated infections (see illustration below)

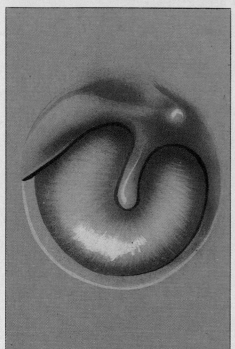

- Impaired hearing from blockage of sound waves by coarse, stiff cilia
- Presbycusis may cause loss of ability to hear high-pitched sounds, progressing to loss of ability to hear normal speech sounds.
- Otosclerosis (fixation of the stapes to the oval window) causing conductive hearing loss. Otoscopic exam won't reveal abnormality, so patient with hearing loss will require both Weber's and the Rinne test. Patient may have *both* presbycusis and otosclerosis. *Note:* For *any* hearing loss, refer the patient for further testing.

 ### Nose

Typical changes
- Possible increased size, from continuing cartilage deposition
- Increased nasal hair (especially in males); coarsening and stiffening of nasal hair
- Olfactory nerve degeneration

Possible problems
- Postnasal drip
- Loss of smell
- Dryness of nasal vestibules
- Vasomotor rhinitis, indicated by smooth, shiny mucous membrane and pale, engorged turbinates (see illustration below)

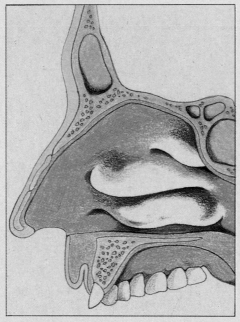

- Sinusitis
- Infection of hair follicle or irritation from clipping nose hairs too closely inside nose
- Itching and sneezing from protruding nasal hairs

 ### Mouth

Typical changes
- Thinning of vermilion borders of lips, lip varicosities (venous lakes), and color changes
- Thinning of mucous membranes
- Atrophic changes of tongue, including loss of papillae (taste buds) with accompanying decreased ability to taste, especially sweetness and saltiness
- Decrease in salivary gland function
- Varicosities (caviar spots) on ventral surfaces of tongue
- Papillary hyperplasia (wartlike lesions on roof of mouth) from suction effect of upper dentures and poor cleaning
- Slowed gag reflex
- Brittle, dry, and stained teeth. Decay at root surface and gingival recession usually increase.

Possible problems
- Malocclusion, from loss of teeth and shifting of remaining teeth
- Derangement of condylar head in glenoid fossa of temporomandibular joint from malocclusion and facial muscular imbalance; can lead to arthritis of this joint
- Cheilosis (fissures at the angles of the mouth)
- Erosion of teeth (enamel loss)
- Abrasions or ulcers from dentures
- Contact dermatitis from acrylic dentures
- Possible loss of three quarters of taste buds by age 70
- Burning sensation of tongue with mouth dryness, from reduced salivary gland function (occurs more often in women)
- Halitosis (bad breath)
- Leukoplakia, a precancerous lesion. Appears on mucous membranes of mouth, tongue, or lips as a white lesion that seems to be painted on membrane surface.
- Keratosis of interior cheek; can be benign or precancerous
- Neuralgia of tongue and throat (affecting ninth cranial nerve)

Respiratory system

Typical changes
- Decreased ciliary activity
- Loss of lung tissue elasticity (compliance)
- Calcification of vertebral cartilage, causing reduced rib mobility and partial contraction of intercostal muscles. This decreases chest expansion.
- Decreased ability to cough
- Respiratory function changes including decreased vital capacity, increased residual capacity, and decreased maximum breathing capacity, from loss of lung compliance and decreased chest expansion
- Decreased PaO_2 (although $PaCO_2$ doesn't increase)
- After activity, increased time for return of respiratory rate to normal
- Increased anteroposterior diameter of chest, which is not associated with chronic obstructive pulmonary disease (COPD)
- Possible tracheal deviation from scoliosis
- Shallow breathing, which may hamper breath sounds assessment
- No change in percussion tones, except for hyperresonance over kyphotic area, or over anteroposterior area in patients with senile emphysema; diaphragmatic excursion may decrease in these patients. No change in auscultation sounds except for decreased sounds over kyphotic area or area of increased anteroposterior distance. Any rales present should clear with coughing.

Possible problems
- Rib fractures caused by patient coughing violently with partially contracted intercostal muscles and reduced rib mobility
- Decreased capacity for exertion, from reduced pulmonary function
- Vulnerability to respiratory tract infection, from decreased ciliary activity, shallow breathing, and decreased coughing ability
- Influenza
- Pneumonia

Cardiovascular system

Typical changes
- Increased systolic pressure
- More pronounced arterial pulses, because of decreased adjacent connective tissue
- Possible slight decrease in heart rate
- Orthostatic hypotension
- Irregular cardiac rhythms, including ectopic beats or arrhythmia from degeneration of conduction system
- Soft systolic ejection murmur (S_4) heard at base of heart early in systole, from sclerotic changes in aortic valve; not a problem in absence of other signs and symptoms
- Decreased cardiac output
- EKG changes such as lengthening of P-R and Q-T intervals and shift of the QRS axis to the left
- Myocardial hypertrophy, including thickened left ventricular wall
- Stiffened, thickened heart valves
- Varicosities, which may be painful
- Reduced cardiac pain sensation
- Increased vasovagal response

Possible problems
- Increase in *both* systolic and diastolic blood pressure. Usually, systolic pressure rises higher, creating wider pulse pressure. Patient with systolic pressure over 160 mmHg and diastolic pressure over 95 mmHg may require blood pressure treatment.
- Clubbing of fingers or cyanosis, indicating circulatory impairment
- Fatigue
- Shortness of breath
- Angina
- Myocardial infarction
- Congestive heart failure
- Cerebrovascular accident (CVA)
- Pulmonary embolism
- Stokes Adams syndrome
- Vertigo or syncope
- Ulcerated, inflamed, or cordlike varicosities (see illustration of calf below)

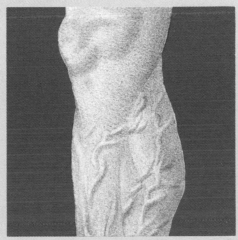

Breasts

Typical changes
- Loss of breast tissue and supportive tissue, which makes breasts pendulous or flaccid. Usually, breast fat increases, but glandular tissues atrophy. Breast tissue atrophy helps make lesions more palpable.
- Cylindrical shape of breasts
- Retraction of nipple, which can be turned outward easily
- Gynecomastia (male breast enlargement), which may be unilateral. Examine breasts for cancer as you would for a female.

Possible problems
- Benign or cancerous breast tumor
- Irreversible nipple retraction, possibly indicating a tumor (see illustrations below)

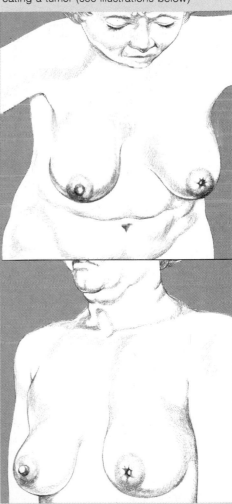

- Discharge from nipple, possibly indicating a tumor
- Gynecomastia in males over age 50 may indicate testicular or pituitary tumor, therapy with steroids or estrogens, or hepatic cirrhosis

Assessment

Performing a physical assessment continued

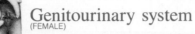
Gastrointestinal system

Typical changes
- Connective tissue and muscle tone loss, which leaves abdominal wall thin and lax (unless patient is obese)
- Abdomen usually feels soft with no organs immediately palpable. However, airway obstruction from chronic obstructive pulmonary disease (COPD) or a low diaphragm may make liver palpable 1 to 2 cm below right costal margin.
- Diminished saliva and gastric acid secretion
- Esophageal nerve degeneration
- Decreased anal tone and sensations

Possible problems
- Difficulty swallowing
- Hiatal hernia
- Peptic ulcer. *Note:* An older adult will express less discomfort in an acute abdominal emergency, from decreased deep-pain sensitivity.
- Diverticulosis
- Fecal incontinence or constipation
- Rectal tumors
- Hemorrhoids (see illustration below)

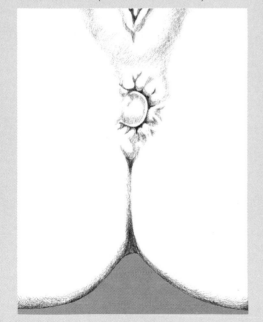

Genitourinary system
(FEMALE)

Typical changes
- Brittleness and decreased amount of pubic hair
- Thin, dry vaginal mucosa
- Decreased vaginal secretions
- Decreased size of vulva, labia minora, and clitoris. Skin over these organs becomes thin and shiny.
- Decreased size of uterus. Uterine mucosa becomes thin, atrophic, and nonsecretory.
- Decreased size of ovaries
- Decreased size of cervix, which normally appears thick, smooth, and shiny. Changes from multiple deliveries, severe atrophy, or hysterectomy may make cervix hard to visualize.
- Scant, thick, cellular cervical mucus
- Narrow, shortened vagina
- No significant physiologic changes sexually, although each stage of sexual act may take longer to perform
- Asymptomatic bladder distention from neural changes

Possible problems
- Vaginitis
- Dyspareunia (painful intercourse) or vaginismus (painful vaginal spasm)
- Itching
- Thickening or hardening of vulva; skin appears leathery and creased
- Uterine prolapse (see illustration below)

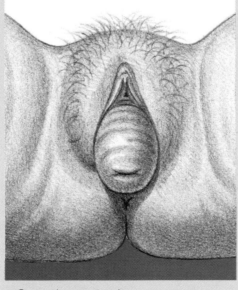

- Cystocele or rectocele
- Benign or cancerous cervical, uterine, or ovarian tumors
- Urinary tract infection
- Urinary incontinence
- Renal calculi

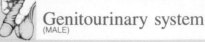
Genitourinary system
(MALE)

Typical changes
- Brittleness and decreased amount of pubic hair
- Low-hanging scrotum with smooth surface
- Decreased size and firmness of testes
- Prostate gland enlargement (see illustration below), with reduced prostate secretion

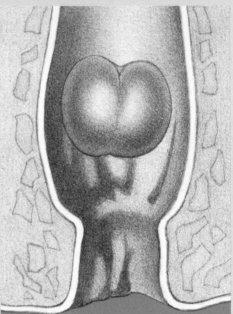

- No physiologic impairment of sexual activity, although each stage of the sexual act may take longer to perform
- Possible decline in testosterone levels late in life
- Decreased anal sphincter tone on palpation

Possible problems
- Prostatitis
- Urinary frequency, nocturia, and dysuria from enlarged prostate
- Prostate cancer, indicated by a hard, irregular nodule palpable on rectal examination of the prostate gland surface
- Urinary tract infection
- Urinary incontinence
- Renal calculi

Musculoskeletal system

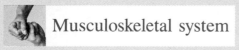

Typical changes
• Decrease in height, from shrinkage of intervertebral discs or osteoporosis
• Increased convexity of thoracic spine (kyphosis) from disc shrinkage. Head tilts backward to compensate for curvature.
• Flexed posture, with slight knee, hip, elbow, and wrist flexion
• Bony structure prominent from subcutaneous fat loss
• Loss of muscle tone; muscle atrophy
• Arthritic joint changes, which may include bony enlargement of distal and proximal finger joints. Fingers may be flexed in lateral or medial deviation. On palpation, you may detect crepitation, joint enlargement, and joint tenderness from synovial effusion.
• Deposition of calcium salts in degenerated tissue, (especially around shoulder joint) which stiffens muscles and limits range of motion

Possible problems
• Dupuytren's contracture (see illustration below), a contraction deformity involving a nodular thickening of the palmar fascia. May be associated with diabetes.

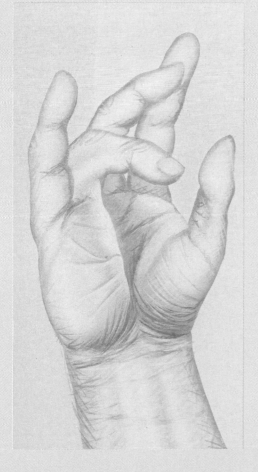

• Calluses and corns
• Hallux valgus, the lateral deviation of the great toe toward the other toes (see illustration below). Usually, it occurs in association with bunions.

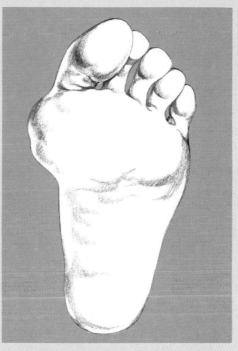

• Hammertoe, a toe deformity involving flexion contracture of proximal interphalangeal joint, with flexion or slight hyperextension contracture of distal interphalangeal joint
• Respiratory problems
• Osteoporosis, osteomalacia, and Paget's disease
• Fractures

Neurologic system

Typical changes
• Altered sleep patterns (see page 14)
• Decreased vocal range, intensity, and duration
• Decreased ability to hear high-frequency sound
• Diminished senses of taste and smell
• Reduced nerve conduction time
• General slowness of movement
• Decreased speed of fine motor movements
• Slight, symmetrical increase or decrease in deep-tendon reflexes, although superficial reflexes remain the same. Arm reflexes may be depressed, but should be present. Eventually, all reflexes decrease.
• Difficulty performing tasks involving coordinated movements or rapidly alternating movements
• Decreased ability to detect vibratory sensation—greater vibration amplitude required
• Diminished sensory perception of deep pain and temperature
• Senile tremors, which occur at a rate of 3 to 7 per second. A senile tremor is coarser than a parkinsonian tremor and involves the head, jaw, and hands. The tremor occurs with movement and doesn't involve limb rigidity or any disability. Fatigue, cold, or emotional stress may aggravate tremor, and alcohol may temporarily relieve it.
• Electroencephalogram shows decreased or slowed alpha rhythms, increased beta rhythms, and some delta rhythms

Possible problems
• Parkinsonian tremors, which occur at a rate of 2 to 5 per second. These tremors are regular, fine or coarse in nature, and occur when a person's at rest. Finger and thumb are flexed and the lower arm is rigid.
• Involuntary movements, indicating motor neuron disease (except for fasciculations in calf muscles of elderly males)
• Senile paraplegia
• Senile chorea
• Senile epilepsy
• Mental dysfunction from organic brain syndrome

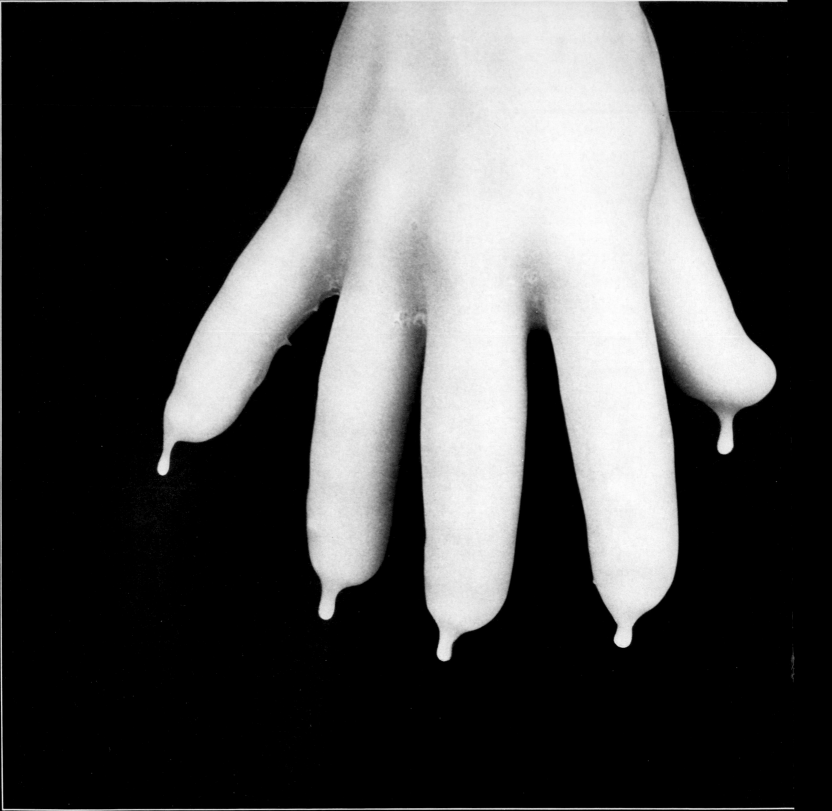

Promoting Hygiene and Mobility

Daily hygiene
Skin care
Joint care

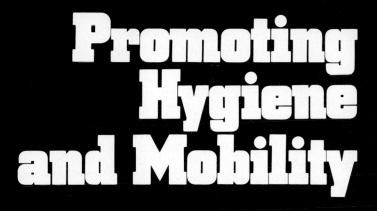

Daily hygiene

Over the years, your geriatric patient has developed his own habits for daily hygiene. If possible, don't suspend his regular routine just because he's been admitted to the hospital. He needs regular care performed (by himself or you) to help him feel and look better and prevent any further health problems.

In the next few pages, you'll find out how to perform some basic procedures, such as giving mouth and denture care, as well as inserting and removing dentures. We'll also tell you how you can promote your patient's hygiene and comfort by giving him a manicure and a foot massage. In addition, we provide tips on how to work hygiene care into your busy schedule; for example, by using a sink bath or giving a quick towel-and-lotion bath. Also, take special note of the home care aid designed to help you promote your patient's independence.

Planning an effective hygiene program

As you know, a person's mobility and lifestyle may change as he ages. But whether your patient's ambulatory or on bed rest, good daily hygiene will help preserve his sense of well-being and self-esteem. And encouraging him to perform as much of his own daily care as possible, in the hospital or at home, will promote independence.

Make sure the following procedures are included in your patient's hygiene program:
• mouth care
• full or partial bath or shower
• hair shampoo and conditioning
• eyeglass or contact lens cleaning
• nail grooming.

He'll perform some of these procedures daily and others weekly.

To give your patient a sense of control over his life, let him schedule his own care (as much as possible), and allow him time to perform it. For example, permit him to choose his bath time. He may prefer an evening bath, to induce sleep, or a morning shower, as a stimulant to begin the day.

To create a more comfortable and familiar setting, encourage your patient's family to bring in his toilet articles from home.

How can you design a practical schedule, considering all the demands on your time? After all, even if your patient performs most of his own care, you'll still need to assist and supervise him. One way to schedule care is to combine hygiene activities; for example, as the sink bath allows. The sink bath is a good alternative to the traditional in-bed partial bath (unless contraindicated by bed rest). While your patient's out of bed for his sink bath, he can also per-

form nail and mouth care and clean his glasses (if he has any). At the same time, you can make his bed and perform other duties.

Your older patient has decreased sweat and oil gland activity, so he'll have less body odor. That's why he'll probably find a daily partial sink bath adequate, rather than a daily complete tub bath or shower.

To organize the patient's hygiene activities around his sink bath, you might have him perform mouth care at the sink before breakfast. Then, he can decide whether to follow through with his partial bath or wait until after his meal. (Either way, he'll probably perform mouth care again, after his meal.) If he has full mobility and enough energy, he can stand and wash at the sink. Or, if he can't stand, he can sit on the toilet seat.

Caution: To help prevent him from slipping, place a bath mat or towel on the floor or toilet seat.

When performing his sink bath, he should wash his face (including the skin around his eyes and his outer ears) and hands with a mild soap. Then, have him wash his underarms and genitalia, and rinse thoroughly with tepid water. He should pat his skin dry with a soft cotton terry cloth towel and sparingly apply deodorant (if he uses it) to his underarms. Recommend lightly dusting his genital area with cornstarch to absorb perspiration and reduce itching.

Before your patient gets dressed, perform back care, including a back rub (see pages 44 and 45), and inspect his skin, nails, and hair.

Note: Avoid confusion and save time by keeping your patient's toilet articles in a labeled container. This also eliminates needless trips back to the bedside.

Encouraging good mouth care

As you know, keeping your patient's mouth—teeth, tongue, palate, and gums—clean and healthy necessitates daily attention. Doing so helps prevent tooth decay and loss and aids in preserving the older adult's normal eating habits and self-esteem.

Remind your patient that good preventive care starts with a semiannual checkup. Dental clinics associated with city hospitals or dental schools may provide this service in your community at low cost. Eating properly can also promote good oral health. Dairy products, such as cheese and yogurt, keep the lower jawbone strong and pliable. Soups minimize mouth dryness and keep gum tissue moist. Daily brushing and flossing help remove plaque buildup, which can lead to tooth decay, gum disorders, and tooth loss.

Teach your patient and his family the importance of good mouth care. Start by teaching them the signs and symptoms of mouth trouble that precede the obvious problems of bleeding and swollen gums. These signs and symptoms include:
• coated tongue
• crusted, thickened saliva
• bad breath
• intolerance of hot and cold fluids
• discomfort when chewing or talking
• decreased appetite or weight loss.

To prevent these problems, encourage your patient to brush and floss his teeth at least twice daily. Educate him in proper brushing techniques. He should brush all tooth surfaces with eight to ten strokes, moving from gum to tooth crowns (see upper illustration). He should use short vibratory strokes where the gum meets the crown (see lower illustration). Provide privacy while he performs mouth care, if possible. Also, supply tooth powder or paste (preferably containing fluoride, if the water supply is not fluoridated), a soft toothbrush, dental floss, and tissues. *Note:* Consider providing an electric toothbrush or a

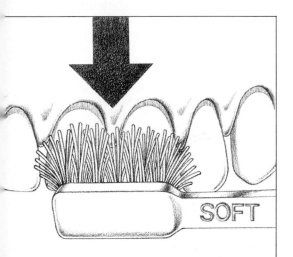

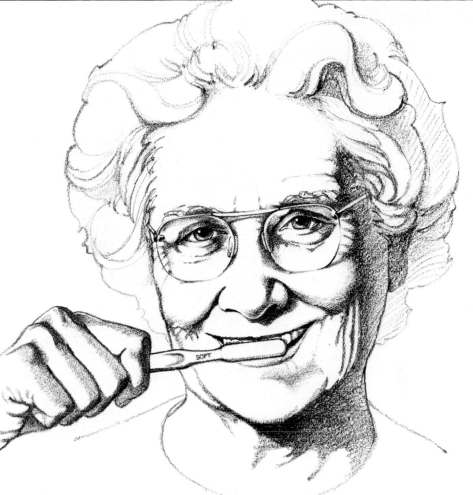

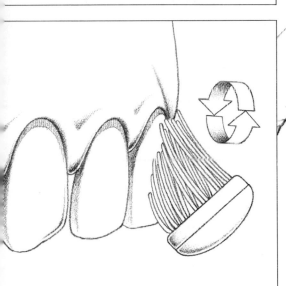

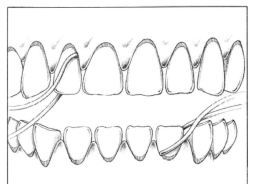

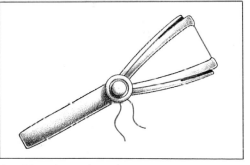

specially adapted brush if your patient has unsteady or weak hands or limited range of motion.

Teach your patient how to remove food particles by flossing between his teeth (see illustration at right). He should introduce the floss between the two teeth and then ease the floss back and forth up between gum and tooth. Provide a floss holder (see illustration at far right), if he finds this helpful. *Caution:* Warn older adults, especially those with cardiac disorders, to avoid using water jet spray appliances, which can force bacteria into the bloodstream through unhealthy gums, causing bacterial endocarditis.

For good mouth care, your older patient must also brush his tongue and the roof of his mouth. This removes thickened saliva caused by decreased salivary activity or

by dentures and bridges. If untreated, the thickened saliva may become a foul-smelling crust called materia alba (sordes), which causes halitosis. Remedy this problem by:
• rinsing his mouth often with tap water.
• increasing his fluid intake.
• offering him sugar-free carbonated beverages or hard candy.
• increasing the humidity in his room.

Encourage your patient to conclude his oral hygiene program by rinsing with

fluoridated mouthwash, warm tap water flavored with lemon juice, or half-strength hydrogen peroxide solution.

Note: Urge your patient to rinse thoroughly after using hydrogen peroxide solution. Warn him that prolonged use may soften gums or decalcify tooth surfaces.

To prevent inner mouth dryness, apply a plain or flavored vegetable-based oil to your patient's tongue and the roof of his mouth. Suggest rinses containing peppermint or lemon juice. However, avoid using lemon-glycerin swabs, which may dehydrate and irritate your patient's mouth tissues.

Your patient can prevent chapped lips by applying lanolin or water-soluble jelly.

Daily hygiene

Denture care

Tooth loss can initiate a chain of complications in your patient's mouth. First, adjacent teeth move out of alignment to fill the vacant space, which increases stress on gums and supporting tissue. Over a long period, this can alter your patient's appearance by hollowing his cheeks. The shifting teeth may cause malocclusion, affecting his speech. They may also trap food particles.

Dentures or bridges can replace missing teeth. But, these substitute teeth can cause temporary discomfort for your patient, because their texture and size may differ from his natural teeth. If your patient acquires dentures while he's in your care, provide support and encouragement during the breaking-in period.

Breaking in dentures

How can you help your patient adjust to his new dentures? Instruct him to use his cheek and tongue muscles to hold them in place when he's speaking or eating. Also, rather than eating three large meals each day, encourage him to eat small amounts of soft food frequently, taking small bites and chewing carefully and thoroughly. Until he's accustomed to his dentures, he must avoid hard foods, foods with a sticky consistency, and foods with seeds. Also, recommend that he cook fruits before eating them, and strain them, if necessary. Suggest that he use such cooking techniques as steaming, which makes food tender and preserves many nutrients.

Inserting and removing dentures

Teach your patient how to insert his dentures properly. First, he should line an emesis basin with a washcloth and half-fill the basin with water, to cushion the dentures if they fall. As he leans over the basin, he should introduce the dentures to his mouth, applying even, gentle pressure on both sides to work the dentures into place. Remind him that inserting the dentures while they're wet helps them form a strong seal with his gums. He'll probably find it easier to insert the top piece first.

Encourage your patient to insert his dentures every morning, unless contraindicated by acute illness. Doing so prevents gum tissue swelling, which could cause a change in his gum line, making the dentures fit poorly.

When removing his upper denture, your patient should grasp the palatal and front surfaces on both sides of the denture (see top photo); insert his forefingers over the denture's upper border; press until he breaks the seal between the denture and his gum; and pull the denture out (see

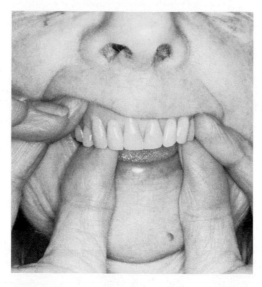

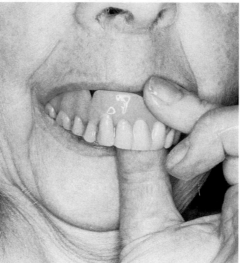

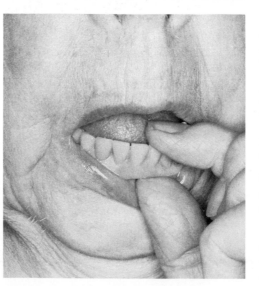

middle photo).

To remove a full lower denture, your patient should grasp the front and lingual (tongue) surfaces of the denture with his thumb and forefinger (see bottom photo).

To remove a partial denture, he should exert equal pressure on both sides of the denture close to his gum.

Caution: Warn the patient not to remove a partial denture by lifting the clasps. Doing so may bend or break the clasps.

Cleaning dentures

Stress the importance of keeping his dentures clean and in good condition. To accomplish this, instruct your patient to:
• handle his dentures carefully.
• brush his dentures after each meal and before going to bed. He should scrub them thoroughly with a hard brush. If your patient can't brush his dentures after every meal, tell him to rinse them with tap water. Encourage him to rinse his mouth when he brushes his dentures, especially after eating foods containing seeds.
• remove his dentures every night, unless otherwise indicated, and soak them in a covered container of tap water freshened with peppermint oil, lemon juice, or a commercial denture cleanser. He should change this solution daily.
• store his dentures in a safe place when he's not wearing them.

Note: His dentures should have permanent identification.

Instruct your patient to perform additional denture care, such as removing hard deposits or stains weekly or when necessary. Soaking dentures overnight in undiluted white vinegar will dissolve hard deposits. He can clean stains by immersing dentures in one of these three solutions: 1 teaspoon (5 ml) of ammonia in 8 ounces (240 ml) of water; 1 tablespoon (15 ml) of Clorox® and 2 tablespoons (30 ml) of Calgon® detergent in 8 ounces of water; or 1 tablespoon of white vinegar in 8 ounces of water. After 30 minutes, your patient should remove the dentures and brush and rinse them thoroughly.

Make sure your patient understands the specific care his dentures require. If he doesn't, have him request information from his dentist. Why is this important? Some toothpastes can discolor dentures made of certain types of plastic. Also, dentures made of chromium, cobalt, or nickel alloys require special cleaning care.

Whether your patient's wearing a complete or partial denture, remind him to continue daily hygiene on his remaining teeth, and on his gums, tongue, and palate.

Home care

Keeping hair healthy

Dear Patient:

Keeping your hair healthy and clean, whether you're at home or in the hospital, will help you feel and look better. To care for your hair properly, follow these instructions closely:

• Stimulate circulation and distribute natural oils to the ends of the hair shaft by brushing and combing your hair twice daily.

• Wash your hair weekly with shampoo that won't sting your eyes or dry your hair. If possible, wash your hair in the shower or use a hose attachment to rinse the shampoo completely out of your hair.

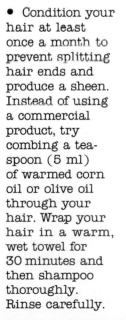

• Condition your hair at least once a month to prevent splitting hair ends and produce a sheen. Instead of using a commercial product, try combing a teaspoon (5 ml) of warmed corn oil or olive oil through your hair. Wrap your hair in a warm, wet towel for 30 minutes and then shampoo thoroughly. Rinse carefully.

• After shampooing, blot your hair dry with a towel. Apply a setting lotion, if you wish, to make your hair easier to comb.

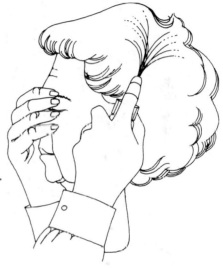

• Do you use hair spray? If you do, use only pump sprays (not aerosol sprays). Apply them in a well-ventilated room, with your eyes and nose covered.

• Chances are, you'll want your hair cut at least once every 8 weeks (if possible, by a professional).

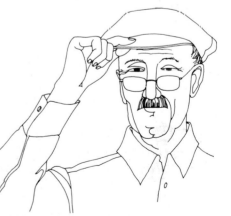

• If your hair is thinning, protect your scalp whenever you go outside. Wear a hat during the winter to keep your head warm and during the summer to prevent scalp sunburn. Also, apply a sunscreening lotion or cream on your exposed skin. Repeated sunburn can lead to serious skin problems.

If you decide to wear a hairpiece or a wig, consult a professional.

Daily hygiene

Giving a towel and lotion bath

1 *The doctor has ordered Bill O'Reilly, an 80-year-old retired teacher, to remain in bed for several days after a heart attack. To bathe him, while providing comfort, give him a towel-and-lotion bath. As you know, a towel-and-lotion bath soothes stiff, aching joints and eases discomfort from dry, itching skin. In addition, this type of bath won't tire your patient as much as a complete bed bath. Follow these steps:*

First, gather three medium-sized cotton terry cloth towels; a bath blanket (warmed); a plastic bag; and a basin. You'll also need a container of lotion warmed to 96° F. to 98° F. (35.6° C. to 36.7° C.). Now, wash your hands, and explain the procedure to your patient.

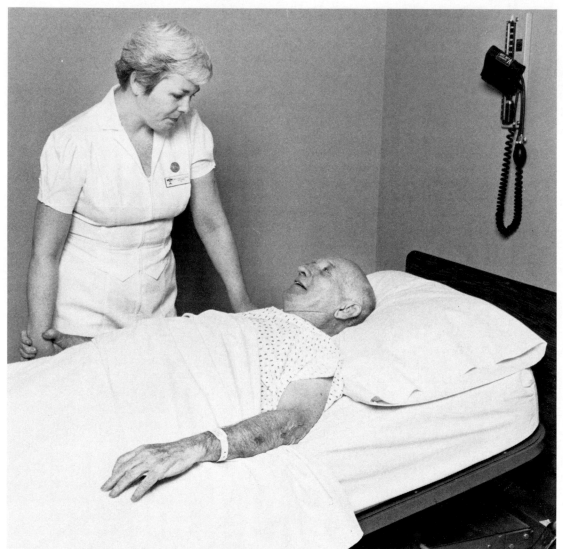

2 Place your patient in the supine position. Then, remove his gown, taking care to preserve his privacy. Take time to inspect his skin, especially bony prominences, for any redness, blisters, abrasions, or open sores. Next, pour the warmed solution into the plastic bag, and saturate the towels in the solution. Then, remove one towel from the bag and wring it out into a basin. Place the towel on your patient's feet and unroll it. Remove the top sheet as you unroll the towel.

📞 *Nursing tip:* To prevent the towel and your patient from cooling as you begin cleansing his legs, place a warmed bath blanket over the top half of his body, as shown.

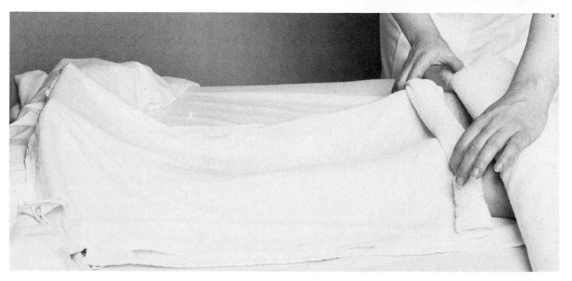

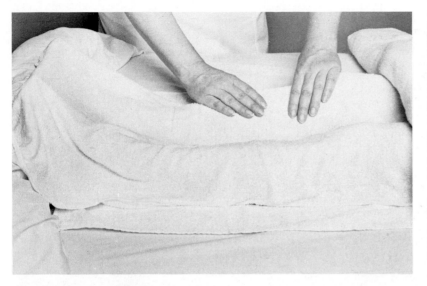

3 Begin cleansing your patient's feet, gently rubbing and massaging them. Cleanse the back, front, and sides of his legs, as the nurse is doing here. *Important:* Do not massage calf areas. Now, cover his legs with a clean sheet or warmed bath blanket.

Note: Because his skin will absorb the lotion quickly, you won't need to dry your patient with a towel, unless he asks you to.

4 Next, wring out a second towel, and place it on his upper body. Continue the bath by cleansing his torso, neck, and face.

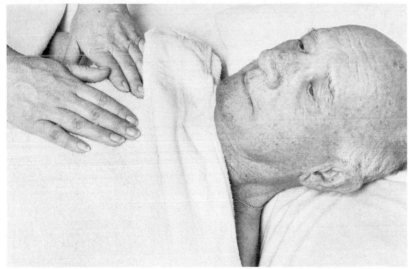

5 Now, turn your patient on his side or stomach, and use the third towel to cleanse his back and buttocks, as shown here.

Finally, put a clean gown on your patient, and change his bed linens.

Document your care in your nurses' notes.

Teaching fingernail care

Even though an older adult's fingernails grow slowly—around 0.5 mm per week (or about half the rate of a younger adult's)—frequent care is still necessary. Instruct your patient to perform daily nail care, including moisturizing and filing, using the procedure given in the following photostory. To keep his nails healthy and properly trimmed, he should supplement this care with weekly manicures. Remind him to perform all nail care in a well-lighted room.

Note: If your patient's hands are unsteady or he has limited vision, diabetes, circulatory problems, or any particular fingernail problems, perform nail care for him. Also, teach his family how to perform his nail care when he goes home. If your patient lives alone, make arrangements for a visiting nurse to care for his nails.

Proper nail care includes protecting the nails from harmful activities and agents. An older adult should:
• keep his hands out of water as much as possible and wear rubber gloves when he immerses his hands in water or cleaning solutions.
• wear a pair of cotton-lined gloves when gardening or doing yard work.
• moisturize his nails and cuticles daily to keep them soft and prevent cracking or tearing.
• buff his nails daily to stimulate circulation.

Daily hygiene

Giving a manicure

1 *If your patient has a slight tremor in her hands, she may not be able to perform nail care for herself. Follow these steps to give her a weekly manicure.*

First, wash your hands and explain the procedure to your patient. Then, gather the equipment you'll need: emery board; cotton-tipped applicators; orangewood stick; basin or container deep enough to submerge the patient's fingers; soap; nail clipper or scissors; towel; baby oil, water-soluble lubricating jelly or cold cream; hand cream or lotion; colorless nail polish; and polish remover.

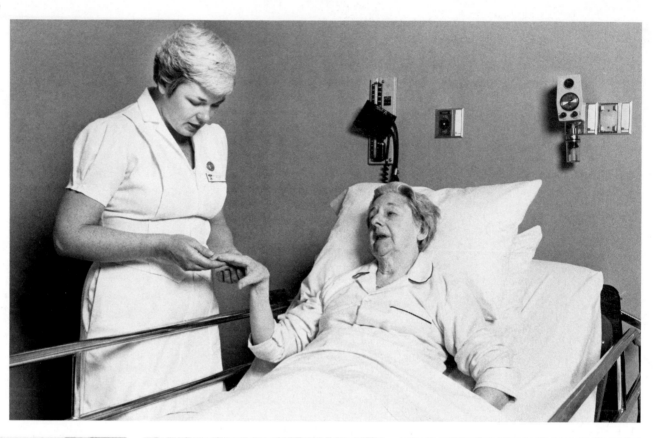

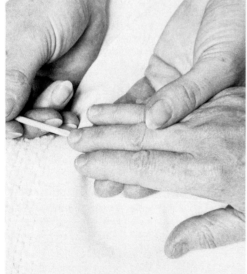

2 If your patient is wearing nail polish, remove it with polish remover or acetone. Wash her hands with warm water. Then, use the pointed end of an orangewood stick to clean under her nails, as shown. Pat her hands thoroughly dry.

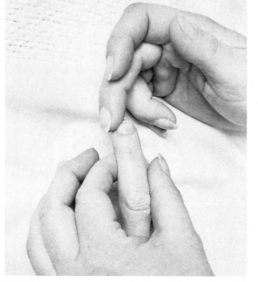

3 Massage your patient's nails and cuticles, using the softener she prefers. Rub the softener into the sides of her nails and where they extend over the fingers, as the nurse is doing here. Massaging these areas stimulates blood circulation to the nail bed and prevents both callus formation and cuticle separation from the nail bed.

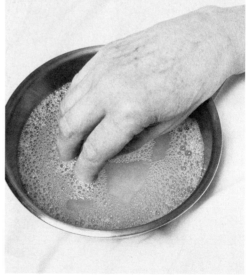

4 Then, soak the nails for 3 to 5 minutes in warm, soapy water. Doing this will both clean the nails and soften the cuticle further.

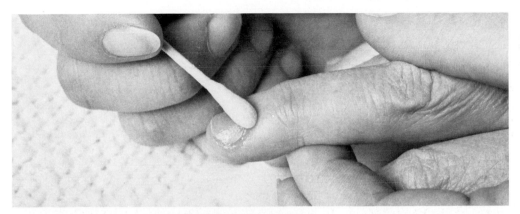

5 Now, using a cotton-tipped applicator (or an orangewood stick with a small amount of cotton wrapped around the blunt side), gently push back the cuticles, as shown.
Caution: Avoid chafing or poking the cuticles; this can cause hangnails or infection.

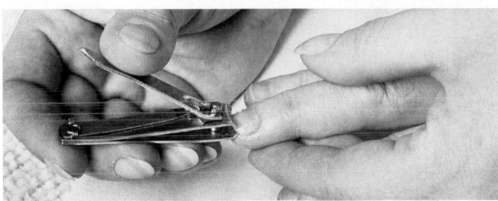

6 Next, you'll use sharp clippers or nail scissors to cut your patient's nails. To do so properly, follow the contour of each nail. If the cuticle's torn, remove the loose skin flap, but avoid cutting any additional skin, which could cause the cuticle to thicken and become infected.

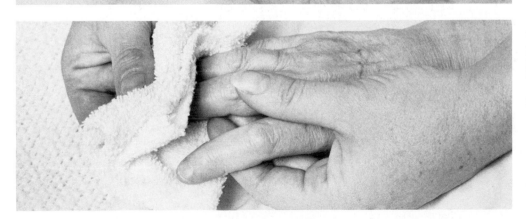

7 Then, remove any rough edges by applying an emery board to the nail, as shown. Hold the emery board at a 45° angle to the nail. When filing, stroke in one direction rather than sawing back and forth.

8 Now, rinse and dry your patient's fingers thoroughly, as shown. Then, if your patient doesn't object, apply colorless nail polish and sealer for added protection. Finally, apply hand cream.
Document the procedure in your nurses' notes.

Caring for your patient's feet

Let's say you're caring for Amelia Rocco, a 79-year-old housewife who was admitted to the hospital with hypertension. Mrs. Rocco tells you she has a foot problem. Until she can be examined by a podiatrist, she may need the following immediate treatment. Be sure to obtain a doctor's order before giving this care.

Suppose she has one of the following problems:
• **Corn or callus.** Apply water-soluble lubricating jelly or cold cream to the affected area. Because friction or pressure can cause a corn or callus, your patient should avoid wearing tight-fitting shoes.
• **Suppurative soft corn.** Apply a continuous cold wet dressing, moistened with normal saline solution. Note: At home, your patient can use a solution of 1 level teaspoon (5 ml) of table salt or boric acid crystals dissolved in 8 ounces (240 ml) of water.
• **Itching or burning sensation between the toes.** Wash and dry the area thoroughly. Then, apply thimerosal (Merthiolate) or fungicidal powder. Finally, cover the foot with a tubular gauze dressing or white cotton sock.
• **Fissure between the toes.** Wash and dry the area thoroughly. Swab the fissure with hydrogen peroxide solution, alcohol, or merbromin (Mercurochrome). Then, place a cotton ball or lamb's wool over it.
• **Painful metatarsal head.** Cut a 2″X2″ (5.1 cm square) pad from a ⅛″ (0.6 cm) thick foam pad or moleskin. Cut out a hole in the middle of the pad to keep pressure off the sensitive area. Place the pad over the affected area, making sure you position the hole directly over the painful area, and secure the pad.
• **General burning or itching, without a rash.** Wash and dry the area thoroughly. Rub the area with witch hazel or a mentholated preparation; then put lightweight cotton stockings or socks on your patient's feet.
• **Abrasion or blister.** Wash and dry the area thoroughly. Dress the abrasion or blister with ½″ (1.3 cm) wide roller bandage, lamb's wool, absorbent lint bandage, or narrow tubular gauze dressing.

Teaching daily foot care

Keeping your older patient's feet healthy and comfortable makes a significant difference in his overall well-being. Why? Because in addition to causing local pain, foot discomfort can cause aches elsewhere in the body, especially if he changes his gait to compensate for discomfort. Also, foot discomfort may make your patient tire more easily and further curtail mobility limited by stiff joints.

What can you teach your patient about proper foot care? Here are some guidelines:
• See a podiatrist or visit a podiatry clinic on a regular basis.
• Always wear cotton socks or nylon stockings with shoes.
• Never wear knee-high nylons, use garters, or tie stockings around your thighs.
• Wear supportive, nonskid, closed-toed shoes or slippers when walking, to prevent foot injury. Wearing shoes also reduces the risk of contracting athlete's foot.
• Wear a different pair of shoes every day or every few days, if possible.
• To promote comfort and accommodate changing foot contour, wear shoes made of naturally ventilating leather or calfskin, with cushioned inner soles.
• Make sure shoes, insoles, socks, and stockings fit correctly and don't pinch, bind, or rub.
• Remove all sources of abrasion, bruising, and blistering, such as pebbles or sand.
• Break in new shoes over a period of several days. Wear new shoes no longer than 30 minutes at a time.
• Massage feet and toes daily to increase blood circulation and alleviate pressure from footwear.
• Provide immediate treatment for any foot problems, as outlined at left.

Your patient should also perform the following foot hygiene regularly:
• Inspecting feet daily (including the soles, the nails, and between and around the toes) for redness, cracking, abrasions, lacerations, scaling, corns, calluses, and ingrown nails. Instruct the patient to perform the inspection in good lighting and to notify you or his doctor of any problems.

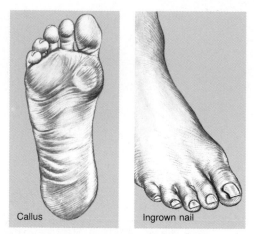
Callus   Ingrown nail

• Changing socks or stockings daily.
• Applying body lotion to his feet daily. Instruct him to apply lotion only after a thorough cleaning and to wipe off any excess with a towel. Remind him to put on clean socks or stockings afterward.
• Applying rubbing alcohol or witch hazel to his feet twice daily if he has profuse perspiration and foot odor. He should always dry his feet thoroughly and wear clean cotton socks each day.
• Soaking both feet weekly in a plastic or metal basin of warm, soapy water. The water temperature should be about 88° F. to 95° F. (31.1° C. to 35° C.). When filling the basin, your patient should begin with cool water and gradually add warm water, as needed. While his feet are immersed, he should perform range-of-motion exercises, such as wiggling his toes, stretching his feet, and flexing and extending his toes and ankles. Then, he should rinse his feet, pat them dry, and dry between his toes.
• Gently rubbing an orangewood stick under each nail, to free any adhering skin.
• Rubbing pumice stone on the heels, soles, and sides of his feet, to remove dry, dead skin.
• Clipping toenails straight across (see illustration), unless contraindicated by foot or nail problems. If problems exist, a podiatrist should cut his nails.

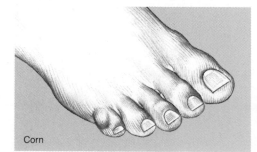
Corn

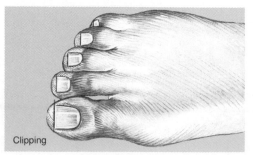
Clipping

How to give a foot massage

1 *Promoting your patient's comfort and general well-being is one of your major nursing goals. A foot massage will help by stimulating blood circulation, reducing foot edema, promoting relaxation, and improving pedal flexibility.*

Caution: Foot lesions or vascular problems in your patient's legs may contraindicate massage.

If massage *is* indicated, teach your patient and his family members how to give one, so they can do so after discharge.

Obtain a container of lotion or oil. Explain the procedure to your patient as you position him comfortably in bed or in a chair. If your patient's in bed, seat yourself at the foot of the bed. If he's seated, sit facing him. Cover your lap with a towel. Support your patient's foot between your knees or rest it on your lap. Apply a generous amount of lotion to your patient's foot.

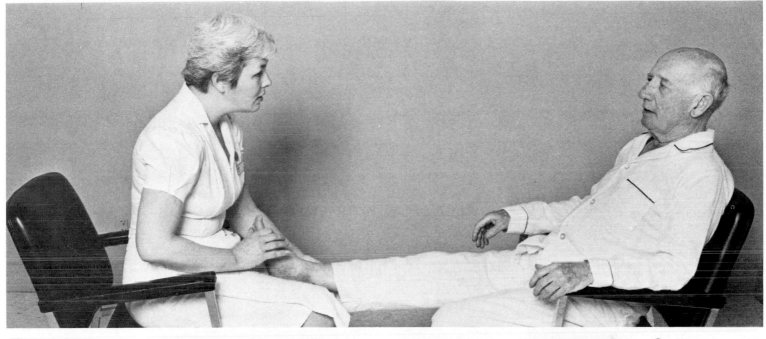

2 To begin the massage, steady his right foot with one hand and use the knuckles of your other hand to make small, firm circles over the entire sole, including the heel, as shown here. Massage firmly; too light a touch could tickle him.

Note: Never suggest to your patient that he'll feel a ticklish sensation. Doing so may cause the sensation to develop.

Avoid applying heavy pressure to an older adult's feet, which are more sensitive than those of a young person. Your patient's general condition and response to pressure as well as the amount of callus present will determine the degree of pressure you'll apply.

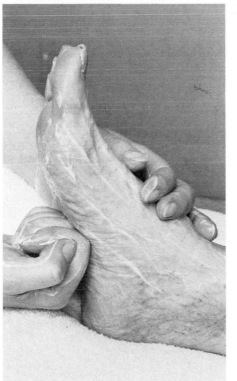

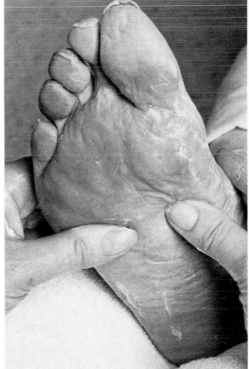

3 Now, support his foot with the fingers of both hands while you use your thumbs to make small circles over the sole, as the nurse is doing here.

Daily hygiene

4 Next, place one hand under his ankle and gently lift his foot. With the other hand, move your fingertips and thumb in small, firm circles over his sole.

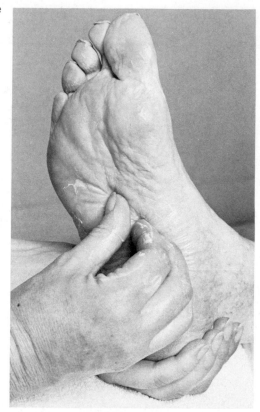

6 Then, grasp your patient's foot with both hands, with your fingers under his sole and the heels of your hands on the top of his foot. Squeeze his foot firmly between your fingers and the heels of your hands, as shown, and then slide your hands toward the edges of his foot. Repeat this motion three times.

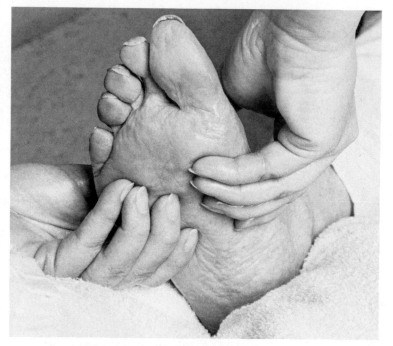

5 Then, locate the long ten dons that run from the base of the ankle to each toe, on his foot's *upper* surface. Now, as you support his heel with one hand, firmly but gently run the thumb of your free hand between each tendon groove and off his foot between the toes, as shown. Adjust the amount of pressure you use, as this manipulation can cause your patient discomfort.

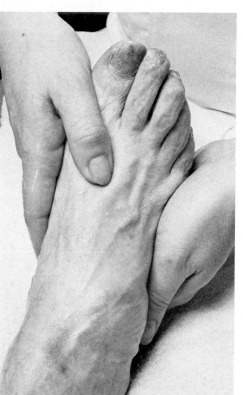

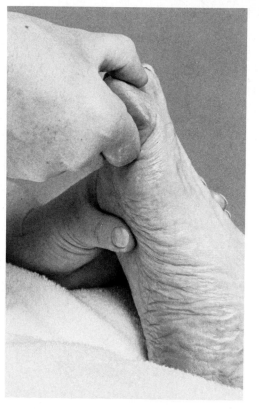

7 Next, use one hand to steady his foot. Grasp the base of his great toe with the thumb and forefinger of your other hand. Gently stretch and rotate the toe, using a corkscrew motion, as shown, until your fingers slide off the tip of his toe. Repeat this procedure on each toe.

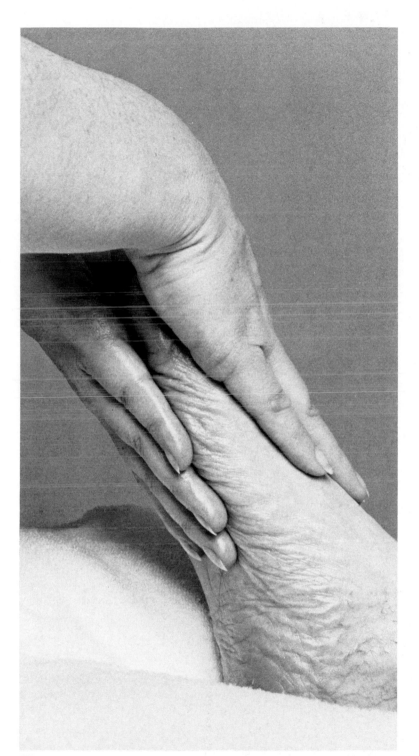

8 Now, complete the massage by cradling his foot between your hands, as the nurse is doing here, and holding it for several seconds. Then, gently place this foot next to his other foot. Repeat the massage on his other foot.

Remember to wash your hands thoroughly after giving a massage. Then, document the massage in your nurses' notes.

Maintaining self-esteem through good grooming

Growing old doesn't necessarily mean looking old. A person can compensate for aging's physical effects by maintaining proper daily hygiene and dressing in clean, neat clothing. If you're caring for an older adult, stress the need for consistent good grooming.

Clean, attractive clothing, for example, promotes dignity and individuality. A daily change of apparel also expresses your patient's control over his life and can signify a link to the outside world. If you're caring for your patient in the hospital, recommend that his family bring nightgowns or pajamas, slippers, and a robe for him to wear. Stress bringing clothing that's easily laundered at the sink and simple to put on and take off. *Note:* When your patient goes home, remind the family to encourage his grooming efforts.

For the male patient

Instruct your patient to pay particular attention to grooming his facial hair. Encourage him to shave his face or trim his mustache, beard, and sideburns regularly. Recommend applying lathering creams before shaving to protect his skin against sharp razors. Make sure he has a styptic pencil or tissue to stop any bleeding from facial cuts. *Note:* If he's unsteady, assist him with shaving, or recommend switching to an electric razor. In addition, suggest that your patient apply after-shave lotions or moisturizers to protect his facial skin. Also, remind him that brushing or combing his eyebrows promotes a neater appearance.

For the female patient

The older female may experience increased facial hair growth. If this embarrasses her, she can remove the hair by shaving, tweezing, waxing, or electrolysis, or she can bleach it with hydrogen peroxide solution and lemon juice.

To protect her skin and prevent dryness, emphasize cleaning her face thoroughly and applying a moisturizer. Recommend soy and almond oils, if available, rather than glycerin and rosewater lotions, which can dehydrate her face. She should apply moisturizers in gentle, upward strokes, especially over her throat and eyes.

Also, encourage your female patient to continue using cosmetics, if she already does so. Suggest that she experiment with new colors and brands (unless you think this may offend her).

Suppose she shows a definite interest in using cosmetics and learning new tips for their application. If so, point out that she can accent her eyebrows with a *light*-colored pencil or brush, applying a soft, feathery stroke. Also, suggest using an eyebrow brush to fluff thinning brows, by running the brush across the eyebrow in the direction opposite hair growth. If she uses eye shadow, tell her to apply a liquid rather than powdered one to avoid accentuating skin dryness. For the same reason, she should avoid frosted makeup and face powder. Using light liquid blusher will give her face a translucent glow. Lip gloss also lends a soft glow and will keep her lips well moisturized.

Stress the importance of daily removing any cosmetics she uses. After removing all makeup, she should wash her face with soap, and apply a skin freshener, such as lemon juice. Next, she should apply a moisturizer; for example, water-soluble lubricating jelly, or soy or almond oil.

Document your teaching in your nurses' notes.

Skin care

The aging changes described in the first section mean your geriatric patient's skin requires special attention. In the following pages, we identify the areas of his skin most vulnerable to pressure when he's in supine, prone, and side-lying positions. We'll also show you how to protect and stimulate circulation in these pressure areas through proper positioning, pressure relief aids, and back rubs.

Suppose your patient does develop a decubitus ulcer, even with good care. We'll show you how to apply a new type of adhesive wound dressing to promote its healing.

Read the following pages for all this and more information, including tips on protecting your patient from hypothermia and heatstroke.

Understanding why a decubitus ulcer develops

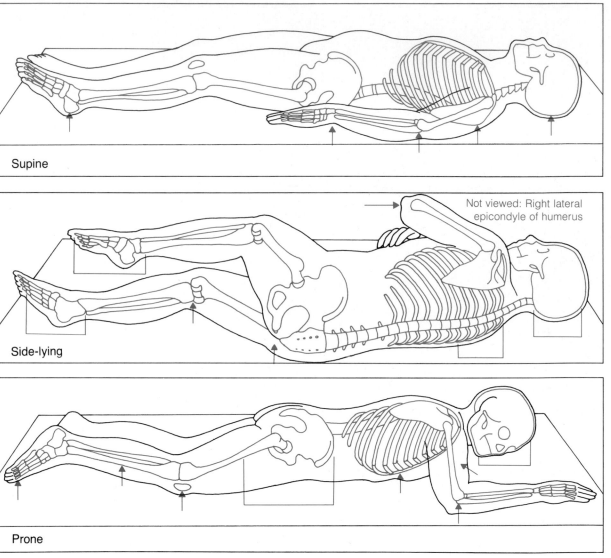

Supine

Not viewed: Right lateral epicondyle of humerus

Side-lying

Prone

As you know, any patient can develop decubitus ulcers from prolonged pressure on vulnerable skin areas. But, this form of skin breakdown most commonly affects the older adult, especially if he sits for long periods or is bedridden. Why? Because he may have one or more of the following predisposing conditions:
• decreased subcutaneous fat
• poor nutrition
• impaired circulation
• impaired sensation
• moisture loss in skin
• immobilization.

Continuous light pressure over a long period causes more skin damage than heavy pressure for a short period. Also, shearing force can create decubitus ulcers; for example, when a patient sits up in bed and gradually slides down or when he's turned or lifted carelessly. Prolonged contact with wet sheets may also cause decubitus ulcers.

Equipment can induce skin breakdown as well. For example, some chair seats apply pressure to the buttocks, and those with plastic cause sweating. Other sources of pressure include X-ray, operating, and examination tables; traction devices; braces; restraints; and irritating objects, such as food crumbs, in the bed.

Do you know how to assess your patient for skin breakdown? Whenever you reposition your patient, observe the body parts most susceptible to pressure, as indicated in the above illustrations. Inspect these areas for dry or chapped skin, which may have been irritated by scratching. Also, look for reddened areas, and note those regions that remain blanched after you've relieved any pressure: both signal early stages of decubitus ulcer formation.

Be sure to relieve existing pressure immediately. Also, gently massage the affected area to improve circulation. If you don't, blistering will develop, leading to local cyanosis, open ulceration, and possibly infection. Document your observations in your nurses' notes.

Positioning your patient

Supine

Side-lying

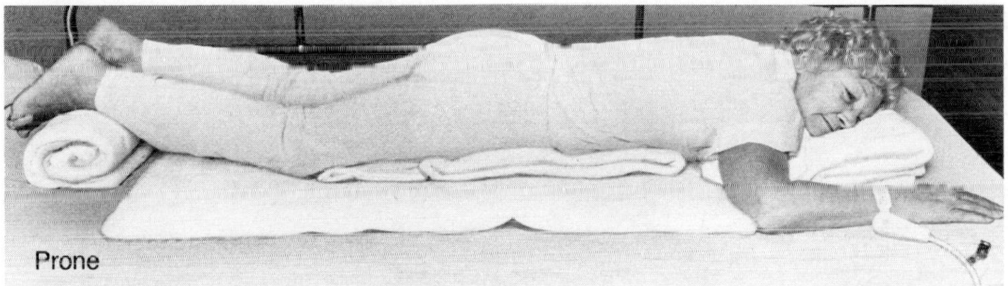

Prone

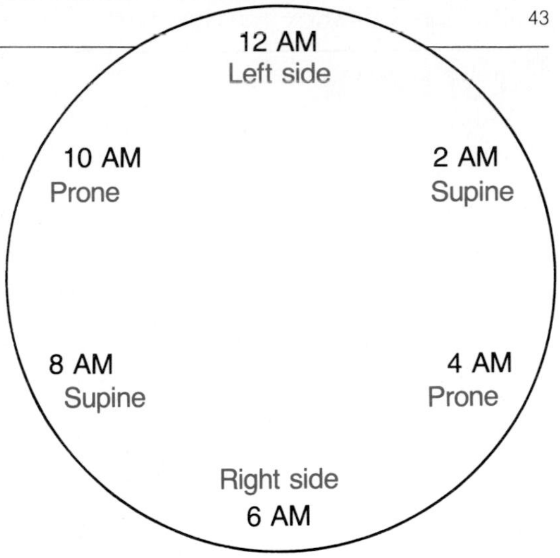

12 AM
Left side

10 AM
Prone

2 AM
Supine

8 AM
Supine

4 AM
Prone

Right side
6 AM

12 PM
Supine

10 PM
Prone

2 PM
Right side

8 PM
Right side

4 PM
Left side

Supine
6 PM

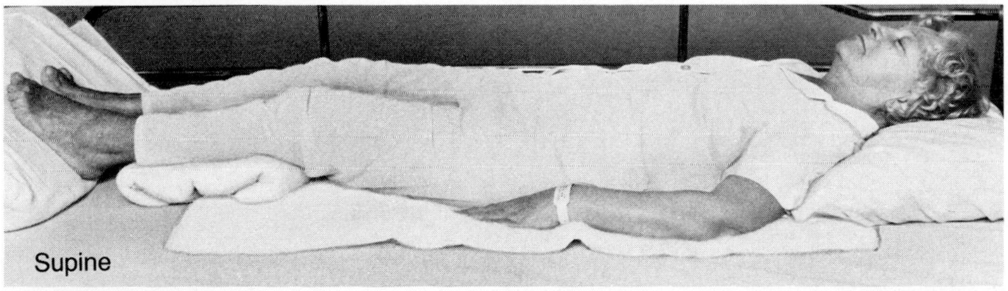

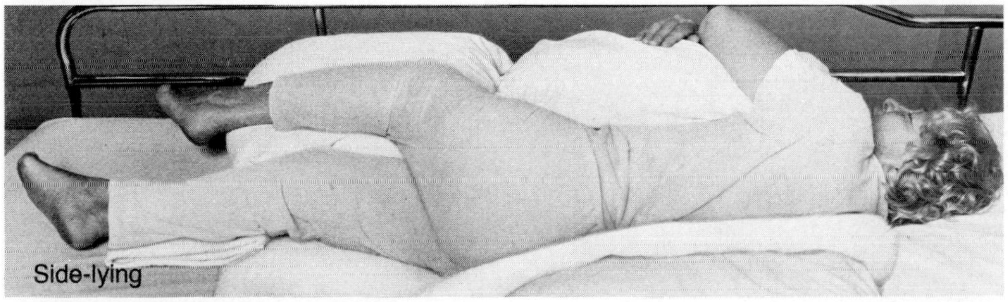

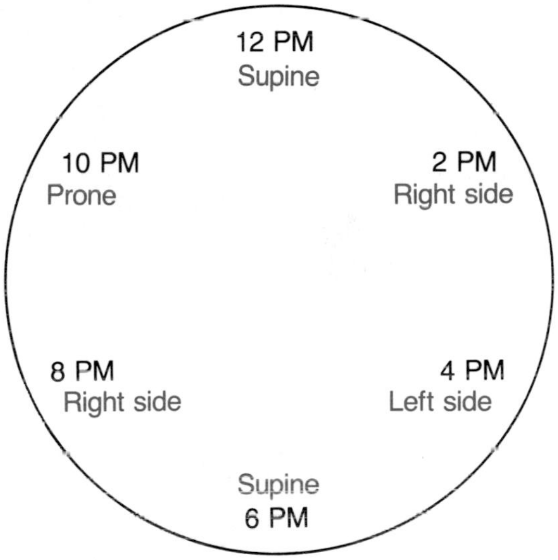

As you know, proper positioning and frequent repositioning can help prevent and alleviate decubitus ulcer formation by stimulating blood circulation and preventing pressure buildup on the skin.

Do you know how to place your patient properly in the supine, side-lying, or prone positions? If not, follow these guidelines.

When positioning your patient supine, make sure you:
• place her head in line with her spine.
• flex her hips minimally and straighten her trunk.
• slightly flex her arms at the elbows, and rest her hands alongside or on top of her abdomen.
• extend her legs.
• support her feet at a 45° angle (with a footboard, for example) and point her toes upward.
• promote comfort and reduce the pressure on your patient's body with adequate padding. Place a pillow under her head, neck and scapulae, a washcloth under her sacrum, and a bath blanket under her lower legs, supporting them from just below the popliteal space to just above her ankles. Also, make sure her heels are off the bed.

When positioning your patient in a side-lying position, make sure you do the following:
• place her head in line with her spine, and support her head and neck with a pillow.
• support her back with a pillow, and wrap her arms around another pillow.
• move her upper leg forward, with her knee flexed. Place a pillow under her legs and keep her heel off the bed.
• slightly flex her lower leg at the knee, and support the lower leg with a towel.

When positioning your patient prone, make sure you:
• turn her head laterally and align it with her body. Place a folded towel under her cheek.
• abduct her arms, externally rotating them at the shoulders and flexing them at the elbows.
• support her shoulders and chest with folded towels.
• place her legs in extension.
• support her abdomen and upper thighs with folded towels, while supporting her ankles with a folded bath blanket to keep pressure off her knees and toes.

You can also redistribute the pressure by using flotation devices, such as a water mattress. Other pressure-reducing devices include sheepskin or wool mattress pads, air or foam mattresses, and gel-filled pads.

■ *Nursing tip:* If you're caring for your patient at home, make an inexpensive water mattress by partially filling a camping mattress with water. To make a small water pad, partially fill several rubber gloves with water and wrap them in a towel or sheepskin.

Reposition your patient at least every 2 hours. If the reddened areas on her skin don't return to normal color after 5 minutes, turn her more frequently; for example, every 1 to 1½ hours. To indicate your patient's position and the length of time she should remain in each position, keep a turning chart (see illustration) at her bedside.

For further information on proper turning and positioning, see the NURSING PHOTOBOOK COPING WITH NEUROLOGIC DISORDERS. For additional information about special beds designed to prevent decubitus ulcer formation, see the NURSING PHOTOBOOK WORKING WITH ORTHOPEDIC PATIENTS.

Skin care

How to perform a back rub

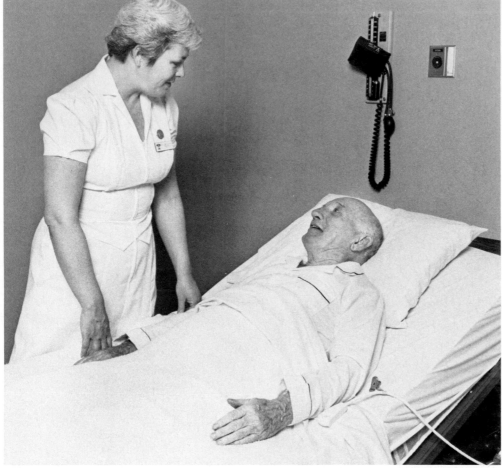

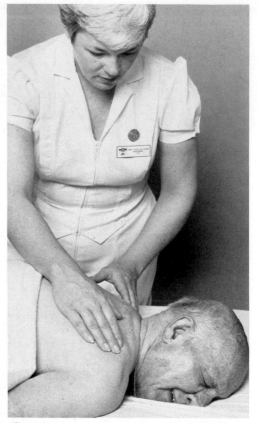

1 *As part of your patient's daily care, you'll administer a back rub. A properly performed back rub stimulates blood circulation, promotes comfort and relaxation, and gives your patient personalized care.*

Never rush through a back rub. Doing so lessens its positive effects. Take this opportunity to talk with your patient and get to know him better. If you are pressed for time, coordinate the back rub with other activities. For example, at the same time, you can turn and reposition your patient and assess his skin.

Nursing tip: Try giving a back rub shortly after administering pain medication, to enhance the medication's effects. Or, give the medication after you've relaxed your patient with a back rub.

2 Wash your hands thoroughly, and obtain a container of lotion. Then, explain the procedure to your patient, and place him in the prone position. If this position's contraindicated or he finds it uncomfortable, place him on his side, as close as safely possible to the side of the bed where you're standing.

Next, adjust the bed to a comfortable height for you to give the back rub. Inspect his skin for signs of breakdown, especially over bony prominences or other vulnerable areas, as the nurse is doing here.

Coping with decubitus ulcers

Helen Rigierri, a 72-year-old homemaker, has been admitted to the hospital with chronic bronchitis complicated by bilateral pneumonia. From prolonged bed rest at home, she's developed decubitus ulcers on her elbows and coccyx. In addition to treating her bronchitis and pneumonia, as ordered by the doctor, you must take steps to promote ulcer healing and prevent new ulcers.

Follow these guidelines:
• Use pressure relief aids to prevent direct pressure on affected areas and bony prominences.
• Change dressings frequently to keep ulcers dry. Doing so discourages bacteria growth.
• Encourage activity and range-of-motion exercises to increase your patient's blood circulation.

• Supply foods and fluids with high calorie, protein, mineral, and vitamin content.
• Protect your patient's *healthy* skin through frequent turning and proper positioning (see page 43).

Are you familiar with the treatments used to heal decubitus ulcers? The doctor may order one or more of the following:
• chemical debridement—debridement with an enzyme preparation of collagenase, proteolysin, and fibrinolysin you apply directly to the ulcer.
• Gelfoam®—a granulation aid you apply to the ulcer and cover with a dry, sterile dressing.
• karaya—a granulation aid you sprinkle into the ulcer after cleaning and irrigating the ulcer with hydrogen peroxide solution. Then, the

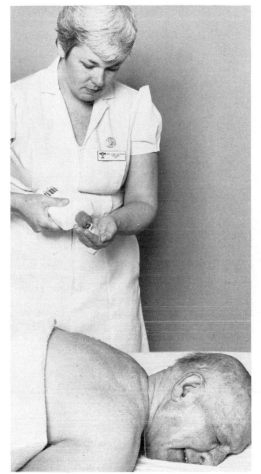

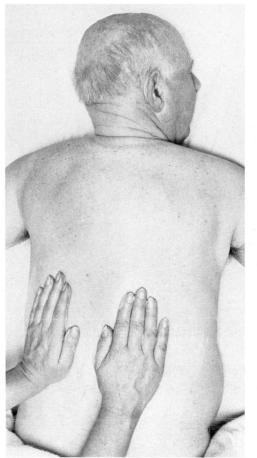

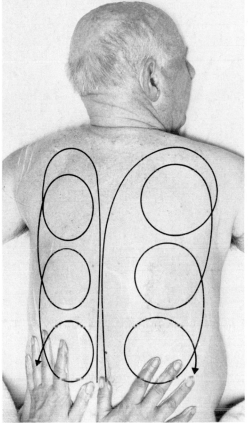

3 To prevent friction and skin injury, apply a moderate amount of lotion to your palm. (Use more as needed.) Close your hand to warm the lotion, or run hot water over the lotion container before use.

Caution: Avoid using talcum powder for a back rub, because it can collect on areas of perspiration in skin folds and may cause skin breakdown.

4 Now, transfer some of the lotion to your other palm, and position your hands side by side, palms down, at the base of your patient's spine. Then, glide your hands along both sides of your patient's backbone, as the nurse is doing here, until you reach his neck. Exert light to moderate pressure, keeping in mind your size and strength relative to your patient's size and condition.

5 Now, separate your hands at his neck, and work them down both sides of his back, toward the base of his spine. Rub in an upward and outward motion, as shown here. Be sure to massage his hips, buttocks, and coccyx, too.

Continue rubbing your patient's back for 3 to 5 minutes, alternating this stroke with a long, stroking motion. When you've finished, help your patient into a clean gown. Document the massage and any observations in your nurses' notes.

---

ulcer is encircled with a karaya ring and covered with plastic wrap.
• wet-to-dry dressings—a debriding procedure you perform using dressings saturated with a cleaning agent, such as Debrisan®. After the dressing dries on the skin, it's replaced with another wet dressing.
• Maalox* suspension and heat lamp—a drying procedure in which you apply a thin coat of Maalox suspension with a cotton applicator or swab (after cleaning the ulcer).
• sugar—a bacteria dehydrating agent you apply to the ulcer in a thin coat, and then cover with a dressing (if indicated).
• whirlpool bath—a debriding method that also stimulates circulation. In most cases, use of the whirlpool bath is combined with one of the above treatments.

*Available in both the United States and in Canada

Other treatments include surgery, electrotherapy, and hyperbaric oxygen therapy.

The doctor may order the ulcer covered with a gauze dressing. If so, secure it with small amounts of nonallergenic tape. When you change the dressing, change the tape placement to prevent skin irritation.

As an alternative to taping, use a tubular net stretch bandage such as Surgifix™ to hold the dressing in place.

📧 *Nursing tip:* To prevent skin irritation, you may apply Stomahesive® around the ulcer before you apply the dressing, and tape the dressing directly onto the Stomahesive.

Or, instead of using a gauze dressing, you may apply an Op-Site® dressing over the ulcer, as explained on the next page.

Skin care

Learning about Op-Site®

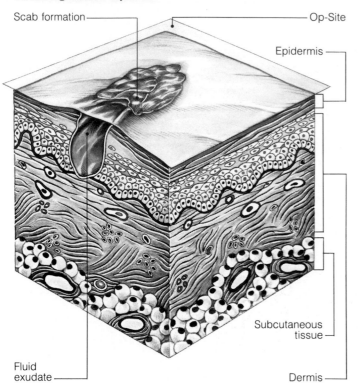

Scab formation

Op-Site

Epidermis

Subcutaneous tissue

Fluid exudate

Dermis

Instead of using a gauze dressing, the doctor may order your patient's decubitus ulcer covered with an Op-Site dressing, after the ulcer's been thoroughly cleaned and dried. (See the photostory at right to find out how this dressing's applied.)

This transparent dressing adheres directly to the skin surrounding the affected area, aiding healing by retaining natural body fluids and shielding the area from bacteria entry.

Being waterproof and elastic, Op-Site allows daily bathing of the area as well as normal mobility. Also, the dressing allows you to see the affected area clearly. Once applied, Op-Site can usually remain in place without being changed, until the ulcer has healed.

After applying Op-Site to your patient's ulcer, follow these guidelines:
• Expect normal fluid formation beneath the dressing.
• Change the dressing only if indicated by excessive drainage, loosening of the dressing, or signs of infection, such as purulent, foul-smelling drainage.
• When changing the dressing, use a 4"x4" sterile gauze pad to clean and thoroughly dry the area before applying a new dressing.
• If the dressing adheres to the wound surface, allow it to loosen naturally rather than by pulling it away. Use a soapy solution if you must remove the dressing.
• Carefully remove the dressing after the ulcer has healed, as ordered.
Caution: Folliculitis can develop under an Op-Site dressing from the pressure of newly grown hair against the dressing film. If so, you may need to remove the dressing. Notify the doctor, and obtain his order for alternative treatment.

Using Op-Site® as a decubitus ulcer dressing

1 *The doctor has ordered you to apply Op-Site wound dressing over your patient's decubitus ulcer. To apply the dressing, follow these steps.*

First, gather the following sterile equipment: gloves, two basins or bowls, water, four 4"x4" gauze pads, and Op-Site wound dressing. You'll also need a bottle of povidone-iodine solution. Next, wash your hands thoroughly, and explain the procedure to your patient.

Note: Remember to observe strict aseptic technique.

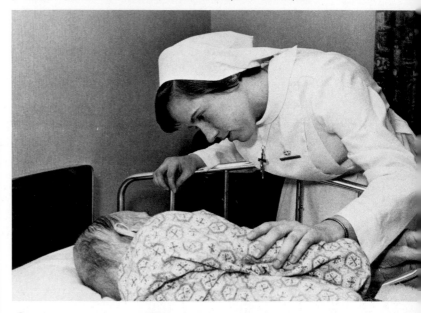

2 Now, pour the povidone-iodine solution and the sterile water into separate sterile basins or bowls. Next, put on your sterile gloves. Then, saturate a gauze pad in the povidone-iodine solution and cleanse the ulcer, as shown here, lightly scrubbing it and the surrounding area with the gauze pad.

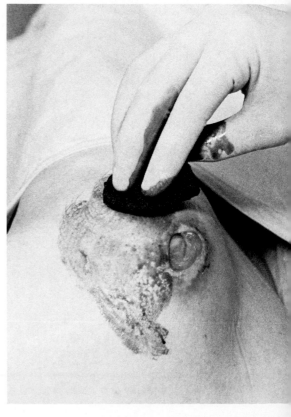

3 Next, saturate a second gauze pad in sterile water and wring it out over the ulcer, as shown.

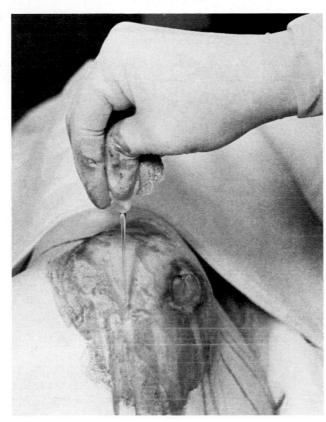

4 Then, use another gauze pad to gently blot dry the ulcer and the surrounding skin.

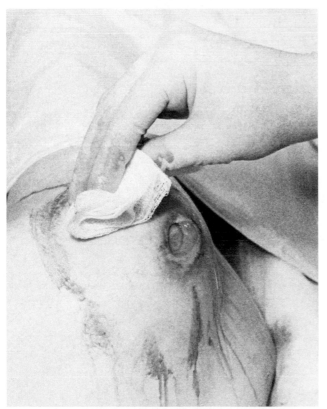

5 Now, take the Op-Site packet, and remove part of the dressing's protective paper. Then, use your thumb to press the dressing on your patient's skin near the wound, as the nurse is doing here.

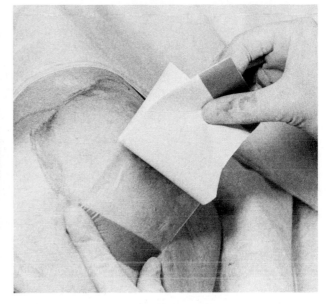

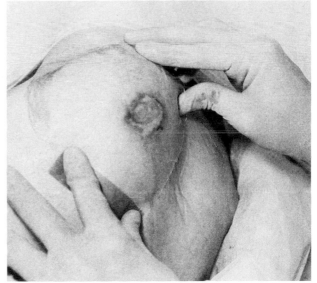

6 Finally, peel the remaining paper off the dressing and smooth the dressing over the wound and surrounding skin. Make sure you anchor the four sides of the dressing securely to prevent leakage. But allow some slack on the skin immediately around the ulcer to accommodate normal drainage.

Note: Avoid placing the dressing too tightly on the skin; doing so may cause irritation.

After you're finished, remove your gloves. Dispose of the pads and gloves, according to hospital policy. Wash your hands thoroughly. Then, document the procedure and the ulcer's appearance, in your nurses' notes.

Skin care

Protecting your patient from temperature variations

Some of the skin changes that occur with age—for example, seborrheic keratosis and slower nail growth—are only cosmetic. However, decreasing glandular activity as well as loss of body fat and body hair leave the older adult vulnerable to much more serious (and possibly fatal) problems, such as hypothermia, heatstroke, and heat exhaustion.

Hypothermia

This condition develops when a person's *internal* body temperature falls to 95° F. (35° C.) or below. It can occur anytime a person is exposed to cold without adequate protection and may occur immediately or over a period of several days. Persons over age 65 may develop hypothermia from exposure to temperatures as mild as 60° F. (15.6° C.).

Signs and symptoms
• Sluggishness
• Lack of coordination
• Slurred speech
• Confusion and disorientation
• Slow, shallow breathing
• Slow and sometimes irregular heartbeat
• Weak pulse and low blood pressure

• Uncontrollable shivering or lack of shivering
• Unusual change in appearance
• Possible coma

Factors increasing risk
• Turning down household heat, without putting on additional layers of clothing
• Immobilization; for example, by arthritis
• Taking such medications as phenothiazines, which alter body temperature
• Chronic illness
• Circulatory disorder
• Defective body temperature regulator. This prevents a person from feeling cold, so his body doesn't receive a signal to produce heat by shivering.
• Living alone, without anyone to

help make sure he stays warm.

Nursing interventions
• If you suspect hypothermia, take the patient's rectal temperature with a special low-reading thermometer. Or, use a regular thermometer, making sure you shake it down thoroughly.
• Notify the doctor immediately if the patient's temperature is below 95° F. (35° C.).
• Until the doctor arrives to treat your patient's hypothermia, you can prevent further heat loss by wrapping the patient in a thermal blanket. Conserving warmth may prevent such complications as kidney and liver dysfunction and ventricular fibrillation.
• If the patient's alert, give him a small amount of a warm *nonalco-*

holic liquid.
• Avoid rubbing the patient's arms and legs, which could cause tissue necrosis.

Patient teaching
To guard against hypothermia, instruct the older adult to:
• set the household thermostat no lower than 65° F. (18.3° C.) in the living and sleeping areas.
• wear adequate clothing when going to bed as well as at other times.
• stay as active as possible.
• eat nourishing foods.
• ask the doctor whether prescribed medications may alter body temperature.
• ask relatives, friends, or neighbors to check on him daily by phone or in person during cold weather.

Heatstroke

Heat and humidity bring the potential for heatstroke, which occurs when heat-regulating mechanisms in the hypothalamus fail to maintain a normal body temperature. This condition requires *immediate* medical attention.

Signs and symptoms
• Faintness
• Dizziness
• Headache and visual disturbances
• Nausea
• Loss of consciousness
• Rectal body temperature of

104° F. (40° C.) or higher
• Rapid (possibly irregular) pulse rate
• Hot, flushed, dry skin
• Severe muscle cramps

Factors increasing risk
• Circulatory, renal, or cerebral disease
• Alcoholism
• History of heatstroke or heat exhaustion

Nursing interventions
• Move your patient out of the sun, or away from the heat source.

• You may give the patient a tepid bath or shower or use ice packs, cool towels, or a sponge bath to lower his body temperature to 102° F. (38.9° C.). If he's hospitalized, you may use a hyper-hypothermia blanket.
• Notify the doctor, or take the patient to the emergency department.

Patient teaching
To guard against heatstroke, instruct the older adult to:
• remain indoors during the warmest part of the day (between noon

and 2 p.m.)
• stay out of direct sunlight and avoid strenuous activity.
• wear lightweight clothing to allow perspiration to evaporate more rapidly, cooling him faster.
• wear light-colored clothing and a hat to help deflect the sun's rays.
• use air conditioners, fans, cool baths or showers, icebags, wet towels, or sitting in the shade to promote coolness.
• drink such liquids as water, fruit and vegetable juices, and iced tea to replenish body fluids lost through perspiration.

Heat exhaustion

Extreme loss of body water and sodium produces heat exhaustion, a slower developing and less severe condition than heatstroke. In heat exhaustion, the patient's body temperature remains normal or nearly normal.

Signs and symptoms
• Weakness
• Dizziness
• Profuse sweating
• Nausea
• Giddiness
• Muscle cramps
• Cool, clammy, pale skin

• Hypotension
• Mental confusion

Factors increasing risk
• Circulatory, renal, or cerebral disease
• Alcoholism
• History of heatstroke or heat exhaustion

Nursing interventions
• Give the patient cool liquids to drink and keep him out of direct sunlight.
• Avoid giving alcoholic beverages or salty fluids because they may

cause fluid and electrolyte imbalance.
• Administer salt tablets only if ordered.
• After recovery, caution the patient to rest sufficiently before resuming his normal daily activities.

Patient teaching
To guard against heat exhaustion, instruct the older adult to:
• remain indoors during the warmest part of the day (between noon and 2 p.m.).
• stay out of direct sunlight and avoid strenuous activity.

• wear lightweight clothing to allow perspiration to evaporate more rapidly, cooling him faster.
• wear light-colored clothing and a hat to help deflect the sun's rays.
• use air conditioners, fans, cool baths or showers, icebags, wet towels, or sitting in the shade to promote coolness.
• drink such liquids as water, fruit and vegetable juices, and iced tea to replenish body fluids lost through perspiration.
• stay alert for such danger signs as nausea, light-headedness, dizziness, and fatigue.

Joint care

As you know, an older adult's joints may deteriorate from degenerative joint conditions, causing him pain, stiffness, and immobility.

In the following pages, we'll deal specifically with arthritis, the most common degenerative joint condition affecting geriatric patients. We'll tell you how the major types of arthritis affect the joints, and we'll review many of the treatments used to relieve the associated signs and symptoms. For example, we'll teach you how to apply paraffin heat therapy, one of the treatments that your patient can use at home to reduce his joint inflammation and pain.

You'll also find information about implements, such as specially adapted eating utensils, that your patient can use to perform everyday tasks. And we'll give you a home care aid with exercises your patient can perform at home to help him strengthen his muscles and joints and improve his mobility.

If you want to know more about caring for an older adult with a degenerative joint disease, read the following pages.

Reviewing common arthritis types

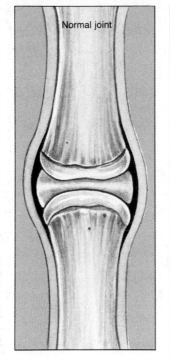

Normal joint

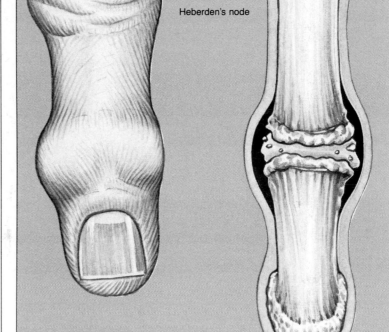

Heberden's node

As aging occurs, an adult's joints are likely to undergo degenerative changes, often causing inflammation, pain, and reduced mobility. The primary cause of this degeneration is arthritis.

Do you know the general early warning signs of arthritis? These include:
• persistent pain and stiffness in one or more joints following exercise or sleep
• intermittent or continuous pain, tenderness, stiffness, or swelling in one or more joints, even while at rest.

Arthritis takes many forms; only some are chronic, but all require ongoing attention. Treatment relieves the symptoms rather than cures the condition. The patient must realize that arthritis can't be eliminated overnight and that a period of remission is likely to be only temporary.

In this chart, we list three forms of arthritis and tell you how to give effective care for them.

For more information, contact the Arthritis Foundation, 3400 Peachtree Road NE, Atlanta, GA 30326.

OSTEOARTHRITIS

Description
A chronic progressive disorder that causes articular cartilage degeneration, bone overgrowth with spur and lip formation, and impaired joint function, primarily in the weight-bearing joints. Osteoarthritis is noninflammatory and affects no other body parts besides the joints. Often, its symptoms are mild; pain is generally moderate. This is the most commonly occurring arthritis type; it's found equally in both sexes.

Signs and symptoms
• Joint pain, particularly following exercise or weight bearing
• Morning stiffness
• Aching or nagging pain, especially during onset of bad weather
• Fluid accumulation in joint
• Muscle weakness in affected area
• Limited joint movement
• Grating of joint during motion
• Appearance of Bouchard's and Heberden's nodes (see illustration), which eventually become red, swollen, and tender, causing numbness and dexterity loss

Nursing interventions
• Reduce joint stress by having patient use ambulation aids, as ordered.
• Assist with supportive measures: physical therapy, massage, and moist heat and paraffin treatments.
• Help patient perform gentle range-of-motion exercises.
• Promote adequate rest, especially after activity. Plan rest periods during the day, and provide for adequate sleep at night.
• Administer antispasmodic, anti-inflammatory, or analgesic medications, as prescribed (see chart on page 56). Teach patient the actions and side effects of all medications he's taking. Observe for side effects and report any to the doctor immediately.
• Provide emotional support to help the patient cope with limited mobility. Explain that osteoarthritis affects individual joints independently, rather than spreading from joint to joint.
• Suggest self-help aids that your patient can use for everyday tasks.
• Provide appropriate preop and postop nursing care, if the patient needs joint surgery.

Joint care

Reviewing common arthritis types continued

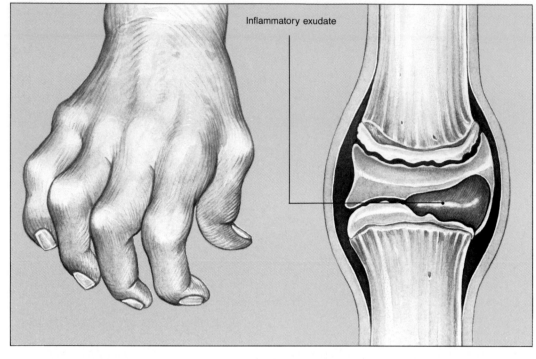

Inflammatory exudate

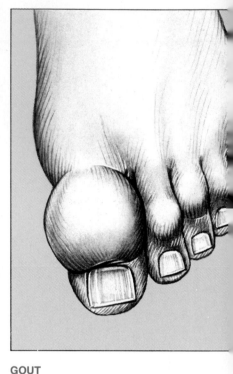

RHEUMATOID ARTHRITIS

Description
A chronic, systemic disease that primarily affects the peripheral joints and their surrounding muscles, tendons, ligaments, and blood vessels. Spontaneous remissions and unpredictable, severe attacks characterize this potentially crippling condition. Rheumatoid arthritis generally affects women more frequently than men.

Signs and symptoms
• Nonspecific signs and symptoms: fatigue; malaise; anorexia; persistent, low-grade fever; weight loss; and lymphadenopathy
• Specific localized signs and symptoms: affected joints are stiff on arising after sleep (may last up to 4 hours); fingers may assume a spindle shape from marked edema and joint congestion; joints become tender and painful following activity, and in later stages, even during rest; joints feel hot to patient; joint function diminishes
• Later signs and symptoms: vasculitis; skin lesions; ulcers; temporomandibular joint problems; numbness, tingling, and loss of sensation in the affected area
• Rheumatoid nodules (subcutaneous, round or oval nontender masses), usually on the elbows

Nursing interventions
• Provide emotional support. The disease's effects may discourage or depress your patient, or make him irritable. Encourage your patient to discuss his fears concerning dependency, sexuality, body image, and self-esteem. Try to keep him relaxed, as stress or tension may precipitate or worsen the symptoms.
• Establish a balanced program of exercise and rest.

• Urge patient to perform as many daily activities as possible.
• Give meticulous skin care. Observe for rheumatoid nodules, pressure areas, and skin breakdown from immobility and vascular impairment. Tell your patient to avoid using excessive soap when bathing and to apply lotion or oil for dry skin.
• Assess your patient frequently. Note vital signs, weight changes, sensory disturbances, and pain level.
• Monitor duration (not intensity) of morning stiffness, which most accurately reflects the disease's severity.
• Carefully apply splints or traction to immobilize joints (as ordered). Observe for development of pressure areas if patient's wearing a splint or is in traction.
• Assist with such supportive measures as hot packs, paraffin baths, and hydrotherapy. Use ice packs, as ordered, during acute episodes.
• Instruct your patient to avoid placing too much stress on joints. Teach him how to support any weak or painful joints by avoiding positions of flexion and by promoting extension; holding any objects close to the center of the body; and sliding objects rather than lifting them, whenever possible.
• Administer antispasmodic, anti-inflammatory, or analgesic medications as ordered. Teach patient the actions and side effects of all medications he's taking. Observe for side effects and report any to the doctor immediately.
• Promote comfort measures. Encourage the patient to take hot showers and baths at bedtime and upon arising, which may decrease the need for pain medication.
• Provide appropriate preop and postop nursing care, if the patient needs joint surgery.
• Suggest self-help aids which will help your patient perform everyday tasks.

GOUT

Description
A hereditary metabolic disease marked by joint inflammation and excessive urate deposits in the joint. This condition, an acute form of arthritis, often occurs after excessive or long-term diuretic use. Gout may affect any joint, but it usually begins in the knee or foot. Primary gout usually occurs in men over age 30 and in women over age 45. Secondary gout (which develops in reaction to another disease, such as multiple myeloma) usually occurs in the elderly.

Signs and symptoms
• Rising serum uric acid levels without associated signs and symptoms
• Warmth, tenderness, inflammation, and dusky-red or cyanotic coloring of joint
• Metatarsophalangeal joint of the great toe usually becomes inflamed first
• Low-grade fever possible
• Mild acute attacks, which subside quickly but recur at irregular intervals
• Severe attacks that may continue for days
• Symptom-free intervals, lasting from 6 months to 2 years, and sometimes for as long as 10 years
• Chronic (final) stage of gout is marked by large, subcutaneous urate crystal deposits in cartilage, synovial membranes, tendons, and soft tissues. Skin may ulcerate and release

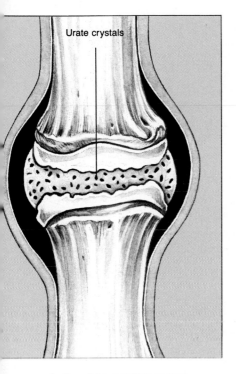

Urate crystals

a chalky-white exudate or pus. Chronic inflammation, secondary joint degeneration, and chronic renal dysfunction may also occur.

Nursing interventions
• Encourage bed rest and joint immobility during acute attack to minimize discomfort.
• Use a bed cradle to keep bed covers off extremely sensitive, inflamed joints.
• Give pain medication, as ordered by the doctor, especially during acute attacks.
• Administer anti-inflammatory medications, as ordered. Teach patient the actions and side effects of all medications he's taking. Observe for side effects (especially gastrointestinal disturbances) and report any to the doctor immediately.
• Apply hot or cold packs to relieve joint inflammation.
• Urge your patient to drink up to 2 quarts of liquid per day (1.9 liters) to prevent kidney stone formation. When forcing fluids, record intake and output accurately.
• Monitor serum uric acid levels regularly. Make sure your patient understands that alcohol (beer and wine) and purine-rich foods (sweetbreads and liver) can aggravate his condition.
• Watch for acute gout attacks from 24 to 96 hours following surgery or any type of emotional trauma that causes stress.

SPECIAL CONSIDERATIONS

Dealing with degenerative joint problems

If you suspect that your geriatric patient has a degenerative joint condition, make sure you inform the doctor. Why? Because if this condition is allowed to continue untreated, the pain and stiffness may make your patient stop moving affected joints. Keeping a joint immobile will cause atrophy of the structures surrounding it and eventually lead to contractures.

Research into a cure for the cause of degenerative joint disease continues. But in the meantime, the doctor can prescribe treatments that will help reduce or alleviate the signs and symptoms, depending on the condition's severity. For example, the doctor might prescribe:

• cold pack application to reduce the swelling caused by joint inflammation.

• rest to reduce joint inflammation.

• lightweight splints or braces to temporarily rest and protect your patient's inflamed joints.

• exercise to promote range of motion. Swimming, for example, is a commonly prescribed exercise.

• physical therapy to restore joint mobility.

• occupational therapy to help the patient perform daily tasks.

• heat treatments, such as hot packs, a whirlpool bath, or paraffin heat therapy, to increase blood circulation to the affected area, ease pain, and promote joint mobility.

• medications to reduce joint pain and inflammation (see the drug chart on page 56).

• joint cap surgery to replace damaged cartilage around the bone with a plastic covering, such as Teflon®

• total joint surgery to replace a joint immobilized by degenerative changes.

• ambulation aids for support. We discuss the two most commonly used ambulation aids in the story that follows at right.

Maintaining mobility through ambulation aids

Suppose the doctor's ordered your patient with a joint problem to use a walker. Do you know how to help him? Follow these guidelines:
• Check your patient's weight-bearing status before he begins.
• Help your patient position himself at the edge of the bed. Closely observe your patient *before* ambulating him, for the following signs and symptoms of orthostatic hypotension: cool, pale, and moist skin; dizziness; weakness; nausea; shortness of breath; decreased blood pressure; and tachycardia. If you detect any of these signs or symptoms, place your patient in a supine position until his condition returns to normal. Then, help him reposition himself at the edge of the bed.
• Instruct your patient to place his palms flat against the bed and lift himself to a standing position. Assist him, if he needs help.
Caution: Never allow your patient to use the walker to pull himself up off the bed.
• Position yourself on your patient's affected or weak side, standing slightly behind him as he ambulates. *Note:* For additional support, use a transfer belt.
• If your patient's using a stationary walker, instruct him to place all four legs of the walker on the ground before taking a step forward. Also, tell him to lead with his affected or weak leg first.
• Assess your patient for signs of fatigue or weakness as he ambulates, especially if he has a past history of cardiovascular or respiratory disease.

When your patient's strong enough, the doctor may recommend he ambulate with a single-point cane. Here are some cane-walking guidelines:
• Find out on which side the doctor wants your patient to use the cane.
• Position yourself on your patient's affected or weakened side and slightly behind him. That way, if he begins to fall, you'll be able to support him.

Assess your patient's actual needs. Don't allow him to become unnecessarily dependent on an ambulation aid. Stress that use of the aid is only temporary, until he achieves independent ambulation. However, if he does *need* the aid, encourage him to use it. Doing so will increase his personal safety and prevent possible injury.

For more information on teaching your patient how to use an ambulation aid, see the NURSING PHOTOBOOK WORKING WITH ORTHOPEDIC PATIENTS.

Document each ambulation session in your nurses' notes.

Joint care

Learning about self-help aids

A variety of self-help aids are available for your patient's use in coping with her day-to-day activities. This equipment makes it easier for her to accomplish tasks made difficult by aging changes or disease. Here are a few of the aids available.

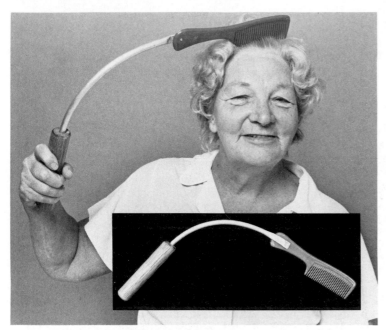

Comb. This special hair grooming utensil is mounted on a long, lightweight handle. It enables your patient to care for her hair while holding her arm at a comfortable level.

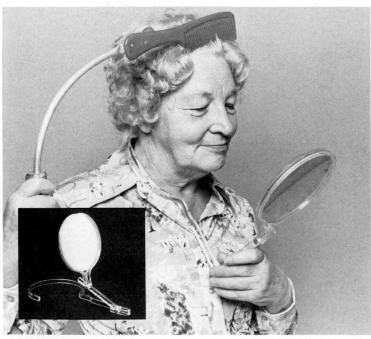

Extension mirror. This mirror fits comfortably around your patient's neck. It can free both hands for combing her hair and performing any other grooming. Some models feature a magnifying mirror on the opposite side.

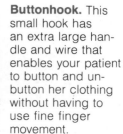

Buttonhook. This small hook has an extra large handle and wire that enables your patient to button and unbutton her clothing without having to use fine finger movement.

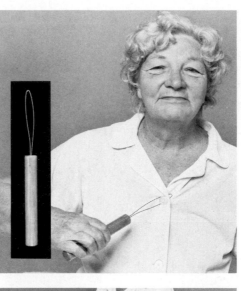

Shoehorn. This shoehorn has a long handle and a special spring that allows your patient to slip on her shoes without bending or moving her ankle unnecessarily.

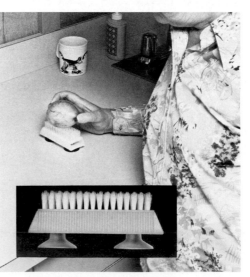

Utility brush. This nylon-bristled brush has suction cups on its base so it can be mounted on most surfaces. Your patient can use this brush to clean her dentures or scrub her nails. In addition, she can use a separate brush in the kitchen to clean vegetables or fruits.

Reacher. This extension tool allows your patient to reach lightweight, nonbreakable items. Some reacher models have magnetized tips which allow your patient to pick up needles and other small metallic objects from the floor.

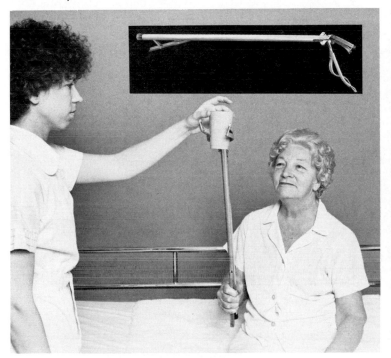

Drinking cup. This cup has a piece cut out at the top, so your patient won't need to flex her neck as much to drink from it as from a regular cup.

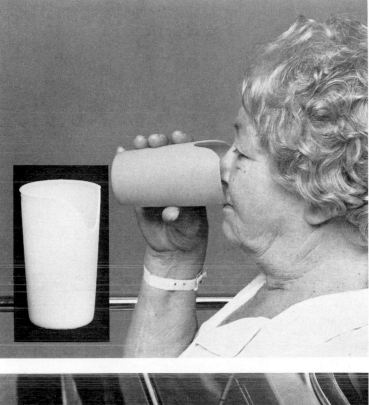

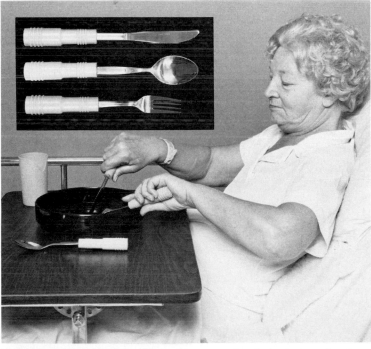

Eating utensils. These utensils have oversized plastic handles to improve your patient's grip, enabling her to feed herself. *Note:* Using a dish with sides rather than a flat plate helps her avoid spilling food.

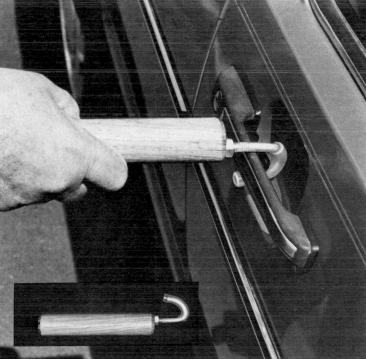

Car utensil. This tool features a hook to help your patient open a car door.

Joint care

When to use paraffin heat therapy

The doctor has ordered paraffin heat therapy for your patient with arthritis. In this therapy, your patient applies melted paraffin to his affected body part. Heat from the paraffin helps relieve pain and stiffness in affected joints and stimulates blood circulation to the affected area.

In addition to treating arthritis discomfort, the doctor may order paraffin heat therapy in the following cases:
• to relieve pain caused by bursitis or other chronic joint inflammation
• to relax the muscles and relieve stiffness and muscle spasms prior to therapeutic exercise or massage
• to stimulate blood circulation.

Caution: You may need to discontinue the treatment if your patient develops dermatitis from the paraffin.

The therapy's contraindicated in patients who have:
• open cuts or wounds in the affected area.
• inflammatory skin conditions, such as a rash or phlebitis, in the affected area.
• peripheral vascular disease with impaired blood circulation.
• cancer.
• skin sensation loss; for example, as a result of diabetes or nerve damage.
• hemorrhagic disorders.

Using the Therabath®

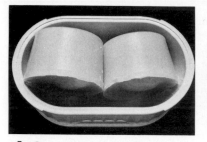 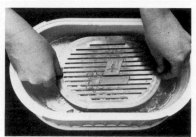 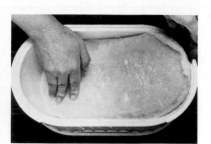

1 *One model of paraffin heat bath is the Therabath®. This portable paraffin bath heats Theraffin® wax to a temperature between 126° F. (52.2° C.) and 130° F. (54.4° C.). Your patient can dip his affected body part, for example, his hand, foot, or elbow, into the tank. Or, he can apply the paraffin with a brush; for instance, to his shoulder or knee.*

Do you know how to set up and dismantle a Therabath? You'll have to set it up about 5 hours before using it to allow enough time for the paraffin cakes to melt completely. Follow these instructions.

To prepare the tank, place it in a secure location next to an electrical outlet. Remove the grille from inside the tank to allow the paraffin to melt faster. Then, position two paraffin cakes in the tank (as shown) and plug in the Therabath. When you do, the red pilot light on the side of the tank should light. After the paraffin cakes melt below the top of the tank, put the lid on the Therabath. Check the cakes periodically to make sure they're melting.

2 When the paraffin melts completely—which takes about 5 hours—place the grille into the tank, flat side up. This grille will prevent your patient from resting his affected body part on the bottom of the tank, which could burn his skin. Then, apply the paraffin to your patient's affected area, as explained in the photostory at right.

If your patient's the only one using the Therabath, he can peel the paraffin off his affected body part after therapy and place it back in the bath for remelting.

However, if a different patient will be using the Therabath next, tell the patient to dispose of the wax he peels off. Then, replace the amount of wax discarded before the next patient uses the bath.

Let's say you're going to clean the tank and replace the old paraffin with two new paraffin cakes. If so, unplug the Therabath following therapy. Next, remove the grille from the tank, and allow the paraffin to solidify into a cake, which should take about 6 hours. Never pour melted paraffin out of the tank.

3 After the paraffin hardens completely, loosen it from the tank's walls by plugging in the Therabath for only a few minutes. Then, unplug the unit. Press firmly on one end of the paraffin with one hand, and carefully lift it out with your other hand.

After removing the paraffin cake, blot up any paraffin residue with paper towels. Then, plug the Therabath in briefly to loosen any residue stuck to the tank's upper walls. *Important:* Never use a knife or any other sharp object to scrape the tank's sides. Doing so may damage the tank's coating.

Again, blot the inside of the tank with paper towels.

Take care not to leave the Therabath plugged in for more than several minutes without paraffin inside. Also, never put water inside the tank to clean it.

Clean the inside of the tank with a soapy cloth. Remove any stains with mild scouring powder. Then, wipe the tank with a clean cloth that you've dipped in hot water and wrung out. Finally, wipe the tank dry.

Using paraffin therapy at home

Is your patient continuing paraffin heat therapy at home with a unit such as a Therabath®? If so, before he leaves the hospital, teach him these guidelines:
• Leave the unit plugged in with paraffin in it at all times. This keeps the paraffin melted and always ready for use. Also, keep the lid on the tank, except during therapy.
• Keep the unit in a safe, secure location, out of any child's reach. Be sure the cord is out of the way.
• To ensure optimum results, keep the room temperature where the unit's located set at about 72° F. (22° C.).
• Before using the bath, wash your hands thoroughly

and check the affected area for cuts or rashes. If you see any, don't use the paraffin bath until they've healed. Notify the doctor, who may prescribe an alternative treatment.
• After removing the paraffin, check the affected area for any rashes, burns, or blistering. If you see any of these conditions, contact the doctor immediately.
• Also, return the paraffin you've used to the tank and remelt it.
• If you use the bath daily, change the paraffin approximately once a month, following the manufacturer's instructions.

Giving paraffin heat therapy

1 *Sister Michael Hogan, a 56-year-old teacher, has an acute case of rheumatoid arthritis. She visits the outpatient clinic three times a week to receive paraffin heat therapy for her hands.*

Here she'll be using a model of paraffin bath different from the Therabath®. But you've prepared the paraffin in the same way.

Now that it's completely melted, you're ready to have her apply it. To do this, first obtain a waxed paper bag or a roll of waxed paper, and two medium-sized terry cloth towels. Then, wash and dry your hands thoroughly, and explain to your patient what she'll be doing.

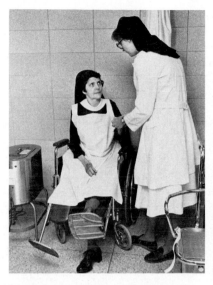

2 Now, have your patient thoroughly wash her hands and wrists with soap and water and dry them thoroughly. Assist her, if necessary. Inspect her hands and wrists for a rash or any open cuts that would contraindicate the paraffin bath. Then, have her momentarily immerse her hands into the tank until the melted paraffin covers them, as shown

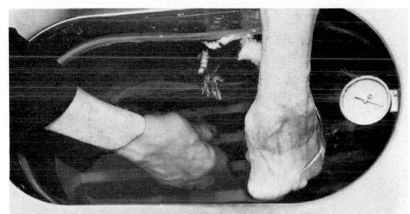

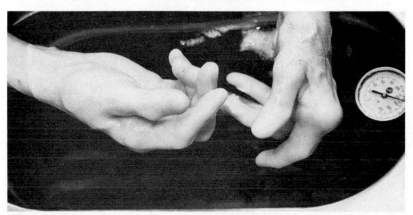

3 Next, tell her to remove her hands from the tank and allow the paraffin to harden. When the paraffin is no longer shiny, have her place her hands in the tank once again and repeat the process.

4 Instruct your patient to dip her hands into the paraffin bath 10 to 12 times, until she's built up a thick paraffin coating around the affected area.

Note: Tell her not to flex her hands during the procedure. Doing so may crack the wax coating, which reduces the therapy's effectiveness and increases the danger of burning sensitive skin.

After building up a thick coating, your patient can immerse her hands in the melted paraffin for 30 seconds more. This will provide additional warmth in the affected area.

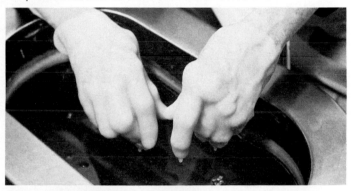

5 After she's finished applying the paraffin, cover her hands and wrists with the waxed paper bag to retain the heat. Or, wrap each arm with a strip of waxed paper and a terry cloth towel.

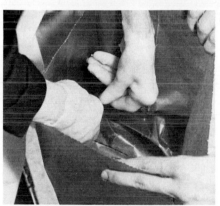

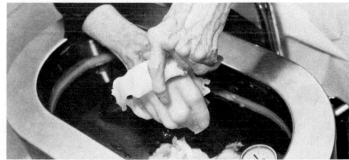

6 Allow the affected area to remain wrapped for 20 minutes. Then, remove the covering and have her peel off the paraffin coating, as shown. Have her wash her hands thoroughly, and inspect her skin. If you see erythema or blistering, notify the doctor immediately.

Finally, to promote joint mobility, instruct your patient to perform any prescribed exercises *immediately* after the paraffin bath. Document in your nurses' notes the procedure, how your patient tolerated it, and any exercises performed.

Joint care

Nurses' guide to antiarthritic drugs

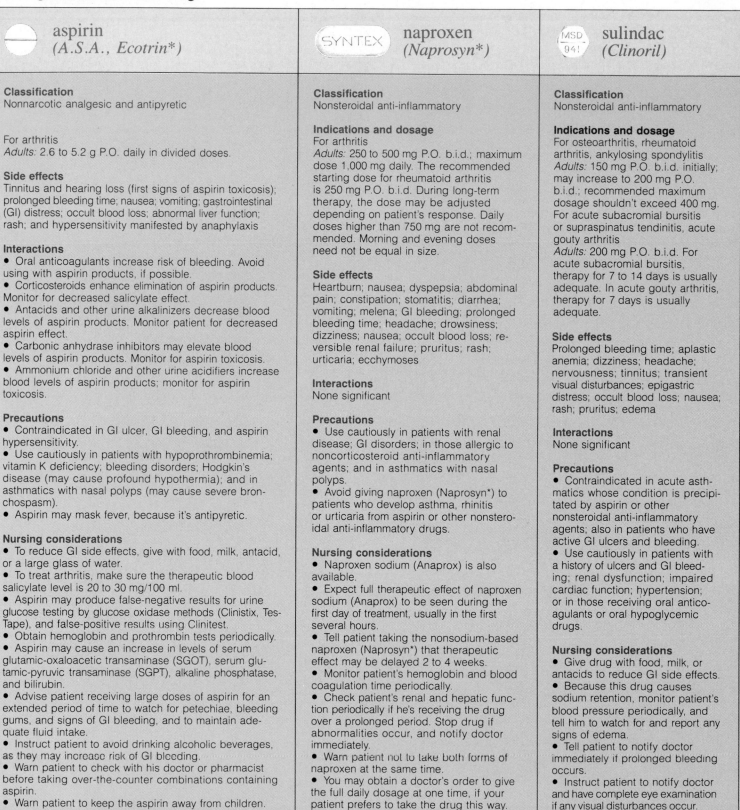

aspirin
(A.S.A., Ecotrin*)

Classification
Nonnarcotic analgesic and antipyretic

For arthritis
Adults: 2.6 to 5.2 g P.O. daily in divided doses.

Side effects
Tinnitus and hearing loss (first signs of aspirin toxicosis); prolonged bleeding time; nausea; vomiting; gastrointestinal (GI) distress; occult blood loss; abnormal liver function; rash; and hypersensitivity manifested by anaphylaxis

Interactions
• Oral anticoagulants increase risk of bleeding. Avoid using with aspirin products, if possible.
• Corticosteroids enhance elimination of aspirin products. Monitor for decreased salicylate effect.
• Antacids and other urine alkalinizers decrease blood levels of aspirin products. Monitor patient for decreased aspirin effect.
• Carbonic anhydrase inhibitors may elevate blood levels of aspirin products. Monitor for aspirin toxicosis.
• Ammonium chloride and other urine acidifiers increase blood levels of aspirin products; monitor for aspirin toxicosis.

Precautions
• Contraindicated in GI ulcer, GI bleeding, and aspirin hypersensitivity.
• Use cautiously in patients with hypoprothrombinemia; vitamin K deficiency; bleeding disorders; Hodgkin's disease (may cause profound hypothermia); and in asthmatics with nasal polyps (may cause severe bronchospasm).
• Aspirin may mask fever, because it's antipyretic.

Nursing considerations
• To reduce GI side effects, give with food, milk, antacid, or a large glass of water.
• To treat arthritis, make sure the therapeutic blood salicylate level is 20 to 30 mg/100 ml.
• Aspirin may produce false-negative results for urine glucose testing by glucose oxidase methods (Clinistix, Tes-Tape), and false-positive results using Clinitest.
• Obtain hemoglobin and prothrombin tests periodically.
• Aspirin may cause an increase in levels of serum glutamic-oxaloacetic transaminase (SGOT), serum glutamic-pyruvic transaminase (SGPT), alkaline phosphatase, and bilirubin.
• Advise patient receiving large doses of aspirin for an extended period of time to watch for petechiae, bleeding gums, and signs of GI bleeding, and to maintain adequate fluid intake.
• Instruct patient to avoid drinking alcoholic beverages, as they may increase risk of GI bleeding.
• Warn patient to check with his doctor or pharmacist before taking over-the-counter combinations containing aspirin.
• Warn patient to keep the aspirin away from children.

naproxen
(Naprosyn*)

Classification
Nonsteroidal anti-inflammatory

Indications and dosage
For arthritis
Adults: 250 to 500 mg P.O. b.i.d.; maximum dose 1,000 mg daily. The recommended starting dose for rheumatoid arthritis is 250 mg P.O. b.i.d. During long-term therapy, the dose may be adjusted depending on patient's response. Daily doses higher than 750 mg are not recommended. Morning and evening doses need not be equal in size.

Side effects
Heartburn; nausea; dyspepsia; abdominal pain; constipation; stomatitis; diarrhea; vomiting; melena; GI bleeding; prolonged bleeding time; headache; drowsiness; dizziness; nausea; occult blood loss; reversible renal failure; pruritus; rash; urticaria; ecchymoses

Interactions
None significant

Precautions
• Use cautiously in patients with renal disease; GI disorders; in those allergic to noncorticosteroid anti-inflammatory agents; and in asthmatics with nasal polyps.
• Avoid giving naproxen (Naprosyn*) to patients who develop asthma, rhinitis or urticaria from aspirin or other nonsteroidal anti-inflammatory drugs.

Nursing considerations
• Naproxen sodium (Anaprox) is also available.
• Expect full therapeutic effect of naproxen sodium (Anaprox) to be seen during the first day of treatment, usually in the first several hours.
• Tell patient taking the nonsodium-based naproxen (Naprosyn*) that therapeutic effect may be delayed 2 to 4 weeks.
• Monitor patient's hemoglobin and blood coagulation time periodically.
• Check patient's renal and hepatic function periodically if he's receiving the drug over a prolonged period. Stop drug if abnormalities occur, and notify doctor immediately.
• Warn patient not to take both forms of naproxen at the same time.
• You may obtain a doctor's order to give the full daily dosage at one time, if your patient prefers to take the drug this way.

sulindac
(Clinoril)

Classification
Nonsteroidal anti-inflammatory

Indications and dosage
For osteoarthritis, rheumatoid arthritis, ankylosing spondylitis
Adults: 150 mg P.O. b.i.d. initially; may increase to 200 mg P.O. b.i.d.; recommended maximum dosage shouldn't exceed 400 mg. For acute subacromial bursitis or supraspinatus tendinitis, acute gouty arthritis
Adults: 200 mg P.O. b.i.d. For acute subacromial bursitis, therapy for 7 to 14 days is usually adequate. In acute gouty arthritis, therapy for 7 days is usually adequate.

Side effects
Prolonged bleeding time; aplastic anemia; dizziness; headache; nervousness; tinnitus; transient visual disturbances; epigastric distress; occult blood loss; nausea; rash; pruritus; edema

Interactions
None significant

Precautions
• Contraindicated in acute asthmatics whose condition is precipitated by aspirin or other nonsteroidal anti-inflammatory agents; also in patients who have active GI ulcers and bleeding.
• Use cautiously in patients with a history of ulcers and GI bleeding; renal dysfunction; impaired cardiac function; hypertension; or in those receiving oral anticoagulants or oral hypoglycemic drugs.

Nursing considerations
• Give drug with food, milk, or antacids to reduce GI side effects.
• Because this drug causes sodium retention, monitor patient's blood pressure periodically, and tell him to watch for and report any signs of edema.
• Tell patient to notify doctor immediately if prolonged bleeding occurs.
• Instruct patient to notify doctor and have complete eye examination if any visual disturbances occur.

*Available in both the United States and in Canada

indomethacin
(Indocin)

Classification
Nonsteroidal anti-inflammatory

Indications and dosage
For moderate to severe rheumatoid arthritis
Adults: 25 mg P.O. b.i.d. or t.i.d. with food and antacids; may increase by 25 mg daily every 7 days, up to 200 mg daily. In patients who have persistent night pain and/or morning stiffness, give a large dose (up to 100 mg) at bedtime to provide relief.
For acute gouty arthritis
Adults: 50 mg P.O. t.i.d. Dose should be reduced and drug discontinued as soon as possible.

Side effects
Hemolytic anemia; aplastic anemia; agranulocytosis; leukopenia; thrombocytopenic purpura; iron deficiency anemia; headache; dizziness; depression; drowsiness; confusion; peripheral neuropathy; convulsions; psychic disturbances; syncope; vertigo; hypertension; edema; blurred vision; corneal and retinal damage; hearing loss; tinnitus; nausea; vomiting, anorexia, diarrhea; severe GI bleeding; hematuria; hyperkalemia; acute renal failure; pruritus; urticaria; hypersensitivity manifested by anaphylaxis

Interactions
• Probenecid (Benemid*) decreases indomethacin excretion. Watch for increased incidence of indomethacin side effects.
• Furosemide (Lasix*) impairs effectiveness of both drugs. Avoid using them together, if possible.

Precautions
• Contraindicated in patients with aspirin allergy and those with GI disorders.
• Contraindicated in patients who have a known allergy to indomethacin or those who have nasal polyps associated with angioedema. Also contraindicated in patients who have a bronchospastic reaction to aspirin or other nonsteroidal anti-inflammatory drugs.
• Use cautiously in elderly patients, or patients with epilepsy; parkinsonism; hepatic or renal disease; infection; or history of mental illness.

Nursing considerations
• Drug is available in sustained release form, requiring only one or two doses daily. The cost, however, is high.
• Give drug with meals to avoid GI distress. Advise patient to notify doctor of any GI problems.
• Periodically test renal function and complete blood cell count (CBC) in patient taking drug over a prolonged period.
• Monitor patient for central nervous system (CNS) side effects, which are more common and severe in elderly.
• Monitor patients with hypertension for increased blood pressure.
• Monitor patient for bleeding if he's also receiving an anticoagulant drug.
• Tell patient that severe headache may occur within 1 hour after taking drug. Decrease dose if headache persists.
• Tell patient to notify doctor immediately if he notices any changes in his vision or hearing. Patients taking drug over a prolonged period should have regular eye examinations and hearing tests.

ibuprofen
(Motrin*)

Classification
Nonsteroidal anti-inflammatory

Indications and dosage
For rheumatoid arthritis and osteoarthritis
Adults: 300 to 600 mg P.O. q.i.d.

Side effects
Prolonged bleeding time; headache; drowsiness; dizziness; visual disturbances; tinnitus; epigastric distress; nausea; occult blood loss; reversible renal failure; pruritus; rash; urticaria; aseptic meningitis; bronchospasm; edema

Interactions
None significant

Precautions
• Contraindicated in asthmatics with nasal polyps.
• Use cautiously in patients who have previously exhibited hypersensitivity to this medication.
• Use cautiously in patients with GI disorders, hepatic or renal disease; cardiac decompensation; known intrinsic coagulation defects and those on anticoagulation therapy; or those with an allergy to other noncorticosteroid anti-inflammatory drugs.
• Anaphylactoid reactions have occurred in patients with aspirin hypersensitivity.

Nursing considerations
• Give drug with meals or milk to reduce GI side effects.
• Monitor patient's renal and hepatic function in long-term therapy. Stop drug at once if abnormalities occur, and notify doctor.
• Tell patient the therapeutic effect of this drug may be delayed for 2 to 4 weeks.
• Tell patient to immediately report to doctor any of the following signs and symptoms: GI distress, unexplained bleeding, visual disturbances, rashes, weight gain, or edema.

colchicine
(Colchicine)

Classification
Anti-inflammatory

Indications and dosage
To prevent acute attacks of gout as prophylactic or maintenance therapy
Adults: 0.5 or 0.6 mg P.O. daily; or 1 to 1.8 mg P.O. daily for more severe cases.
To prevent attacks of gout in patients undergoing surgery
Adults: 0.5 to 0.6 mg P.O. t.i.d. 3 days before and 3 days after surgery.
To treat acute gout, acute gouty arthritis
Adults: initially, 1 to 1.2 mg P.O., then 0.5 to 0.6 mg every hour, or 1 to 1.2 mg every 2 hours until pain is relieved or nausea, vomiting, or diarrhea begins; 2 mg I.V. followed by 2 mg I.V. in 12 hours if necessary. Total I.V. dose should not exceed 4 mg in 24 hours.

Side effects
Nausea; vomiting; abdominal pain; diarrhea; urticaria; dermatitis; severe local irritation if extravasation occurs; alopecia; peripheral neuritis; aplastic anemia and agranulocytosis with prolonged use; nonthrombocytopenic purpura

Interactions
None significant

Precautions
• Use cautiously in elderly or debilitated patients or in those with hepatic dysfunction, cardiac disease, renal disease, or GI disorders.

Nursing considerations
• Store in tightly closed light-resistant container.
• Precede therapy with baseline laboratory studies, including CBC, and repeat them periodically.
• Don't administer by I.M. or subcutaneous routes, because drug causes severe local irritation.
• Give with meals to reduce GI side effects.
• Monitor fluid intake/output. Keep output at 2,000 ml daily.
• Change needle before administering I.V.
• Reduce dosage if patient shows weakness, anorexia, nausea, vomiting, or diarrhea. Observe for the following signs and symptoms of acute overdose: GI symptoms, followed by vascular damage, muscle weakness, and ascending paralysis. Delirium and convulsions may occur without the patient losing consciousness.
• For chronic gout, other drugs may be prescribed, such as allopurinol (Zyloprim*) or phenylbutazone (Butazolidin*).

Joint care

Home care

Exercises for your joints

Dear Patient:
Now that you're ready to return home, you'll need to keep affected joints active and to strengthen the muscles around them. Performing everyday activities such as cooking and cleaning is a start. But, you'll also need some form of regular exercise, such as daily walking, swimming, or joint exercises, to make sure you work out *all* joints.

The following exercises should help increase joint movement and reduce stiffness and pain. Follow the exact directions for performing these exercises. Make sure you complete the number of repetitions required. If you can't, notify the doctor. He may prescribe a different exercise.

Important: If you feel severe pain when performing any of these exercises, stop immediately. If the pain continues, notify your doctor. Never force or overstretch a muscle or joint, or you may cause further damage.

To get the most out of this program, try to work the exercises into your daily routine; for example, exercise as you bathe, or while you're sitting in a chair watching television. Begin each exercise session by briefly limbering up and stretching, and pause between exercises to relax. Perform each exercise slowly and carefully.

Note: If you're performing the exercises in a bed or chair with wheels, make sure the wheels are locked before you begin.

For your wrists and hands: While either sitting or standing, extend one arm out in front of you, keeping it slightly bent at the elbow, with your palm down. Using your other hand, gently push your fingers back toward your forearm. Then, push your fingers down, as shown. Perform this exercise five times. Then, switch hands and repeat the exercise five times.

For your fingers: While either sitting or standing, extend both arms out in front of you at shoulder level, with your palms down. Spread your fingers apart as much as possible; then bring them back together. Perform this exercise five times.

For your shoulders and arms: Sitting upright, extend your arms out to the sides, keeping your elbows straight and your palms down. Rotate your arms from the shoulders, making small circles. Do this five times, rotating forward. Then reverse the procedure, and rotate your arms backward five times.

For your neck: While either sitting or standing, slowly move your head back as far as possible. Then move it to the right, toward your shoulder. From that position, lower your chin toward your chest. Then, complete the exercise by moving your head toward your left shoulder. Perform this exercise five times; then change direction, and perform it five times.

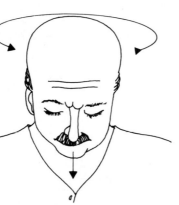

For your posture and back: Obtain a wooden stick (for example, a broom or mop handle) long enough for you to grasp with both hands. Hold it in your hands, and rest it on your lap. Then, slowly extend the stick straight out in front of you, raise it over your head (with arms straight), and place it behind your neck. Next, return the stick to its starting position in your lap. Perform this exercise five times.

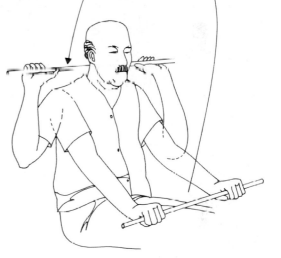

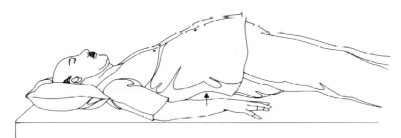

For your hips: Perform this exercise while lying flat on your back. Place your arms at your side, palms down. Then, use your hands and arms to lift your hips a maximum of 6″ (15.2 cm) off the bed. Hold this position momentarily; then relax. Perform this exercise five times.

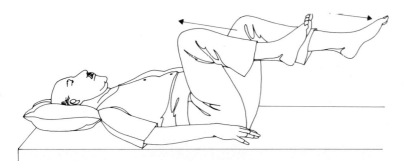

For your hips and legs: Perform this exercise while lying flat on your back. Place your arms at your side, palms down. Lift both legs and slowly pump them, as if you were riding a bicycle. Do this exercise five times.

For your ankles and feet: Sit in a rocking chair and rock back and forth. The constant pushing movement of your feet and ankles will stimulate blood circulation and reduce joint stiffness.

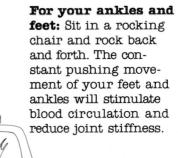

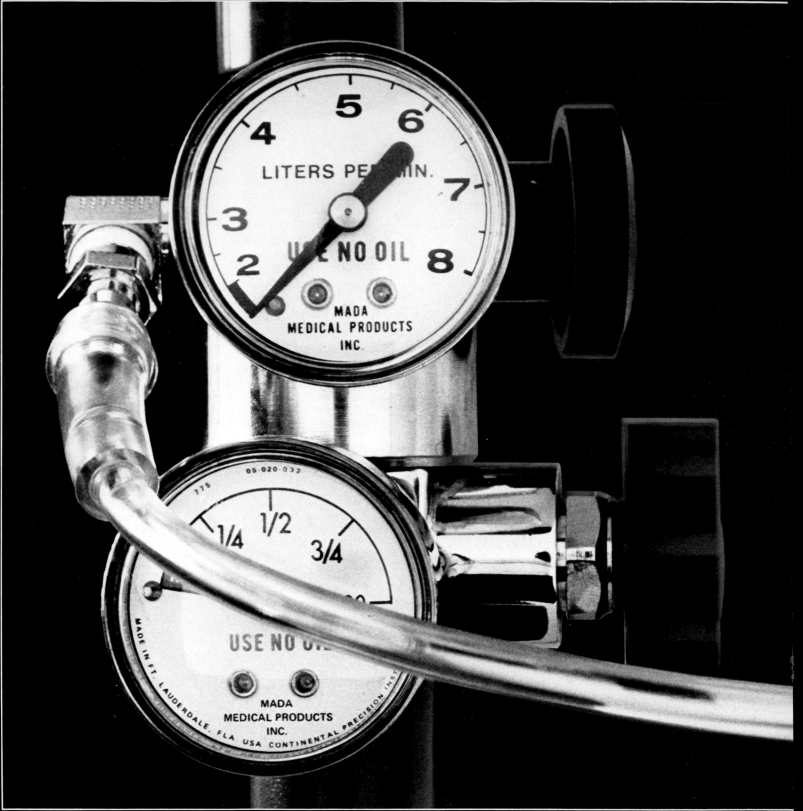

Maintaining Respiratory and Circulatory Function

Breathing exercises
Home oxygen use
Antithrombotic measures
Stroke rehabilitation

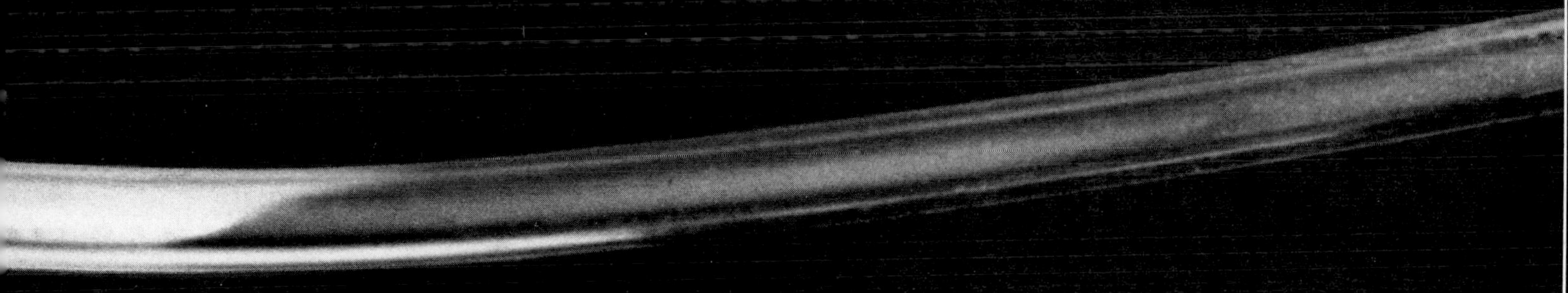

Breathing exercises

Your geriatric patient will probably experience reduced respiratory function. That's why you must take special precautions when he's confined to bed rest at home or in the hospital. To find out how to help prevent respiratory problems and how to teach him deep-breathing and coughing exercises, study the next few pages.

Also, while your patient's in the hospital, give him a copy of our self-care aid on incentive spirometer use. When he goes home, give him a copy of our home care aid, which offers some tips on avoiding fatigue.

Preventing respiratory problems

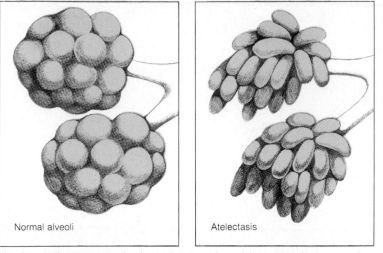

Normal alveoli

Atelectasis

You know that your geriatric patient's vulnerable to respiratory problems. So, no matter why he's in the hospital, take the following steps—unless contraindicated by his condition—to help him:
• Teach your patient proper deep-breathing and coughing techniques (see instructions at right and on the next page). Deep breathing encourages lung expansion, and coughing prevents secretion retention. Both help prevent atelectasis (see illustrations).
• Help your patient deep breathe by using an aid such as an incentive spirometer.
• Give oxygen as necessary.
• Turn and reposition your patient at least every 2 hours. Encourage him to help as much as possible. Check to be sure his position enhances respiration. For example, don't allow your patient to slump in bed or in a chair.
• Promote early ambulation. Increase ambulation gradually but steadily as soon as your patient is able. Encourage him to walk to the window, bathroom, hall, or nurses' station at least once every 4 hours. Be ready to assist, as needed. Have the patient's family help him ambulate, as much as possible.
• Encourage good posture to promote maximum lung expansion. Have your patient stand straight and breathe deeply while walking.
• Urge your patient to eat small, frequent meals. Overeating at one sitting may make breathing more difficult.
• Have your patient drink plenty of fluids and avoid milk products, to help keep mucus thin. Monitor his intake carefully. *Caution:* Be sure you don't give excessive fluids to a patient with congestive heart failure.
• Use intermittent positive pressure breathing (IPPB) treatments, as ordered, to help loosen secretions. Be sure you don't schedule IPPB treatments close to a meal, or your patient may experience nausea and vomiting. Also, after eating, his heart will have to work harder, so he'll require more oxygen. Have your patient sit up straight during treatment to allow adequate chest expansion. Also, make sure he coughs after the treatment, to expel any secretions. *Note:* In some hospitals the respiratory therapy department may administer these treatments.
• For long-term prevention, encourage your patient to have a yearly physical exam. The doctor may want him to have an annual influenza vaccine and a pneumococcal vaccine every 3 years. *Caution:* Receiving vaccinations more frequently may cause severe reactions at the injection site.

For more information, see the NURSING PHOTOBOOKS PROVIDING RESPIRATORY CARE and CARING FOR SURGICAL PATIENTS.

Teaching deep breathing

To help prevent lung problems, your patient needs to deep breathe every 1 to 2 hours while she's awake. Doing this will help expand her lungs, improve oxygenation, and prevent atelectasis. Deep breathing may also help your patient relax.

To deep breathe correctly, your patient must use her diaphragm and abdominal muscles—not just her chest muscles. To teach this technique, follow these steps:
• Position your patient comfortably so she's lying supine (see upper photo). Place one of her hands on her chest, and the other over her upper abdomen, at the base of her breastbone. Flex her knees slightly and support them with a small pillow. Encourage her to *relax*.

Remember: If your patient's just undergone chest or abdominal surgery, have her splint her incision.
• Instruct her to exhale normally. Then, tell her to close her mouth and inhale deeply through her nose. As she does this, have her concentrate on feeling her abdomen rise, *without expanding her chest*. Tell your patient that if the hand on her abdomen rises as she inhales, she's breathing correctly. *Note:* After your patient's learned this technique, she should be able to perform it without placing her hand on her abdomen.
• Tell your patient to hold her breath and slowly count to five.
• Now instruct your patient to purse her lips, as though she were whistling, and exhale completely through her mouth, without puffing her cheeks out (see lower photo). Have her use her abdominal muscles to squeeze all the air out, as her ribs sink downward and inward. Tell her that exhalation should last twice as long as inhalation.
• Instruct her to rest several seconds and then continue the exercise until she's performed it correctly five times. Encourage her to gradually increase the number of repetitions until she can perform the exercise ten times.
• After she's learned the exercise, inform your patient that she can perform it whether she's sitting, standing, or lying in any position in bed.
• Document your teaching in your nurses' notes.

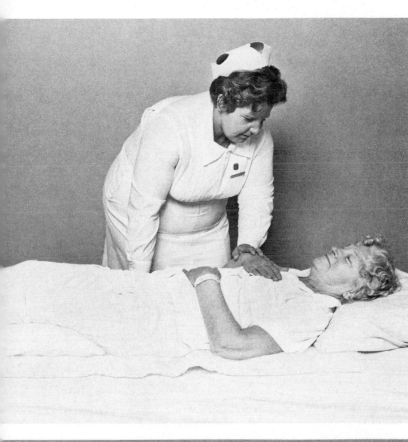

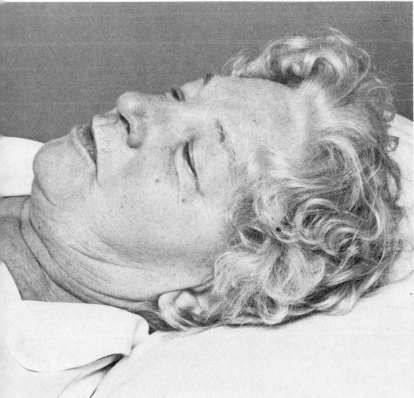

Teaching effective coughing

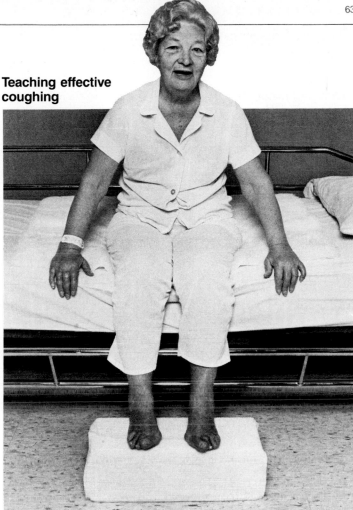

Teach your patient to perform coughing exercises at least every 2 hours. Careful, controlled coughing helps keep her lungs free of secretions. To teach her the proper technique, follow these steps:

• Have your patient sit on the edge of the bed. If her feet don't touch the floor, give her a stool to rest them on. She should bend her body slightly forward (see photo)

 Nursing tip: If your patient's not very strong, you may provide a bedside table with a pillow on it for her to rest her arms on.

• Tell your patient to take a slow, deep breath, and exhale (using the breathing technique on the previous page). Doing this will help stimulate her cough reflex. Then, have her take a second breath and exhale.

• Now, have her inhale again, hold her breath, and then cough twice vigorously. *Note:* Coughing twice will help control the cough and prevent a coughing spasm.

As she coughs, she should concentrate on trying to force out all the air in her chest.

• Tell your patient to pause for a moment's rest and breathe normally. She may take a sip of water to help her keep from coughing again. When she's rested, have her repeat the exercise at least five times.

• Don't allow your patient to cough excessively, because it expends too much energy.

• If your patient *can't* cough effectively (for example, because of chronic obstructive pulmonary disease), have her cough three times gently instead of twice vigorously. *Note:* You may administer hypertonic saline solution through a nebulizer (as ordered) to stimulate coughing in a patient who can't cough effectively.

Document the teaching in your nurses' notes.

Breathing exercises

Exercising accessory breathing muscles

1 *Does your geriatric patient suffer from chronic obstructive pulmonary disease (COPD)? If so, teach him the breathing exercise described below. This exercise strengthens his accessory breathing muscles.*

Position your patient comfortably; for example, in semi-Fowler's position with his knees slightly bent (at about a 10° angle). Bending his knees decreases tension on abdominal muscles. Support his knees with a pillow.

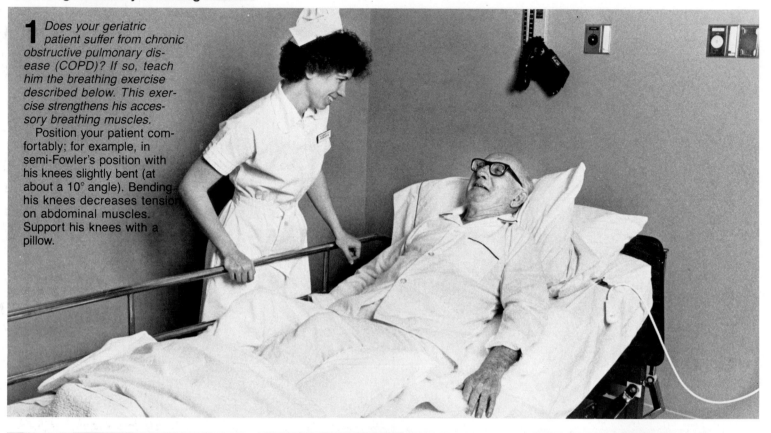

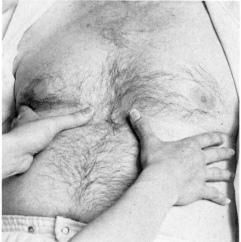

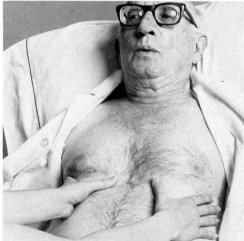

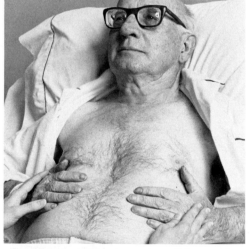

2 Firmly place your hands on each side of his lower rib cage, with your little fingers resting on his lowest ribs. Encourage him to relax. If he's in a sitting position, ask him to keep his shoulders lowered throughout the exercise.

Have him inhale through his nose, taking a slow, deep breath, and expand his lower rib cage outward against your hands. Urge him to avoid using his shoulder muscles as he inhales.

3 Now, ask him to purse his lips, as though whistling, and exhale slowly through his mouth. Discourage him from exhaling forcefully, which may cause his alveoli to collapse.

As he exhales, urge him to concentrate on feeling first his chest, then his lower ribs, sink. As you feel his lower ribs sink inward, gently squeeze his rib cage with your hands to force all the air out from the base of his lungs.

4 When he's able to perform this exercise properly, encourage him to practice it with his own hands placed bilaterally over his lower rib cage.

Instruct your patient to do this exercise for 5 to 10 minutes every hour, or less if he becomes tired or short of breath.

Document your teaching in your nurses' notes.

Self-care

How to use an incentive spirometer

1 Dear Patient:
The doctor wants you to use a breathing aid called an incentive spirometer. Using this aid will expand your lungs, to help you breathe in more oxygen and avoid lung complications.

First, hold the spirometer upright in your hand. Be careful not to tilt it at an angle.

3 Inhale deeply, until the ball in the chamber rises to the top. Hold your breath for a count of three (even though the ball drops).

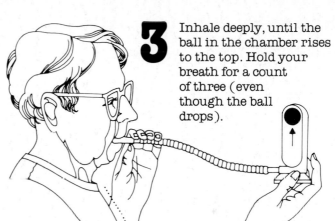

2 Now, exhale normally, and place your lips tightly around the spirometer's mouthpiece.

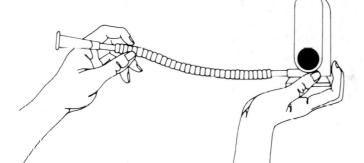

4 Finally, take the mouthpiece out of your mouth, and exhale normally. Relax and rest for a moment. Repeat the exercise several times, resting after each time.

Use the spirometer to deep breathe at least once every 2 hours while you're awake.

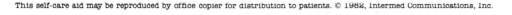

Breathing exercises

Home care

How to avoid tiring easily

Dear Patient:
The nurse taught you various deep-breathing exercises while you were in the hospital. Now that you're going home, observe the following guidelines to help you breathe better and tire less quickly.
• Avoid rushing by planning your day carefully. For example, if you have a scheduled activity, get up a little earlier. That way, you'll have time to get ready for the activity without any hurry.
• Spread your activities out over the day. For example, don't do *all* your chores in the morning. Save some for the afternoon or the next day.
• Rest between activities.
• Practice deep breathing regularly, at least every 2 hours while you're awake. Remember to use your abdominal muscles. Breathe out with your lips pursed. Breathing out should last twice as long as breathing in. Also, use an incentive spirometer if you have one.
• Use deep breathing while performing any active movement, such as sweeping or mopping, or with any activities that require you to raise your arms, such as lifting packages or combing your hair. Coordinate your movement with breathing, as shown at right.
   Note: Whenever possible, avoid working with your arms raised, which can tire you more quickly. Work with objects at waist level instead.

1 Inhale deeply, using your abdominal muscles.

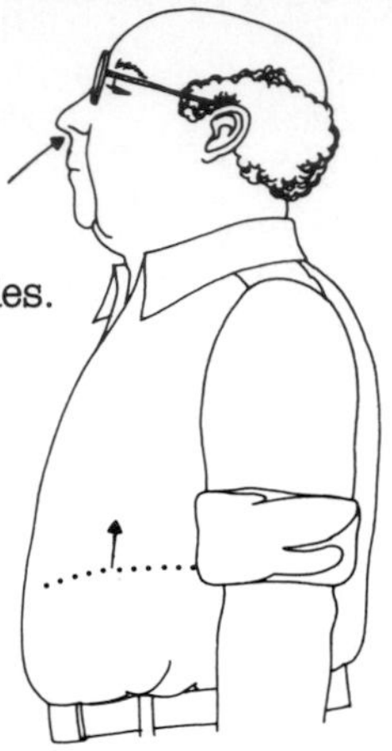

2 Exhale through pursed lips, lift your arms, and put a package on the shelf.

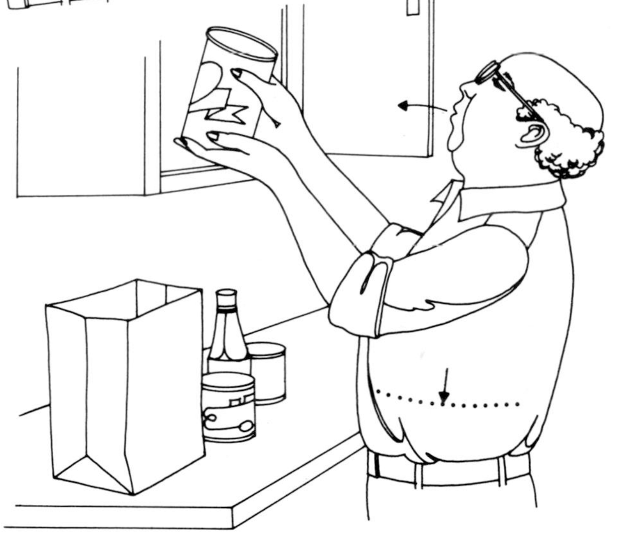

3 Lower your arms and inhale *again.* Then, raise your arms while exhaling, and put another package on the shelf.
   Repeat these steps as necessary. *Remember:* Always perform the activity while exhaling.

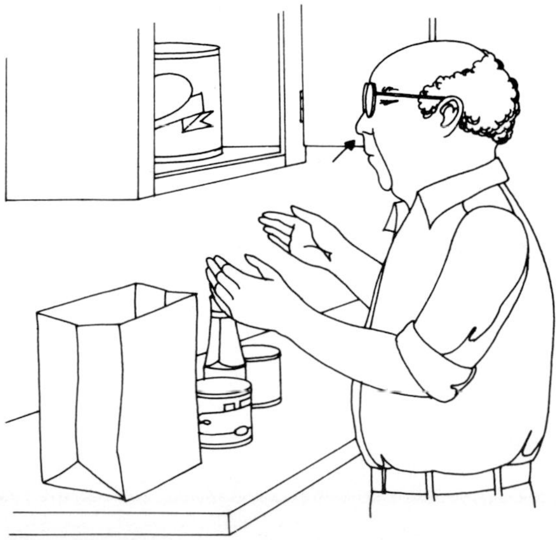

Home oxygen use

The doctor's ordered oxygen for your patient's use at home. Naturally, you'll be concerned about safety. To protect both your patient and his family, you'll need to teach them proper administration, equipment handling, and patient care, as well as safety precautions. In the following pages, we've provided text, photostories, and home care aids for you to use as teaching tools.

We'll also introduce you to some new equipment. You're probably very familiar with oxygen tanks as a source of oxygen. But, how much do you know about liquid oxygen, or about oxygen concentrators? Study the information we give here on liquid oxygen use. Then, read about the Healthdyne BX-4000® model oxygen concentrator, including the step-by-step photostory that explains how to operate it.

Using oxygen at home

If you're teaching your patient how to use oxygen at home, you'll need to cover a number of important points.

First, he'll need instruction on oxygen hazards (see text below). Then, consider which oxygen source he'll use: tank or liquid oxygen, or an oxygen concentrator.

If he's using tank oxygen, give him the safe-handling guidelines below and the home care aid on page 68. Be sure to fill in your patient's prescribed flow rate on the home care aid. To teach him about liquid oxygen, see page 69. For instructions on use of an oxygen concentrator, see pages 70 to 72. Also, remember to inform your patient using tank oxygen or an oxygen concentrator about a small portable oxygen tank that he can use when he's away from home (see page 74).

Your patient using oxygen outside the hospital almost always receives it through a nasal cannula. Teach him how with the help of the home care aid on page 73. Again, be sure to fill in the prescribed flow rate on the home care aid.

Your patient and his family will also need to monitor the oxygen's effects. Tell them how to determine whether he's receiving too much or too little oxygen by observing for the signs and symptoms described on page 74.

When you've completed this teaching, you can feel more confident that your patient's prepared to use oxygen for maximum benefit, with minimum risk.

Reducing oxygen hazards

As you know, a high oxygen concentration will make a fire burn hotter and more rapidly. And, it can make smoldering objects, such as cigarettes, burst into flame. Also, oxygen under pressure may explode when subjected to heat. To help protect your patient and his family from these hazards, give them the following safety instructions:
• Notify the local fire department that oxygen is in the house.
• Keep the oxygen source (usually a tank or concentrator) at least 5' (1.5 m) from a heat source. If the patient's confined to bed and the heat source is stationary (for example, a radiator or baseboard heater), turn it off, if possible, and place an alternate heat source at a safe distance from the oxygen. *Never* use a fireplace for heat.
• Take stringent measures to prevent smoking. Post large, clearly printed *No smoking* signs on the front door of the house and on the door of the patient's room, as well as inside his room. Doing so will alert visitors not to smoke. Also, make sure they don't give the patient any smoking materials or matches.
• Avoid creating static electricity during oxygen use by having the patient wear all cotton garments and use all cotton sheets and blankets, if possible. As a second choice, have the patient wear garments made of 85% cotton and 15% synthetic fabric.

• Keep electrical devices such as radios, televisions, and vaporizers at least 5' (1.5 m) away from the oxygen source. Use a straight razor instead of an electrical razor when shaving during oxygen use. Avoid using electric heating pads and electric blankets.
• Remove all candles from the patient's room. Give him a flashlight to keep at his bedside in case of power failure, or if a light bulb burns out.
• Keep all aerosol cans out of the patient's room.
• Prohibit use of lotions, creams, or other products containing oil or alcohol during oxygen therapy and for 3 to 6 hours after oxygen use is discontinued. Alcohol and oil are both flammable. And, oxygen remains in linens and clothing for as long as 3 to 6 hours after use. Substitute glycerin when giving body rubs. Instead of a temperature-reducing alcohol bath, use ice bags or towels moistened with cool water.
• Keep the patient's hands oil- and grease-free.
• Don't use petroleum jelly or other oil-based moisturizers on patient's mouth and facial skin to relieve dryness. Use water-soluble lubricating jelly instead.
• Never lubricate any oxygen delivery equipment.
• Keep an all-purpose fire extinguisher on hand. Make sure *all* family members (including the patient) know how to use it.
• Apply these rules when using *portable* oxygen equipment as well as stationary equipment.

Using an oxygen tank safely

If your patient uses a tank as a source of oxygen, he'll need to observe certain guidelines for safe handling. Teach him the following:
• Keep at least a 3-day supply of oxygen available.
• Obtain tanks designated *patient-ready*. These are preequipped with a flow meter, a regulator, and a humidification bottle.
• Keep the tank away from heavily trafficked areas, so it won't get knocked or bumped.
• Secure the tank in place by positioning it in a stand rented from a supplier. Or, as a temporary stopgap, use a sturdy belt to fasten the tank securely to the head of the bed or some other sturdy piece of furniture.

Tipping it over could release oxygen under extremely high pressure, increasing risk of fire as well as injuring anyone in the path of a detached tank valve.
• Label full and empty tanks with appropriately marked adhesive tape.
• If you must move the tank, obtain a special carrier with wheels from the supplier, or have the supplier move it for you.
• Suspect a leak if you hear an unusual hissing sound or notice that the tank's emptying quickly. *Remember:* Oxygen is both colorless and odorless.

If you suspect a leak or any other problem, call the supplier right away. Ventilate the area, if possible.

Home oxygen use

Home care

Setting up an oxygen tank for use

Dear Patient:
The doctor has instructed you to use oxygen at home. Follow these steps to set up your equipment:

First, obtain from your supplier an oxygen tank that's *patient-ready*. It will have a flow meter, a regulator, and a humidifier bottle attached to it.

Now, unscrew the humidifier bottle, fill it with distilled water, and reattach it to the flow meter. *Note:* Be sure to change the water every day. Also, check the water level throughout the day's oxygen use. Whenever you need to refill the bottle, first pour out all the water.

Open the tank by turning the knob on top of the tank counterclockwise (as shown in the illustration), until you see the needle on the regulator gauge move, registering pressure. Now, attach the nasal cannula to the humidifier bottle. The nurse will give you another aid to teach you how to do this.

Then, turn the flow meter knob counterclockwise and adjust it to ____liters per minute (see inset). You should see the water bubbling in the humidifier bottle.

Continue oxygen therapy for the prescribed period. When you're finished, turn off the oxygen. Make sure the needle on the regulator drops to zero. Then, turn off the flow meter.

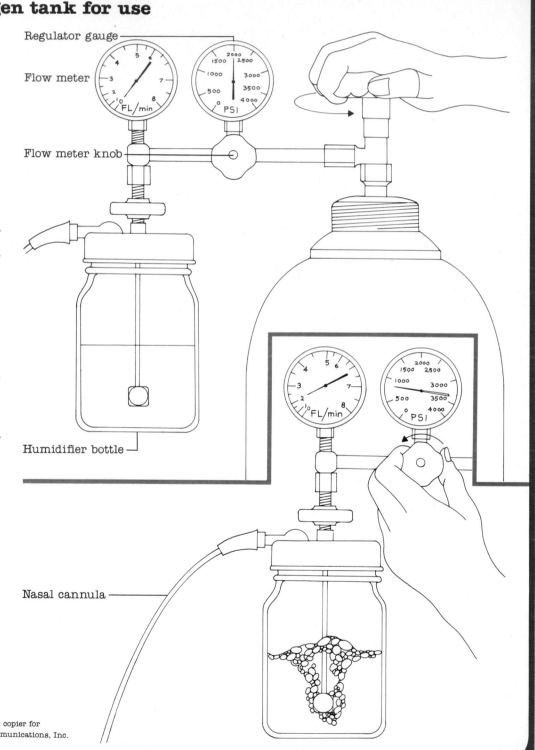

Regulator gauge

Flow meter

Flow meter knob

Humidifier bottle

Nasal cannula

Learning about liquid oxygen use

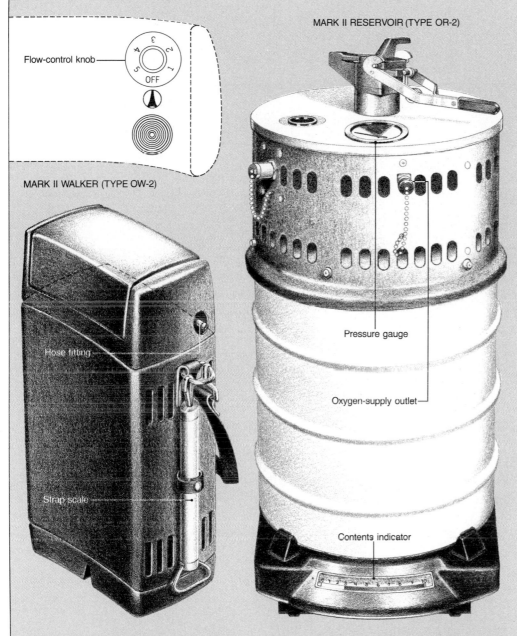

MARK II WALKER (TYPE OW-2)

Flow-control knob

MARK II RESERVOIR (TYPE OR-2)

Pressure gauge

Oxygen-supply outlet

Hose fitting

Strap scale

Contents indicator

Many patients use oxygen gas tanks at home. But, oxygen's also available in liquid form. This way, it takes up much less space. Also, it doesn't need to be kept under high pressure, so containers don't have to be as heavy and strong as gas tanks.

However, oxygen remains liquid only at very low temperatures, around −300° F. (−184.4° C.), so it requires vacuum-insulated storage containers. During oxygen use, the liquid warms up outside the vacuum insulation. It's then dispensed as a gas, at about room temperature.

Above, we've illustrated the Linde® Oxygen Walker System-Mark II, which consists of a reservoir unit (above right) for storage and nonambulatory use and a portable unit (the Walker; above left) for use during ambulation. *Note:* Containers are also available *without* the portable unit, for nonambulatory patients.

Important: Here we provide only an introduction to liquid oxygen use. Be sure your patient consults the supplier for more detailed instructions.

Using the reservoir or Walker for breathing

Your patient can use the reservoir as a source of oxygen for breathing *or* filling the portable Walker unit. If necessary, he can do both at once.

If he'll be using the reservoir for breathing, tell him always to make sure the pressure indicator is in the colored zone. If it isn't, he must call the supplier immediately. However, he may continue to use the reservoir until the supplier arrives.

To use the reservoir, your patient will remove the cap from the oxygen supply outlet. Then, he'll securely attach a filled humidifier bottle and a nasal cannula to the flow meter. He'll connect the flow meter to the oxygen supply outlet. Have him double-check all connections for tightness. Then, he'll set the flow meter at the prescribed rate. *Important:* Caution him never to increase the liter flow above the prescribed rate. Also, warn him to consult the supplier if the oxygen gas coming from the cannula feels uncomfortably cool.

The reservoir comes with a special base that indicates how full or empty it is. Make sure this scale is calibrated with the accessory breathing equipment in place. Have your patient contact the supplier when the reservoir needs refilling.

Using the Walker

Is your patient using the Walker for breathing? Then, he'll connect the nasal cannula to the small hose that fits into the case side, just above the strap attachment. Before each use, he should check hose connections at both the Walker and the breathing device to make sure they're securely attached. He should also make sure that the hose isn't kinked.

To start the oxygen flowing, he'll turn the knob located under the Walker's hinged cover until it clicks into position at the proper flow-rate setting. Caution him never to set the control knob *between* the marked positions, or no oxygen will flow. *Note:* Inform your patient that during use he'll hear a continuous hissing sound, from the venting of liquid oxygen through a pressure-relief valve.

The Walker has a handle with a built-in scale. When your patient suspends the unit by the handle, the scale will indicate how full the unit is. Have him consult the supplier for detailed instructions on filling the Walker from the reservoir.

Home oxygen use

Using liquid oxygen safely

In addition to the general safety precautions on page 67, teach your patient the following safety measures for liquid oxygen:

• Keep oxygen supply valves turned off when equipment's not in use.

• Always keep the portable Walker unit and reservoir units upright. Never lay them on their sides.

• Keep the Walker and reservoir in a well-ventilated area (rather than in a drawer, cupboard, or closet), because they continually vent a small flow of pure oxygen through their pressure-relief valves. Confining them in a small space may create an oxygen-rich atmosphere. For the same reason, never carry the Walker under your coat or other clothing.

• Don't run oxygen tubing under your clothing, bed covers, furniture, or carpets.

• In a car, always keep windows or vents open for adequate ventilation; never place the oxygen container in the trunk.

Note: Consult the supplier for information on traveling with the Walker.

• If you must move the reservoir, handle it carefully. Always lift it with two hands. Don't tip it or try to roll or walk it.

• Hold the Walker by its shoulder strap. Never lift it by the hose or by the hinged cover.

• Because liquid oxygen's so cold, piping and other metal parts can cause frostbite injury on contact, especially during filling. Never touch frosted fittings or piping with your bare hands. Be particularly careful if you have a circulatory problem.

• Open doors and windows to ventilate the room while you're filling the Walker. If liquid or cold gas escapes from the fill couplers, stand clear of it, and call the service representative immediately.

• Have the service representative maintain the units regularly. Follow his instructions for connecting breathing equipment, dealing with condensation problems, and filling the Walker from the reservoir. Contact him immediately in case of an emergency. Remember to keep his phone number taped to your telephone.

• Use only warm water and household detergent for cleaning the Walker. Don't use alcohol, solvents, polishes, or any oily substances on the Walker or reservoir. Never try to sterilize the Walker or the reservoir.

• Keep oxygen equipment out of the reach of unsupervised children.

Introducing the Healthdyne BX-4000® oxygen concentrator

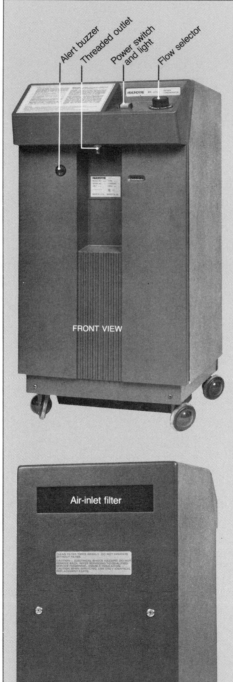

FRONT VIEW

Alert buzzer — Threaded outlet — Power switch and light — Flow selector

Air-inlet filter

REAR VIEW

Suppose your patient has a condition such as chronic obstructive pulmonary disease (COPD) that means he'll require low-flow oxygen for an extended period—perhaps for the rest of his life. If so, you might recommend that he use an oxygen concentrator, such as the Healthdyne BX-4000® shown at left. The concentrator draws in room air through filters that remove particulate matter; removes nitrogen from the air; and stores the remaining oxygen. The patient breathes oxygen through a nasal cannula at the prescribed liter flow.

Important: This model supplies oxygen flow rates of 4 liters per minute (LPM) or less. Never use an oxygen mask with this model, because the mask requires a flow rate of 5 LPM or more for maximum efficiency.

The oxygen concentrator has several advantages over oxygen tank use. For one thing, the patient need no longer store or move cumbersome tanks or worry about frequent tank changes. Also, except for power failure, the oxygen supply is guaranteed. And the concentrator may be safer, because the oxygen it contains isn't under high pressure.

Caution: A patient using an oxygen concentrator should keep an alternate oxygen source available, such as a portable oxygen tank. He'll need to use it in case of power failure (as this model has no backup battery), equipment failure, or during equipment cleaning.

For proper care and maintenance, teach your patient to do the following:

• Place the concentrator in an area free from traffic, to prevent damage. Position the concentrator at least 4" (10.2 cm) away from a wall, and well away from draperies, to avoid obstructing air intake.

• Clean the AIR-INLET FILTER in the rear of the cabinet twice each week and the outside of the cabinet as needed. Always unplug the unit before cleaning. To clean the filter, take it out and wash it in mild soap and water. Then rinse, pat dry, and replace it. *Caution:* Never operate the oxygenator without an AIR-INLET FILTER, or with a dirty AIR-INLET FILTER.

To clean the outside of the cabinet, wipe it with a cloth dipped in a solution of water and a household cleaning agent and wrung almost dry.

• Have the supplier check the oxygen flow after the first 60 days of operation. Have him check it again every 6 months, or any time the ALERT BUZZER activates (except during a start-up or power interruption.) Remember to keep the supplier's phone number taped to the telephone, in case of emergency.

• Have annual maintenance and repair performed by the supplier.

Using the Healthdyne BX-4000® oxygen concentrator

1 *You're helping your patient use the oxygen concentrator at home for the first time.* Explain the procedure to him. Then, as you perform each step, teach him what to do.

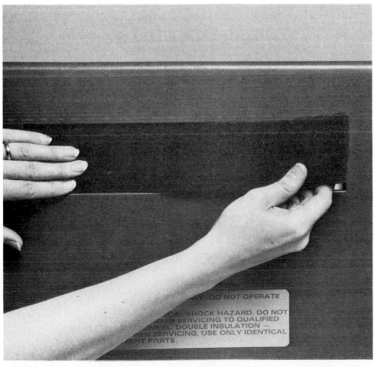

3 Then, depress the POWER SWITCH to check operation of the POWER INTERRUPTION ALERT SYSTEM and condition of the battery. The ALERT BUZZER, which warns of power interruptions and certain machine malfunctions, should sound. *Important:* If it doesn't sound, turn the unit off, use an alternate oxygen source, and immediately notify the supplier. If it does sound, turn it off by depressing the POWER SWITCH.

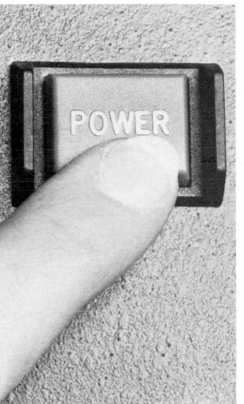

4 Next, set the prescribed oxygen flow by turning the FLOW SELECTOR dial to the appropriate number (1; 1.5; 2; 3; or 4 liters per minute—LPM). Align the number with the white INDEX DOT, and let the FLOW SELECTOR click into place. If you don't set it at exactly the right spot, no oxygen will flow.
Caution: Never try to force the FLOW SELECTOR dial past the 4 LPM setting.

2 Before you plug in the unit, be sure to check the air filter. You want to make certain it's clean and in place. If it's dirty, clean it very carefully, following instructions on the preceding page.

Home oxygen use

Using the Healthdyne BX-4000® oxygen concentrator continued

5 Now, attach the humidifier filled with distilled water to the THREADED OUTLET in the center of the console. *Important:* Use only a bubble-type humidifier. Dual-purpose or nebulizer types won't work properly with this model of oxygen concentrator. Also, instruct the patient to change the water in the humidifier bottle daily. He should check the level periodically during oxygen use.

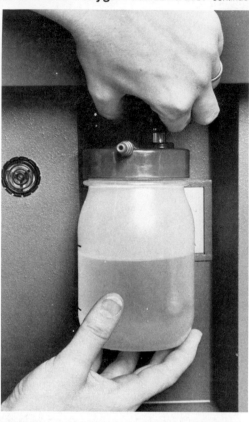

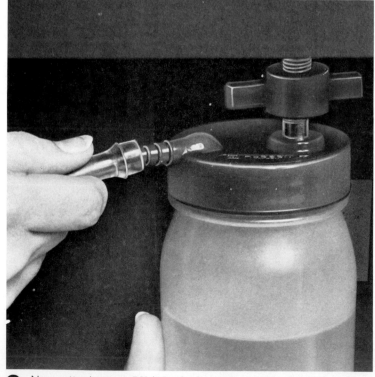

6 Now, attach up to 50' (15 m) of standard delivery tubing with an inside diameter of ³⁄₁₆" (4.7 mm) to the humidifier nipple.

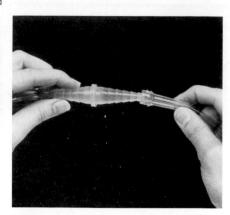

7 Then, attach a nasal cannula to the delivery tubing.

Next, plug the power cord into an ordinary household electrical outlet. *Note:* You can plug the Healthdyne BX-4000 directly into a wall outlet without an adapter, because it's double-insulated. However, Canadian units require a three-prong connector.

8 Now, to turn on the unit, depress the POWER SWITCH as you did in step 3. The POWER LIGHT should come on. Also, the ALERT BUZZER will sound for 60 seconds. If it doesn't, turn off the unit and switch to an alternate oxygen source until the supplier can check the unit.

Note: If the green power light goes out during operation, the ALERT BUZZER will sound. If this happens, check for accidental disconnection at the wall outlet. If the power supply's been interrupted temporarily, turn off the unit and use an alternative oxygen source until the power comes on again. If the ALERT BUZZER comes on during use, even though the power supply *hasn't* been interrupted, switch to an alternate oxygen source and notify the dealer.

However, if the ALERT BUZZER sounds for 60 seconds and then goes off, the unit's functioning properly and will supply the prescribed liter flow within a few minutes.

If all's well, put the nasal cannula on your patient, as the nurse is doing here. Administer the oxygen. Be sure to document the procedure.

To turn off the unit when you're finished, simply depress the POWER SWITCH.

Home care

How to use a nasal cannula

Dear Patient:
Because the doctor's ordered a low oxygen concentration for you, you'll be using a *nasal cannula* to receive it. To use it, follow these steps:

1 First, check the distilled water level in the humidifier bottle attached to your oxygen source. If you need to fill it, first dispose of all water already in the humidifier. *Note:* Be sure to change the water at least once daily.

2 Attach the end of the oxygen tubing to the humidifier nipple, as shown here.
Next, turn on the oxygen.

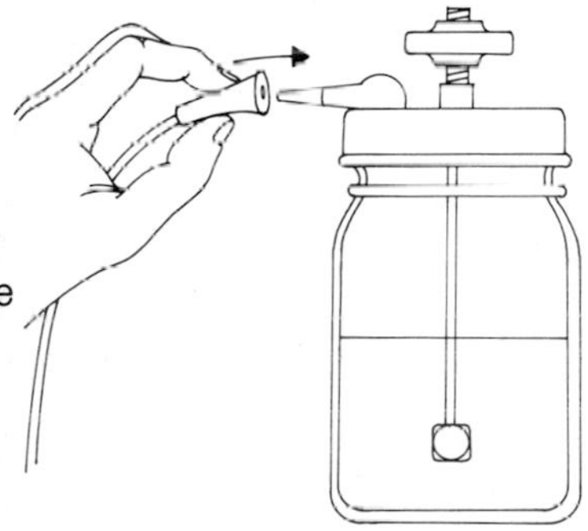

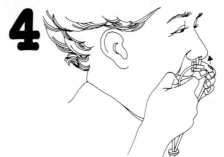

3 Now, set the liter flow rate at _____ liters per minute (LPM). *Important:* Never change the oxygen flow rate without the doctor's permission.
If you're receiving oxygen at 2 LPM or more, you should feel it flowing from the prongs. If you can't, briefly turn up the flow rate. Then, turn it back to the prescribed level. *Note:* At the same flow rate, you should see bubbling in the humidifier. If you don't, see if the oxygen source is open.

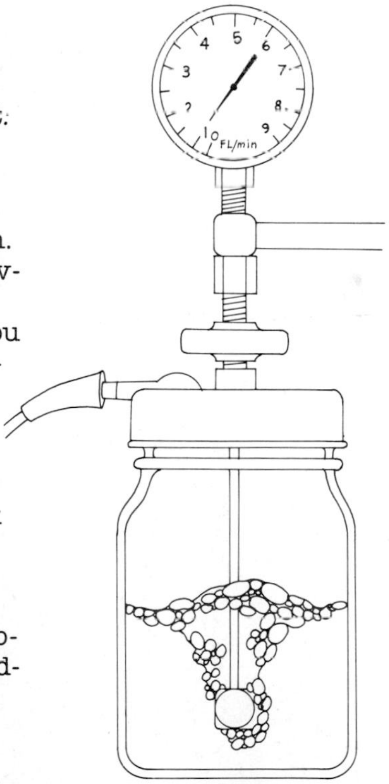

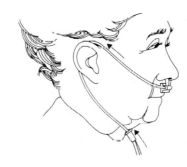

4 Next, insert the two prongs of the cannula in your nostrils, with the tab facing up. Make sure the prongs follow the curve of your nose.

5 Then, position the tubing over and behind each ear. Secure it by sliding the adjuster under your chin. But be careful not to adjust it too tightly.

6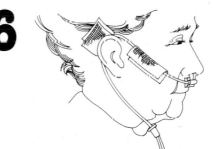

To guard against skin irritation, pad the tubing with 2"x2" gauze pads, placing them against your cheeks and behind your ears. Every 2 hours, check for reddened areas under your nose and around your ears. Massage these areas if you see redness. Notify the doctor if you develop any skin problems.
You may moisten your lips and nose with a water-soluble lubricating jelly (such as K-Y Brand Lubricating Jelly), but take care not to plug the cannula.
Every 8 hours, remove the cannula and wipe it clean with a wet cloth.
Important: Keep emergency phone numbers taped to your phone, in case you have any problems with oxygen use.

Home oxygen use

Assessing the effects of oxygen use

If your patient will be using oxygen at home, he and his family need to know when he's not getting enough oxygen and when he's getting too much.

Teach them to recognize the signs and symptoms of hypoxia, which include air hunger (fast, labored breathing), apprehension, change in patient's normal skin color, restlessness, and confusion. Warn the patient or family to notify the doctor at once (or call a local emergency service if he can't reach the doctor immediately), if he experiences any of these symptoms. Your patient may be tempted to increase the flow rate if he feels he's not getting enough oxygen. However, he should never change the oxygen flow rate, unless the doctor orders.

Note: If you're checking on a patient at home, and notice that he's changed the flow rate, find out why he's done so. Discourage him strongly from doing it again. If he feel's he's not receiving enough oxygen, or is having some other difficulty, contact the doctor immediately. If he continues to change the flow rate, suggest that the family obtain a locking flow meter.

Receiving *too much* oxygen can be a problem for your geriatric patient because many older people have age-related respiratory changes. This prevents normal oxygen diffusion into the blood, causing decreased PaO_2. When this happens, low oxygen levels replace high carbon dioxide levels as a respiratory stimulus. If your patient receives too much oxygen, he could develop carbon dioxide narcosis. Signs and symptoms include headache, lethargy, slurred speech, difficulty being aroused, reduced respiratory rate, shallow breathing, coma, and apnea. He or his family should notify the doctor or other emergency assistance immediately.

Using a portable oxygen tank

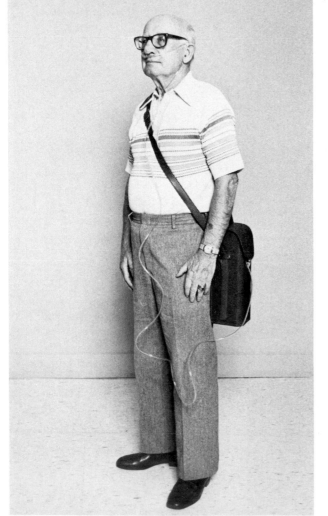

Suppose your patient's using tank oxygen or an oxygen concentrator 20 to 24 hours each day, but desires more independent movement. Then, you might suggest he use a portable oxygen tank, such as the one shown here, when he's away from home. As an alternative, your patient may use a wheeled carrier or have a family member carry the tank for him.

A portable tank allows your patient greater mobility combined with a continuous oxygen supply.

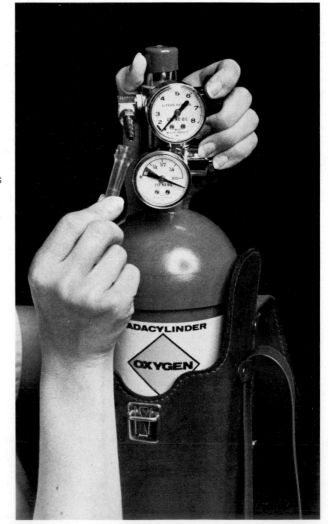

Antithrombotic measures

Do you know why your older patient's vulnerable to thrombus formation? How to assess him for a thrombus? What you can do to prevent or treat a thrombus? If not, read the following pages. We'll tell you all this, as well as how to use antiembolism stockings properly and how to administer anticoagulant medication safely. In addition, we'll give you tips on teaching your patient how to prevent a thrombus and how to take anticoagulant medication.

Reviewing vascular changes

Your geriatric patient may experience the following vascular changes that could cause circulatory problems:
• diminished blood vessel elasticity, muscle tone, and valve efficiency
• damaged blood vessels from prolonged high blood pressure
• diminished blood flow to heart, kidneys, and liver from above changes, possible arteriosclerotic problems, and decreased myocardial performance.

These changes affect your patient by reducing his venous blood return,

which results in venous stasis (pooling of venous blood). Problems associated with venous stasis include dependent edema, hypoxia of organs, and phlebothrombosis (venous blood clot without vein inflammation), or thrombophlebitis (venous blood clot with vein inflammation). And remember, a thrombus can be dislodged, leading to pulmonary embolism.

To find out how a clot actually forms in your patient's blood vessels, read the text below.

Understanding blood clotting

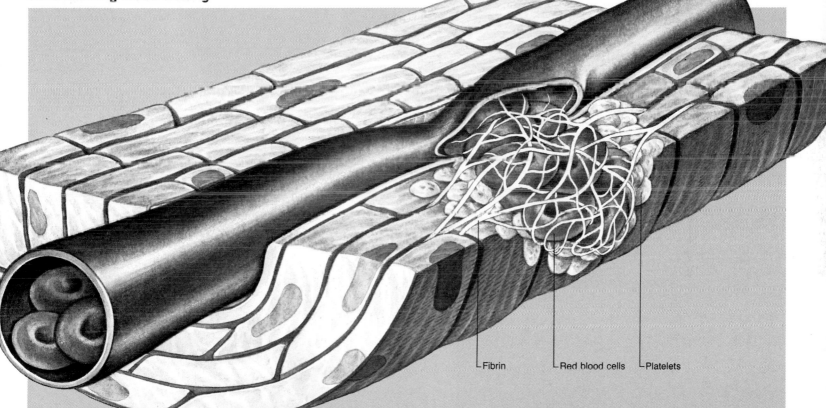

Fibrin   Red blood cells   Platelets

You're probably aware that blood clotting is a very complicated process. At least 35 blood factors participate in clot formation. To give you a basic working knowledge, we've summarized the four major stages as follows:

Stage 1:
Release of platelet factors
When blood flowing through a blood vessel comes in contact with a rough area on the blood vessel endothelium (for example, from a cut or an arterial plaque), platelets

begin to adhere to the rough area within a few seconds. Next, the platelets rupture, releasing a factor that initiates clotting.
Stage 2:
Thromboplastin formation
Platelet factors combine with calcium ions and other anticoagulant factors present in blood to form thromboplastin.
Stage 3:
Conversion of prothrombin to thrombin
Thromboplastin catalyzes conversion of prothrombin (an inactive circulating

blood protein) to thrombin. Participating substances include calcium ions and accelerator factors. *Note:* Vitamin K is an essential factor in prothrombin synthesis, which occurs in the liver.
Stage 4:
Fibrin formation
Thrombin catalyzes conversion of fibrinogen, another inactive circulating blood protein, to fibrin, which enmeshes red blood cells, platelets, and white blood cells to form the clot (see illustration above).

MINI-ASSESSMENT

Assessing your patient for thrombus development

When is your patient likely to develop a thrombus? When he's inactive or on bed rest (for example, when he's recovering from surgery); or when he has leg trauma such as a hip or leg dislocation or fracture; cardiovascular problems such as congestive heart failure, arteriosclerosis, hypertension, or varicose veins; clotting disorders; dehydration; or obesity. Also, consider him predisposed to develop a thrombus if he has any history of these conditions.

A thrombus is most likely to occur in your patient's pelvis and legs, although it may occur in his upper body. Signs and symptoms vary, depending on whether the thrombus forms in the superficial veins, the deep small veins, or the major veins. See the chart at right for signs and symptoms associated with each location.

Notify the doctor immediately if you detect any of these. He may order such conservative measures as putting the patient on bed rest with his legs elevated; applying warm, moist compresses; measuring leg circumference once every 8 hours; and applying antiembolism stockings. In addition, after evaluating baseline blood coagulation studies, he may order anticoagulant drug therapy.

The chief danger from a thrombus is that it may not remain in place in the vein. A portion of it could become dislodged and travel through the venous blood system as an embolus. If it does, it may eventually block a branch of the pulmonary artery. This condition's called a pulmonary embolism. The patient may show no signs and symptoms, or he may have some combination of the following: dyspnea, substernal chest pain, hemoptysis, tachycardia, anxiety, restlessness, electrocardiographic changes, fever with elevated leukocyte count and elevated erythrocyte sedimentation rate, convulsions, shock, syncope, and right-sided heart failure.

Notify the doctor immediately of any such signs and symptoms. Administer oxygen using a nasal cannula or mask, treat shock if necessary, and provide reassurance to allay the patient's fear and apprehension.

Suppose your patient shows no present signs or symptoms of any problems. If he has a predisposing history or condition, the doctor may order antiembolism stockings or anticoagulant therapy as preventive measures. In addition, always have your geriatric patient take the precautions listed below.

Thrombus signs and symptoms by vein site

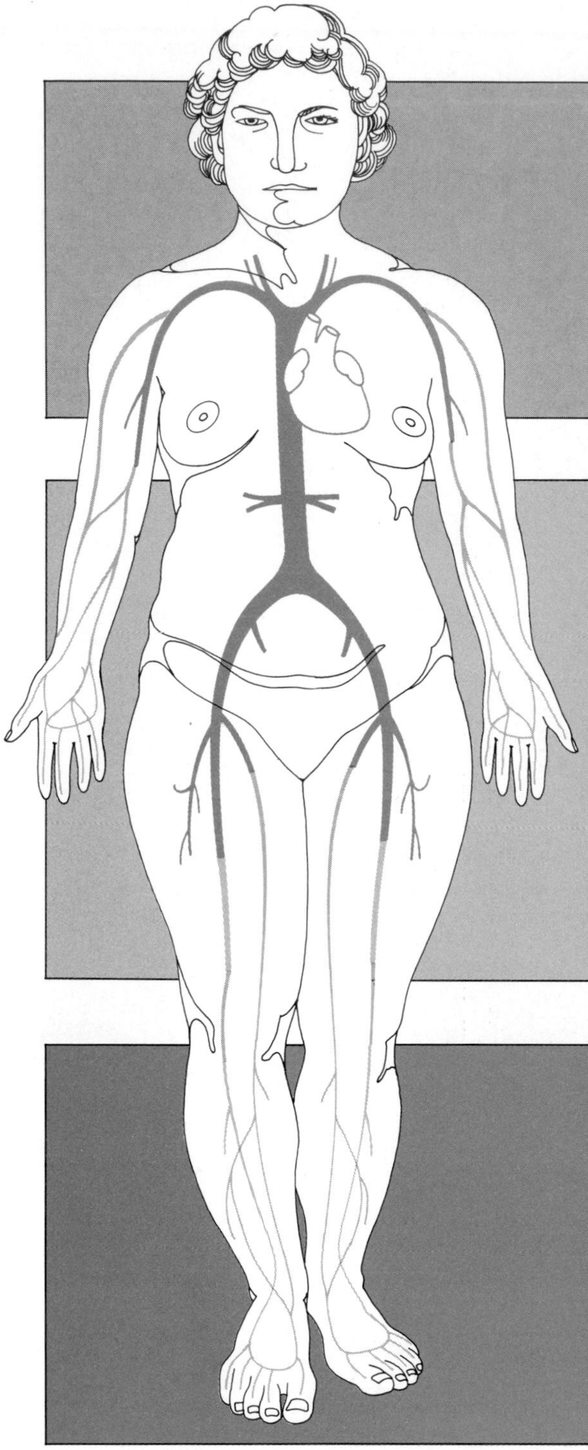

SUPERFICIAL VEINS
Cephalic, basilic, saphenous

Signs and symptoms
Local tenderness, induration, and redness; visible and palpable cord along vein

DEEP SMALL VEINS
Anterior tibial, posterior tibial, popliteal

Signs and symptoms
Swollen, congested muscles over tender area on affected vein; deep muscle tenderness; minimal or no vein engorgement; warmth of affected limb; pain on foot dorsiflexion (Homans' sign); possible fever, which rarely exceeds 101° F. (38.3° C.)

MAJOR VEINS
Subclavian, superior and inferior vena cava, axillary, iliac, femoral

Signs and symptoms
Changes in skin color, such as cyanosis or mottling; edema; venous engorgement in affected limb; no local signs of inflammation

Tips on thrombus prevention

Whether or not your geriatric patient's using antiembolism stockings or anticoagulant medication, make sure he observes the following preventive measures. Tell him to:
• avoid crossing his legs or wearing constrictive clothing, especially garters and knee-length stockings.
• keep pressure off popliteal spaces when lying in bed, sitting, or dangling his legs over the edge of the bed.
• turn and reposition himself every 1 to 2 hours.

• elevate his legs for 5 to 10 minutes after walking, dangling, or sitting in a chair.
• flex and extend his feet and legs, and rotate his feet to the left and right several times each, every 2 hours.
• ambulate frequently, if allowed.
• drink plenty of fluids and eat nourishing meals.
  Remember: If your patient *is* taking anticoagulant medication, make sure you explain why, and how the medication works.

Learning about antiembolism stockings

Antiembolism stockings help prevent blood clot formation by compressing the capillaries and small veins of the patient's legs. This forces blood into the large veins, accelerating the flow so the blood can't pool and clot.

For optimum benefit, the stockings must fit correctly. If they're too tight, they could restrict circulation, encouraging blood clot development rather than preventing it. If they're too loose, they'll have no effect. So measure and apply the stockings very carefully, using the measuring and application instructions in the following stories. But keep in mind that measurement, application, and care methods vary from brand to brand. Always follow the manufacturer's specific instructions.

To care for your patient wearing antiembolism stockings, follow these general guidelines:
• Remove the stockings every 8 hours.
• After removing the stockings, assess your patient's legs for circulation, sensation, and skin integrity (see opposite page). Also, examine the skin between his toes for any developing pressure sores. Document your assessment.
• If your circulatory system assessment reveals any problems, first make sure the stockings fit correctly. If no constriction is present, suspect other problems and notify the doctor.
• After assessing, wash and dry your patient's legs. You may apply powder or lotion sparingly, but do so without vigorously massaging your patient's legs or feet.
• Wait 1 hour before re-applying the stockings.
• Put a clean pair of antiembolism stockings on your patient each day.

Measuring for antiembolism stockings

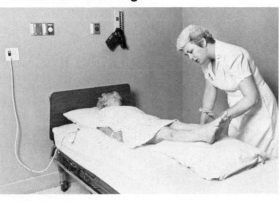

1 *Suppose the doctor's ordered antiembolism stockings for your patient. To obtain the correct size stocking, measure her accurately. Here's how:*

First, position your patient lying on her back or side. If she's just been walking, or sitting with her legs in a dependent position, elevate her lower legs and feet for 5 to 10 minutes. This position assists venous blood return and reduces leg vein engorgement so you can obtain accurate measurements.

Note: When you elevate her legs, avoid applying pressure beneath her knees.

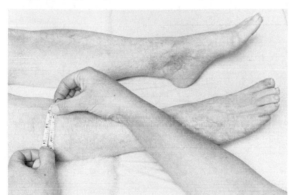

2 Now, position your patient's legs flat on the bed. To fit knee-length stockings, measure the largest part of her calf.

3 Then, position the patient on her side. Measure the distance from the back of her knee to the bottom of her heel.

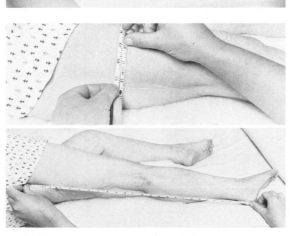

4 If the doctor's ordered thigh- or waist-length stockings, *first* measure the largest part of her calf as shown in step 2. Then, measure the largest part of her thigh (see top photo). Finally, position the patient on her side and measure the distance from her gluteal furrow to her ankle (see bottom photo).

Establish baseline measurements for your patient by noting them in her care plan. Then, to obtain the correct stocking size, compare the patient's measurements with those given in the table on the stocking package.

Note: Is your patient obese, very thin, or long-legged? If so, you may have to obtain a special size stocking from an orthopedic or medical-surgical supply store.

Antithrombotic measures

Applying antiembolism stockings

1 *Now you're ready to apply knee-length stockings. Elevate your patient's legs for 5 to 10 minutes, as you explain the procedure to her. Then, just before applying the stockings, check the circulation in her legs. Also, make sure her legs are clean and dry.*

To apply the stockings, first turn one stocking leg inside out. Then, slip your hand into the stocking up to its heel. Grasp the center of the heel and turn the stocking's foot right side out as far as the heel.

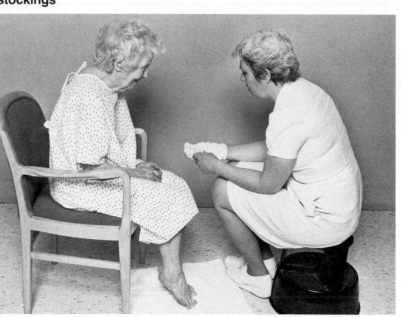

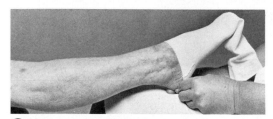

2 Next, center the patient's heel in the stocking heel band.

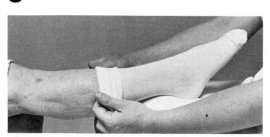

3 Then, pull the stocking foot over her foot.

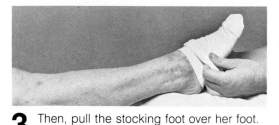

4 Now, gather the rest of the stocking and fit it *smoothly* over her leg. Avoid wrinkling it, which creates pressure points and can impair local circulation. To avoid putting pressure on the patient's popliteal space, make sure the stockings fit approximately 2″ (5.1 cm) below her knee.

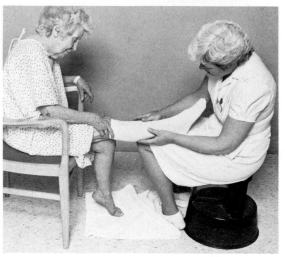

5 Finally, have your patient insert her finger between the stocking and her leg to make sure the stocking doesn't fit too tightly.

Now, apply the other stocking in the same way. *Caution:* Warn your patient never to turn down the tops of her stockings, because this may cause constriction or venous stasis.

If you're applying waist-length stockings, make sure you fit your patient with an adjustable belt. Check to be sure the belt's waistband or side panels don't press against any external devices, such as a catheter or drainage tube. Attach the stockings to the belt.

📖 *Nursing tip:* If your patient's stockings have toe holes, tell her to frequently check for normal toe color, if she's able. Or, ask a family member to do so. Tell her to alert you if she detects a problem.

Document the procedure in your nurses' notes.

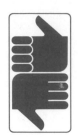

Does your patient need anticoagulant therapy?

Your older patient may receive anticoagulant therapy in the following circumstances:
• if he has phlebothrombosis or thrombophlebitis or a history of such problems
• during prolonged bed rest
• if he has congestive heart failure
• if he has a hip fracture
• after surgery, especially bone replacement surgery.

Because anticoagulant therapy increases the risk of hemorrhage, the doctor won't order it if your patient has any of the following conditions:
• hemorrhagic blood dyscrasias
• recent or impending central nervous system surgery or eye surgery
• active ulcers or hemorrhage in his gastrointestinal, genitourinary, or respiratory tract
• cerebrovascular hemorrhage
• aneurysm
• subacute bacterial endocarditis.

Reviewing anticoagulant drugs and an antagonist

The doctor's ordered you to give your patient anticoagulant medication. Are you familiar with these drugs? To find out how to use them safely, as well as how to administer a heparin antagonist, study the chart below.

heparin sodium *Lipo-Hepin*

Classification
Anticoagulant

Indications and dosage
Treatment of deep vein thrombosis
Adults: Initially, 5,000 to 7,500 units I.V. push. Then, dose is adjusted according to partial thromboplastin time (PTT) results.
I.V.: usually 4,000 to 5,000 units every 4 hours.
I.V. bolus: 5,000 to 7,500 units, then 1,000 units/hour by I.V. infusion pump. Hourly rate will be adjusted 8 hours after bolus dose according to PTT.
Treatment of pulmonary embolism
Adults: Initially, 7,500 to 10,000 units I.V. push. Then, dose is adjusted according to PTT results.
I.V.: usually 4,000 to 5,000 units every 4 hours.
I.V. bolus: 7,500 to 10,000 units, then 1,000 units/hour by I.V. infusion pump. Hourly rate will be adjusted 8 hours after bolus dose according to PTT.
Embolism prevention
Adults: 5,000 units subcutaneously every 12 hours
  Note: These dosages are only approximate guidelines. Dosage is prescribed on an individual basis, depending on patient's disease, age, and renal and hepatic status.

Side effects
Hemorrhage with excessive dosage; overly prolonged clotting time; thrombocytopenia; local irritation and mild pain; hypersensitivity reactions, including chills, fever, pruritus, rhinitis, burning feet, conjunctivitis, lacrimation, arthralgia, urticaria

Interactions
• With salicylates, anticoagulant effect increases. Don't use these drugs together.
• With oral anticoagulants, anticoagulant effect increases. Monitor prothrombin time (PT) and PTT.

Precautions
• Conditionally contraindicated in active bleeding; blood dyscrasias; bleeding tendencies, such as hemophilia and thrombocytopenia; hepatic disease with hypoprothrombinemia; suspected intracranial hemorrhage; suppurative thrombophlebitis; inaccessible ulcerative lesion (especially of GI tract); open ulcerative wound; extensive denudation of skin; ascorbic acid deficiency and other conditions causing increased capillary permeability; subacute bacterial endocarditis; shock; advanced renal disease; severe hypertension; during or after brain, eye, or spinal cord surgery; and during continuous tube drainage of stomach or small intestine. Although heparin use is clearly hazardous in these conditions, the danger must be weighed against risk from failure to treat the thromboembolic disorder.
• Use cautiously in mild hepatic or renal disease, alcoholism, and in patients whose occupations have a high risk of physical injury or who have a history of allergies, asthma, or gastrointestinal (GI) ulcers.

Nursing considerations
• Elderly patients should usually begin therapy at lower doses.
• Drug requirements are higher in early phases of thrombogenic diseases and febrile states and decrease when patient's condition stabilizes.
• Because heparin comes in various concentrations, check the order and vial carefully. Concentrated heparin solutions (greater than 100 units/ml) can irritate blood vessels.
• Give doses on time.
• Avoid administering I.M.
• Use I.V. administration whenever possible because of long-term effect and irregular absorption associated with subcutaneous administration. If possible, use an infusion pump to administer heparin I.V., for maximum safety.
• Check constant I.V. infusion rate regularly, even when pumps are in good working order, to prevent over- or underdosage.
• Never piggyback other drugs into an infusion line while infusing heparin. Many antibiotics and other drugs deactivate heparin. When using bolus therapy, never mix any drug with heparin in syringe.
• Give low-dose injections sequentially between iliac crests in lower abdomen, deep into subcutaneous fat. Inject drug slowly subcutaneously into fat pad. Leave needle in place for 10 seconds after injection; then withdraw needle. Alternate site every 12 hours—use the right side in the morning and the left side in the evening. Don't massage after subcutaneous injection. Watch for signs of bleeding at injection site. Rotate sites and keep an accurate record.
• When using intermittent I.V. therapy, always draw blood ½ hour before next scheduled dose, to prevent falsely elevated PTT.
• Wait at least 8 hours after initiating continuous I.V. heparin therapy before drawing blood for PTT. Never draw blood for PTT from the I.V. tubing you're infusing heparin through or from the vein you're infusing heparin into. Falsely elevated PTT will result. Always draw blood from opposite arm.
• Place notice above patient's bed to inform I.V. team or lab personnel to apply pressure dressings after drawing blood.
• Monitor platelet counts regularly. Thrombocytopenia caused by heparin may be associated with arterial thrombosis.
• Measure PTT carefully and regularly. PTT values of one and one half to two times control values indicate an anticoagulation effect. Numerical PT values depend on procedure and reagents used in an individual laboratory.
• Avoid excessive I.M. injections of other drugs, to prevent or minimize hematomas. If possible, don't give any I.M. injections.
• Regularly assess your patient for bleeding gums, bruises on arms or legs, petechiae, nosebleeds, melena, tarry stools, hematuria, hematemesis. Tell patient and family to watch for these signs and notify doctor immediately.
• Abrupt withdrawal from heparin may cause increased blood coagulability. Usually, the doctor orders an oral anticoagulant after heparin therapy to prevent blood clotting problems.
• Tell the patient to avoid nonprescription medications containing aspirin or other salicylates or other drugs that may interact with heparin.

protamine sulfate

Classification
Heparin antagonist

Indications and dosage
Heparin overdose
Adults: Dosage based on venous blood coagulation tests. Usual dose is 1 mg for each 78 to 95 units heparin. Give diluted to 1% (10 mg/ml), slow I.V. injection over 1 to 3 minutes. Maximum dose is 50 mg in 10 minutes.

Side effects
Blood pressure drop; bradycardia; transitory flushing; feeling of warmth; dyspnea

Interactions
• None significant

Precaution
• Use cautiously with patients who are allergic to fish.

Nursing considerations
• One mg protamine sulfate neutralizes 78 to 95 units heparin.
• Be aware that protamine sulfate in very high doses may act as an anticoagulant.
• Depending on hospital policy, the doctor rather than the nurse may administer this drug. He'll give it slowly to reduce side effects. Have equipment available to treat patient for shock.
• Monitor patient continually. Check vital signs frequently.
• Watch for spontaneous bleeding (heparin *rebound*), especially in patients undergoing dialysis and those who have had cardiac surgery.

Antithrombotic measures

Reviewing anticoagulant drugs and an antagonist continued

warfarin potassium *Athrombin-K** warfarin sodium *Coumadin**	anisindione *Miradon*

warfarin potassium *Athrombin-K** / warfarin sodium *Coumadin**

Classification
Anticoagulant

Indications and dosage
Prevention and treatment of deep vein thrombosis; treatment of pulmonary emboli
Adults: 10 to 15 mg P.O. for 3 days.
Then, give ordered dosage based on daily prothrombin time (PT) determinations.
Maintenance dose—
P.O.: Initially 2 to 10 mg daily
Alternative regimen—
P.O.: Initially, 40 to 60 mg daily. Then, 2 to 10 mg daily based on PT determinations.
I.V.: Rarely used; available in vials of 50 mg with sterile water for injection.

Side effects
Hemorrhage with excessive dosage; leukopenia; paralytic ileus or intestinal obstruction resulting from hemorrhage; diarrhea; vomiting; cramps; nausea; excessive uterine bleeding; dermatitis; urticaria; rash; necrosis; alopecia; fever

Interactions
• Prothrombin time may increase with allopurinol, clofibrate, dextrothyroxine, thyroid drugs, heparin, anabolic steroids, cimetidine, disulfiram, para-aminosalicylic acid, glucagon, inhalation anesthetics, metronidazole sulfinpyrazone, sulindac, and sulfonamides. Monitor patient carefully for bleeding. Remind the doctor to consider reducing anticoagulant dosage.
• Prothrombin time may increase with ethacrynic acid, indomethacin, mefenamic acid, oxyphenbutazone, phenylbutazone, and salicylates. Also, the combination may have ulcerogenic effects. Don't use these drugs with warfarin.
• Prothrombin time may decrease with griseofulvin, haloperidol, paraldehyde, and rifampin. Monitor patient carefully.
• Prothrombin time may increase or decrease with glutethimide, chloral hydrate, and triclofos sodium. Avoid using these drugs with warfarin. If you must use them together, monitor patient carefully.
• With barbiturates, inhibition of hypo-prothrombinemic effect may occur. If the doctor instructs you to discontinue barbiturates, remind him about reducing the anticoagulant dose. The inhibition effect may last for several weeks after the barbiturate is discontinued, so the patient may be vulnerable to bleeding.
• With cholestyramine, anticoagulant effect diminishes if you give drugs too closely together. Give cholestyramine 6 hours after giving oral warfarin.

Precautions
• Elderly patients and patients with renal or hepatic failure are especially sensitive to warfarin effect.
• Contraindicated in bleeding or hemorrhagic tendencies from open wounds, visceral cancer, GI ulcers, severe hepatic or renal disease, severe uncontrolled hypertension, subacute bacterial endocarditis, and vitamin K deficiency; and after recent eye, brain, or spinal cord surgery.
• Use cautiously in diverticulitis, colitis, mild or moderate hypertension, mild or moderate hepatic or renal disease; if your patient has a drainage tube in any orifice; or in any condition increasing risk of hemorrhage.
• Be aware that PT determinations are essential for proper control. Patient has high risk of bleeding when PT exceeds two and one half times control values. The doctor usually tries to maintain PT at one and one half to two times control values.

Nursing considerations
• Warfarin half-life is 36 to 44 hours.
• Give preferentially over other anticoagulants when patient must receive antacids or phenytoin.
• Because onset of action is delayed, the doctor may order heparin sodium given during the first few days of treatment. If you give heparin sodium simultaneously, don't draw blood for PT within 5 hours before or after I.V. heparin administration.
• You may divide large doses to reduce GI distress.
• Give doses at the same time daily.
• Have patient carry a card and wear a necklace or bracelet that identifies him as a potential bleeder. Make sure he keeps follow-up appointments. Stress the importance of complying with recommended dosage.
• Fever and skin rash signal severe complications.
• Regularly inspect patient for bleeding gums, bruises on arms or legs, petechiae, nosebleeds, melena, tarry stools, hematuria, and hematemesis. Tell patient and family to watch for these signs and notify doctor immediately if they occur.
• If necessary, neutralize warfarin effect with vitamin K injections.
• Warn patient to avoid over-the-counter products containing aspirin or other salicylates or drugs that may interact with warfarin.
• Tell patient to use an electric razor when shaving to avoid scratching skin and to brush teeth with a soft toothbrush.
• Light to moderate alcohol intake doesn't significantly affect PT, but have the patient check with the doctor before consuming alcoholic beverages.

anisindione *Miradon*

Classification
Anticoagulant

Indications and dosage
Deep vein thrombosis (prevention and treatment); pulmonary embolism
Adults: 300 mg P.O. first day; 200 mg P.O. second day; 100 mg P.O. third day.
Maintenance dose—
P.O.: 25 to 250 mg daily, based on prothrombin time (PT).

Side effects
Hemorrhage with excessive dosage; agranulocytosis; leukopenia; leukocytosis; eosinophilia; headache; myocarditis; tachycardia; conjunctivitis; blurred vision; paralysis of ocular accommodation; diarrhea; sore mouth and throat; nephropathy with renal tubular necrosis; albuminuria; jaundice; rash; severe exfoliative dermatitis; fever

Interactions
• Prothrombin time may increase with allopurinol, clofibrate, dextrothyroxine, thyroid drugs, heparin, anabolic steroids, disulfiram, para-aminosalicylic acid, glucagon, inhalation anesthetics, and sulfonamides. When using anisindione with any of these drugs, monitor patient carefully. Remind doctor to consider reducing anticoagulant dosage.
• Prothrombin time may increase with ethacrynic acid, indomethacin, mefenamic acid, oxyphenbutazone, phenylbutazone, and salicylates. Also, the combination may have ulcerogenic effects. Don't use these drugs with anisindione.
• Prothrombin time may decrease with antipyrine, carbamazepine, antacids, griseofulvin, haloperidol, paraldehyde, and rifampin. When using anisindione with any of these drugs, monitor patient carefully.
• Prothrombin time may increase or decrease with phenytoin, glutethimide, chloral hydrate, triclofos sodium, alcohol, and diuretics. Avoid using these drugs together. If you do use them, monitor patient carefully.
• With barbiturates, inhibition of hypoprothrombinemic effects of anisindione may occur. If the doctor instructs you to discontinue barbiturates, remind him of the need to reduce the anisindione dose. The inhibition effect may last for several weeks after the barbiturate is discontinued, so the patient will be more vulnerable to bleeding.
• With cholestyramine, anisindione effect diminishes when drugs are given closely together. Give cholestyramine 6 hours after oral anisindione.

Precautions
• Use with extreme caution (if at all) in psychiatric or debilitated patients.
• Contraindicated in hemophilia, thrombocytopenic purpura, leukemia with pronounced bleeding tendency, open wounds or ulcers, impaired hepatic or renal function, severe hypertension, acute nephritis, and subacute bacterial endocarditis.
• Use cautiously in a patient with a drainage tube in any orifice or in whom slight bleeding is dangerous.
• Start or stop any other drug cautiously during anisindione therapy.

Nursing considerations
• Give drug at same time daily. The doctor schedules doses according to PT. He usually tries to maintain PT at one and one half to two times control values.
• Because onset of action is delayed, the doctor may order heparin sodium given during the first few days of treatment. If you give heparin sodium simultaneously, don't draw blood for PT within 5 hours before or after I.V. heparin sodium administration.
• Have patient carry a card or wear a necklace or bracelet that identifies him as a potential bleeder. Make sure he keeps follow-up appointments. Stress importance of complying with recommended dosage.
• Fever and skin rash signal severe complications.
• Regularly inspect patient for bleeding gums, bruises on arms or legs, petechiae, nosebleeds, melena, tarry stools, hematuria, and hematemesis. Tell patient and family to watch for these and notify the doctor of them immediately.
• Warn patient to avoid over-the-counter products containing aspirin or other salicylates or any drugs that may interact with anisindione.
• Tell patient to use an electric razor when shaving to avoid scratching his skin and to brush his teeth with a soft toothbrush.
• If patient's urine is alkaline, it may turn reddish-orange for 1½ to 5 days.
• Light to moderate alcohol intake does not significantly affect PT, but have your patient check with the doctor before consuming alcoholic beverages.

*Available in both the United States and in Canada

Home care

Taking anticoagulant medication

Dear Patient:
The doctor's ordered that you take a medication called _____. This medication affects your blood's clotting mechanisms to keep clots from forming inside your blood vessels. Take it ____ times a day. While you're taking this medication, you may experience such side effects as:

_____

_____ .

Because this medication reduces your blood's ability to clot, you must take special precautions to keep from bruising or cutting yourself. Also, you must be careful to avoid a bad reaction from combining this medication with other medications. To avoid any such problems, be sure to follow these guidelines:
• Wear a Medic Alert™ bracelet with the information that you're taking anticoagulants stamped on it.
• Take your medication at the same time each day, as prescribed.
• Keep all appointments for blood tests. You may have blood taken at home by a visiting nurse, or at the hospital by laboratory personnel.
• Increase or decrease your medication only as directed by the doctor.
• Prevent getting bruised, by placing furniture out of pathways and by putting a rubber bath mat and safety rails in your bathtub.
• Never walk barefoot.
• Don't cut your toenails, unless they grow very long. If they need cutting, have a family member, visiting nurse, or podiatrist cut them.
• Don't shave with a straight razor. Use an electric razor or a depilatory.
• If you do cut yourself, immediately apply pressure directly to the wound with a clean, dry dressing or cloth. If you cut your arm or leg, elevate it above heart level. Maintain pressure for 5 to 10 minutes. If the bleeding doesn't stop, go to the emergency department of a hospital immediately.
• If you have any dental work done, tell your dentist that you're taking an anticoagulant.
• Always check with your doctor before taking any new medication. Other medication might react badly with your anticoagulant medication.
• *Never* take aspirin or over-the-counter preparations that contain aspirin. Read all labels carefully.

• Avoid alcoholic beverages. They may alter your blood clotting time. Because the effect varies from patient to patient, ask your doctor for specific advice.

In addition, immediately report any of the following signs or symptoms to your doctor:
• nosebleeds
• coughing up red to black mucus
• bruises that persist longer than usual or that increase in size
• bleeding gums
• blood in your urine or stool (which may be bright red or tarry)
• weariness
• dizziness, faintness
• anxiety and apprehension
• irritability
• confusion.

Stroke rehabilitation

Your patient who's had a stroke needs special care to help him regain the fullest possible function in affected body parts. Do you know how to proceed?

In the following pages, we give you guidelines on communicating with an aphasic patient, tips on proper positioning, and exercises to help your patient recover motor function.

As he progresses, we'll show you how to help him regain his balance while sitting and standing and give you special tests for assessing his readiness for ambulation.

Read these pages to find out how to best guide your patient through the early stages of convalescence. *Remember:* Stroke rehabilitation is a challenging but often frustrating process. To help your patient recover successfully, you'll need all the working knowledge you can absorb.

Understanding cerebrovascular accident (CVA)

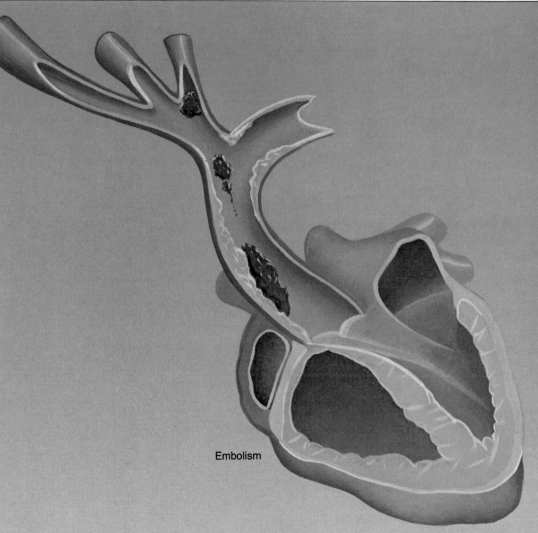

Embolism

A cerebrovascular accident (stroke) may occur when a thrombus or embolism occludes a blood vessel supplying the patient's brain. Or, stroke may occur from hemorrhage; for example, from a leaking or ruptured aneurysm.

The risk of stroke increases with:
• hypertension
• history of cerebrovascular or coronary artery disease
• diabetes
• obesity
• family history of stroke
• anticoagulant medication therapy
• heavy smoking and drinking
• sedentary lifestyle.

Thrombotic stroke
By far the most common cause of stroke, particularly in the elderly, is a thrombus from

atherosclerotic changes. The stroke may be preceded by a series of transient ischemic attacks or TIAs (see text at right), which may occur from months to hours before actual stroke onset. Symptoms may develop slowly, over a period of hours or even days. The stroke usually begins while the patient is asleep or shortly after he awakens.

Embolic stroke
In geriatric patients, embolic stroke usually develops from atherosclerotic heart changes. An embolus originating from a heart thrombus lodges in a cerebral artery, causing an infarction. Embolic stroke usually occurs rapidly. Although it may occur when the patient's either resting or active, it's more likely to occur during activity. The patient may suffer abrupt onset of hemiplegia or impaired vision, with no loss

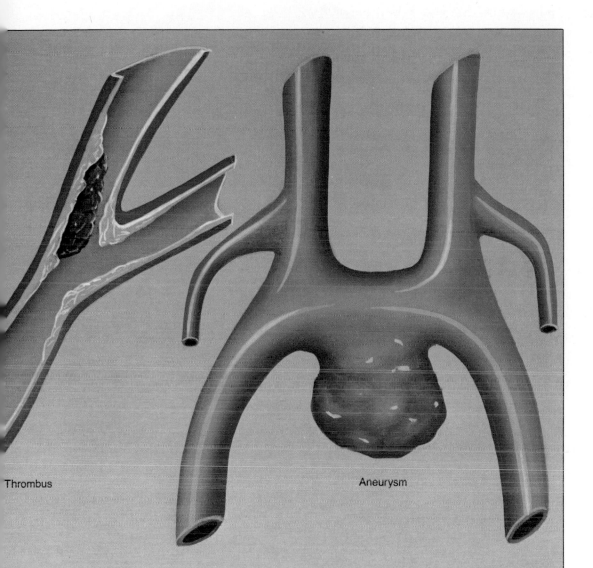

Thrombus

Aneurysm

Recognizing stages of cerebrovascular disease

If you know or suspect that your patient has cerebrovascular disease, you can assess his condition according to the onset and severity of his symptoms. Use the following stages of cerebrovascular disease as a guide.

For convenience, we've presented each stage in order from least severe to most severe. Your patient may progressively experience each stage as his condition worsens, or he may experience only one or two of them.

Premonitory phase: Patient experiences generalized warning symptoms which include drowsiness, dizziness, headaches, and occasionally, mental confusion.

Transient ischemic attack (TIA): Neurologic signs and symptoms, caused by temporary interruption of blood supply to the brain, appear and disappear within 24 hours. Most attacks are over within 30 minutes. After an attack, the patient regains complete control of normal functions.

Recurring intermittent neurologic deficit: Neurologic signs and symptoms may last from 12 hours to days or even weeks. The patient will recover completely after the attack, but remains susceptible to relapse. *Important:* Consider a TIA or recurring intermittent neurologic deficit to be a warning sign of stroke from a thrombus or leaking aneurysm.

Progressive stroke: Signs and symptoms evolve slowly over hours or days. At first, the patient shows only a few neurologic signs and symptoms. Then, as his condition worsens, one particular sign or symptom worsens, or new ones appear. He may have such generalized signs and symptoms as headache, vomiting, mental impairment, convulsions, nuchal rigidity, fever, and disorientation. Progressive stroke may be caused by a thrombus extending along an artery to block collateral circulation.

Completed stroke: When the patient's neurologic condition stabilizes, his stroke is considered complete. Neurologic signs and symptoms won't increase or worsen. But they may persist for a long time, and recovery can be slow.

of consciousness. He may be alert and able to understand explanations, but have a headache on the affected side.

Hemorrhagic stroke
Cerebral hemorrhage may occur from hypertension or rupture of an aneurysm. Hypertension causes bleeding into the brain tissue, whereas a ruptured aneurysm bleeds into the subarachnoid space. Stroke onset from hypertensive hemorrhage most often takes place very rapidly, while the patient's up and active. But the stroke episode can last from minutes to days, depending on the bleeding rate. The patient usually has a severe headache and may vomit initially.

An aneurysm is an arterial-wall pouch developing at a weak spot. Aneurysm ruptures usually occur during physical exertion.

The patient may have sudden severe headache with or without loss of consciousness, or loss of consciousness with no other symptoms. This kind of stroke can be immediately fatal, or the patient may recover within a few minutes, depending on the amount of bleeding. If bleeding's confined to the subarachnoid space, the patient will not have *focal* neurologic signs and symptoms (those indicating the affected brain area). However, if an intracerebral clot or cerebral infarction's associated with aneurysm rupture, he may have focal signs and symptoms.

To find out how cerebrovascular disease develops, see the text at right. Keep in mind that signs and symptoms vary, depending on stroke type and severity, as well as lesion location. (For focal signs and symptoms, see the chart on the following page.)

Stroke rehabilitation

Stroke signs and symptoms by lesion location

A stroke lesion's location determines your patient's signs and symptoms. Read the following chart to find out what to expect.

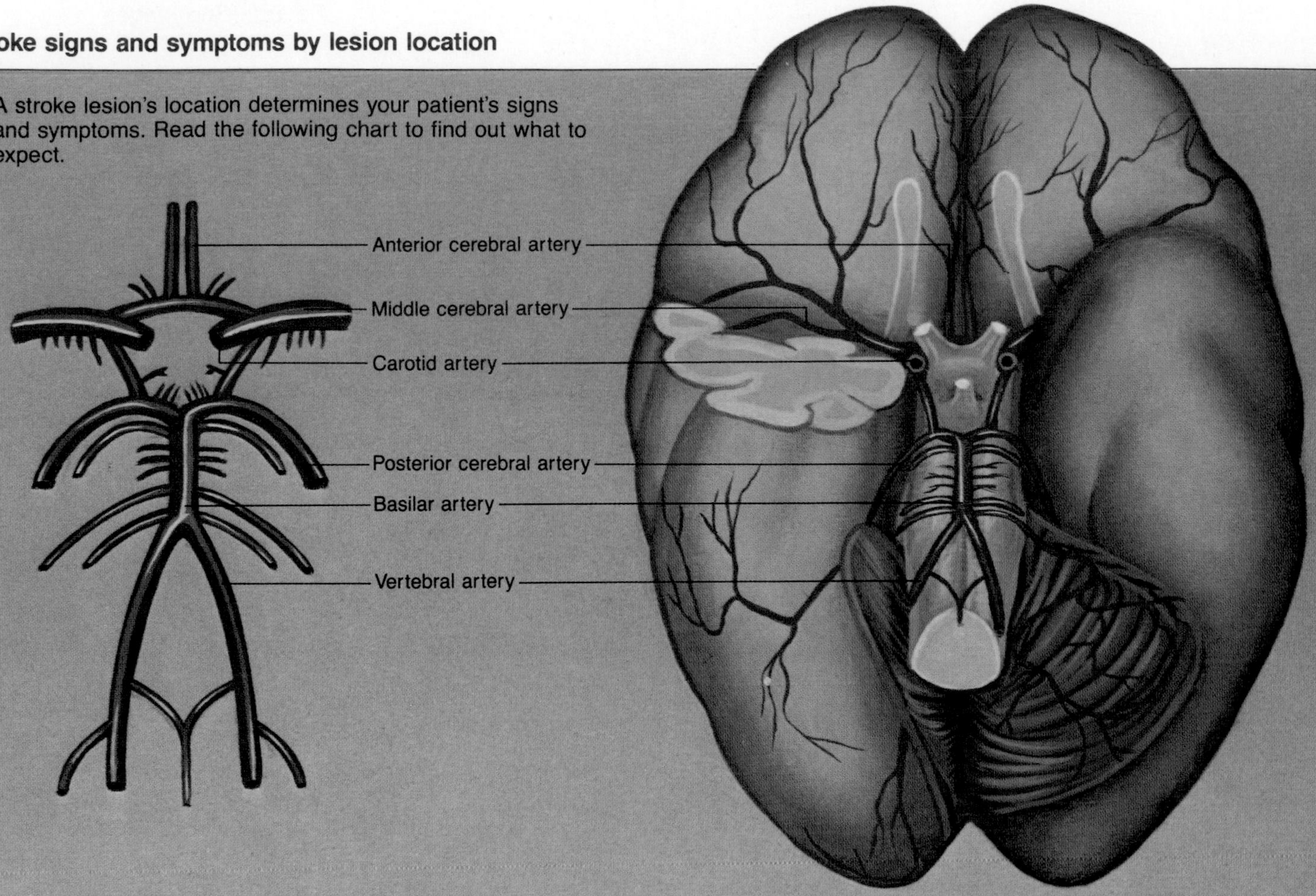

Anterior cerebral artery

Middle cerebral artery

Carotid artery

Posterior cerebral artery

Basilar artery

Vertebral artery

Lesion location	Signs and symptoms
Carotid artery	Contralateral hemiplegia; hemianesthesia; speech disturbance if lesion occurs in dominant hemisphere; neglect of half his body and space surrounding it; headache; ptosis; bruits; homonymous hemianopia or other visual disturbances on the affected side
Anterior cerebral artery	Contralateral hemiplegia with cortical sensory loss over leg (arm may also be affected, but less so); incontinence; flat affect; gait apraxia; personality change
Middle cerebral artery	Most signs and symptoms are the same as for carotid artery
Posterior cerebral artery	Homonymous hemianopia; sensory impairment; motor disability; dyslexia; coma. Paralysis is usually absent.
Vertebral artery	Lateral medullary syndrome, including numbness, pain, and impaired facial sensation; ataxia; vertigo; nausea and vomiting; nystagmus; diplopia; dysphagia; hoarseness; impaired gag reflex; contralateral diminished pain and temperature sensation
Basilar artery	*With partial occlusion:* Cerebellar ataxia; nausea and vomiting; slurred speech; contralateral pain and temperature sensation loss; sensation loss over face, trunk, and extremities; Horner's syndrome; dizziness; nystagmus; tinnitus; deafness; ocular movement disorders; hemiplegia *With total occlusion:* Quadriplegia; diplopia; paralysis of gaze; nystagmus; blindness or impaired vision; visual field defects; bilateral cerebellar ataxia; coma

Caring for a patient with a stroke

Mrs. Molly Carney, your 80-year-old stroke patient, has just been transferred to your unit from the intensive care unit (ICU). To give proper care, observe the following guidelines:

• Maintain a patent airway. To do so, place her in a side-lying or semiprone position. *Note:* She may need an artificial airway to keep her tongue from blocking her air passage.

Suction secretions as necessary. If ordered, use a humidifier to keep them thin.

• Assess oxygenation by checking for cyanotic skin color (especially of nailbeds), faster respiratory rate, restlessness, or apprehension. Give oxygen, as ordered, either by nasal cannula or face mask.

• Assess neurologic function by checking pupil response (including size, shape, symmetry, and light reaction); level of consciousness; motor response, response to stimuli, and vital signs.

Important: Test responsiveness to painful stimuli only as a last resort, when your patient shows no other signs of response.

• Assess your patient's neurologic and respiratory status every hour after transfer from the ICU, until her condition's stabilized. Then, check her every 2 hours. As you perform each assessment, note changes, and immediately notify the doctor of them.

• Check your patient's temperature even more frequently than other vital signs, to detect hyperthermia. The stroke may have affected her temperature-regulating mechanism. To lower her temperature, use antipyretic medications, sponge baths, a cool-mist vaporizer, or a hyper-hypothermia blanket, as ordered. *Caution:* Use a hyper-hypothermia blanket only as a last resort. Because the blanket's hard and has ridges, it can contribute to skin breakdown.

• Turn and reposition your patient at least every 2 hours to prevent respiratory problems and contractures (see guidelines on pages 86 and 87). At the same time, provide skin care to prevent skin breakdown.

• Since your patient's on bed rest, observe her for signs and symptoms of thrombus and pulmonary embolism (see page 76).

• Provide meticulous eye care. Remove secretions with a moist cotton ball. Instill eyedrops or ointment as ordered. If your patient can't close her affected eyelid, place a patch over her eye.

• Maintain fluid and electrolyte balance. If your patient can take liquids by mouth, offer them as often as fluid limitations permit. (Always check her gag and swallow reflexes before offering fluids or food.) Administer fluids I.V., as ordered (at a slow rate to avoid increasing intracranial pressure). Monitor intake and output.

• Provide adequate nutrition to help her regain her strength and prevent infection and decubitus ulcer formation. Encourage her to eat by frequently offering small amounts of food. *Note:* If your patient can't tolerate food by mouth (for example, because of her impaired gag or swallow reflex, or a decreased level of consciousness), the doctor will order tube feedings or total parenteral nutrition (TPN).

• If possible, position your patient sitting upright for each meal. Be sure to place foods within her visual field, and document this tray arrangement on her care plan. If you must lower the head of the bed shortly after she eats, position her lying on her side to reduce risk of aspiration.

• Perform meticulous oral hygiene after each meal, or every 4 hours. Remember, food will tend to collect on the affected side of her mouth. After mouth care, apply water-soluble lubricating jelly to her gums, tongue, lips, and the roof of her mouth.

For guidelines on mouth care for a comatose patient, see the NURSING PHOTOBOOK COPING WITH NEUROLOGIC DISORDERS.

• If your patient's aphasic, follow the communication guidelines on the next page.

• Help her cope with bowel incontinence by following the guidelines on page 101.

• Take measures to control urinary incontinence, as recommended in the fourth section. Avoid indwelling catheterization, especially since your stroke patient may experience only brief intervals of urinary incontinence. And remember to assess the cause of incontinence. Don't just assume that it results from specific neural damage. She may simply be unable to get out of bed or to undress herself quickly enough.

• Encourage self-care as early as possible. As soon as your patient's able, have her feed herself. (But, don't let her become hungry and frustrated if she can't do it. Assist as necessary.) Teach her to perform daily hygiene, including mouth care and sponge baths. As she improves, teach her to use the self-help aids on page 52, which will make daily living activities easier.

• Involve family members in teaching self-care. Their participation is crucial. Remember, they may fear that the patient will be permanently helpless. Give them relevant reading material and provide reassurance.

• Be aware of your patient's emotional changes (see page 89), and give support to both patient and family.

• Involve both patient and family in any decisions about long-term rehabilitation.

Rehabilitation: A continuing process

Begin stroke rehabilitation the day you begin patient care, regardless of your patient's condition. Early rehabilitation helps your patient compensate for neurologic and other body system losses so she can make the most of remaining function.

During rehabilitation, you'll encourage your patient to become as independent as possible, as well as help her cope with aphasia, paralysis, and incontinence. In addition to the daily nursing care you provide, your patient's rehabilitation program should include:

• physical therapy for improving muscle weakness, balance, coordination, and ambulation.

• occupational therapy for mastering activities of daily living, such as taking a bath, dressing, housecleaning, and cooking.

• speech therapy, if the patient's aphasic.

• psychological counseling (for the family as well as the patient) to help cope with emotional and sexual difficulties.

When the doctor determines that your patient's neurologically and medically stable and ready for discharge, he may refer her to a rehabilitation center, so she can continue her program. But, this depends on the degree of neurologic deficit. Many patients go directly home and continue rehabilitation through outpatient agencies. Others go to a convalescent center or nursing home for more intensive daily rehabilitation.

Important: At discharge, instruct the patient and family to report any premonitory signs and symptoms of stroke, such as severe headache, drowsiness, confusion, and dizziness. Stress the importance of regular follow-up visits.

Stroke rehabilitation

Coping with aphasia

As you probably know, aphasia can take a number of forms. Two of the most common include *expressive* and *receptive* aphasia. In expressive aphasia, which involves motor disturbance, your patient is unable to express his ideas with the appropriate words, although he understands what you say to him. In receptive aphasia, which involves sensory disturbance, he can't understand what you say to him. Many patients have some combination of these problems. Whatever your patient's particular problem, he'll probably need speech therapy. This should begin as soon as his condition's stabilized and may continue long after discharge from the hospital.

How can you best help your patient? Follow these general guidelines:
• Maintain continuity in nursing care by seeing that the same

nurses are regularly assigned to him. Familiar faces will make him feel secure and aid his recovery.
• Try to find out as much as possible about your patient, his personality before the stroke, and his previous ability to speak. In the past, did he become frustrated easily? How did he react to frustration? Before his stroke, was he fluent in the language you're using with him? This information can help you determine how much of his behavior after the stroke is normal for him.
• Reduce his frustration by arranging articles in his room conveniently. For example, place the call button, bedpan, and water pitcher and glass within easy reach.
Important: If your patient suffers from hemiplegia, make sure all articles are within reach of his *unaffected* arm.

• Encourage all types of communication, including watching TV, listening to the radio, and using the phone. Urge family members to maintain daily telephone contact with the patient, even if he can't respond clearly.
• Plan ample time each day to allow your patient to communicate in a relaxed, unhurried atmosphere.
• Speak in a normal tone of voice at a normal volume. Don't use baby talk or jargon, or your patient may feel that you're condescending to him.
• But do speak slowly, using short, simple sentences. You want to avoid overstimulating him or you may confuse or frustrate him.
• Don't start a conversation you can't finish, or abruptly change the subject.
• Be aware of feelings you're communicating nonverbally. Your patient will immediately

pick up negative *or* positive messages in your glance, tone of voice, or posture.
• If he becomes frustrated or tired, postpone your attempts at communication until he relaxes or rests. But don't leave him abruptly, without any explanation, or he may assume you're angry or frustrated with him.
• Be generous with praise and encouragement, because the rehabilitation process is slow and tedious. Your patient needs all your support to avoid becoming discouraged.
• Enlist the family's continuing involvement in attempting to overcome aphasia.

In addition to the above guidelines, here are some specific tips for a patient who clearly has either expressive or receptive aphasia:

If your patient has expressive aphasia, encourage *all* attempts at speech. Accept whatever

Preventing shoulder problems

Your patient may develop either of the following two shoulder problems:

Shoulder dislocation. This occurs from gravitational pull on an unsupported affected arm, as well as pulling and tugging on the affected shoulder during turning, repositioning, and transfer.

For prevention, always support your patient's arm in a sling when she sits or walks (see upper photo). This keeps the humerus positioned securely in the glenoid fossa. *Note:* While your patient's lying in bed or sitting up in a bed or chair, you can use two pillows to support her arm, instead of a sling.

When turning her in bed, prevent stress on the affected shoulder by using proper turning technique. Or, use a drawsheet (turning sheet) to turn her. When helping her to sit or stand, always place your arms *under* her arms and around her trunk (see lower photo). *Never* turn or lift her by pulling on her arms.

Assess your patient for shoulder dislocation by checking for shoulder pain, deformity, and edema. Your patient may also have pain along the entire extremity. Also, note any lack of resistance during shoulder range-of-motion (ROM) exercises. Report these symptoms to the doctor immediately, and elevate the affected arm. The doctor will reduce the dislocation and may immobilize the shoulder in a sling or wrap. Give pain medication or muscle relaxants, as ordered.

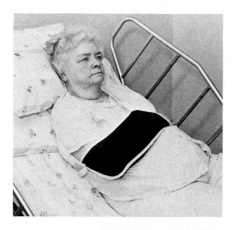

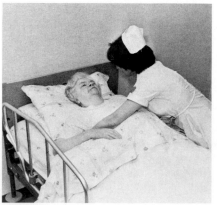

Shoulder-hand syndrome. This is a form of compartment syndrome from neurovascular impairment. The patient will have pain in her shoulder, as well as generalized hand and arm edema, pain, pallor, diminished-to-absent pulse, paresthesia, and decreased mobility. *Note:* Keep in mind that you may have difficulty distinguishing these signs and symptoms from the effects of stroke.

To prevent shoulder-hand syndrome, elevate the affected arm, including the elbow, above heart level, as much as possible. *Also, never use the patient's affected arm to draw blood or to start an I.V. infusion.*

If you detect signs and symptoms of shoulder-hand syndrome, immediate intervention will help prevent full-blown reflex sympathetic dystrophy syndrome, with atrophy of subcutaneous tissues, contractures, and osteoporosis. Intervene (as ordered) by performing passive ROM exercises for the shoulder. For edema or redness, the doctor may instruct you to apply heat locally and give contrast baths (using cool water first, and following it with warm water) to increase vasodilation. Also, he may order analgesics to help alleviate pain. Have your patient perform active ROM exercises as soon as she's able.

If your patient has advanced signs and symptoms of shoulder-hand syndrome, the doctor may have to surgically relieve compression to increase blood circulation.

speech sounds he's able to make, without criticism. However, don't pretend you understand him when you don't. He'll respond better to an honest approach. Use flash cards with simple words, phrases, or images to help him communicate and to minimize his frustration. Be sure to let him know that you empathize with his frustration.

Does your patient have receptive aphasia? Then, he'll benefit from your treating him *as if* he understands you. But, keep in mind that he can't understand everything you say, so he may not always respond appropriately. When you speak to him, be sure to stand well within his visual range. Talk slowly, and use gestures to clarify your meaning. Try to interpret *his* gestures. Also, keep in mind that his comprehension level may vary from day to day.

Preventing contractures through positioning

Your patient with a stroke may have some form of paralysis. With this loss of voluntary muscle control, some muscle groups exert more control than others; for example, flexor muscles dominate extensor muscles, and adductor muscles dominate abductor muscles. This makes the patient more vulnerable to certain contractures.

You can help protect your patient from contractures with proper—and regular—repositioning. Follow these guidelines:
• Post an illustration of proper positioning, as well as a positioning schedule, where other staff members and family members can see them. This way, an improper position change can be quickly corrected.
• To prevent hip flexion, keep the head of the patient's bed flat, except when he's performing daily living activities.
• Turn and reposition him every 2 hours, unless you last turned him to his affected side. He should remain on his affected side for no more than 20 minutes at a time. When he's able, encourage self care by having him turn himself.

Note: Have your patient use his unaffected leg to lift his affected leg when he repositions himself.

Put your patient in a prone position for at least 15 minutes each day. Doing this promotes hip hyperextension, which is necessary for walking, and helps prevent hip and knee flexion contractures.
• Use a bed board under the mattress for firm support.
• Protect bony prominences from pressure with a sheepskin, water-filled mattress, or other pressure-relief device.
• Elevate all extremities (especially those affected). Paralysis decreases or eliminates muscle pumping, slowing venous flow and causing edema. Elevating the extremities above heart level helps prevent edema and promotes venous blood return.

Important: Prevent application of direct pressure on the popliteal area. Direct pressure impedes venous blood return and contributes to knee flexion contractures.
• Use a footboard to keep your patient's feet at a 70° angle. Or, use laced, high-topped sneakers.
• Use trochanter rolls or sandbags to help prevent hip adduction and shoulder rotation.
• Use a handroll to keep fingers in a functional position.

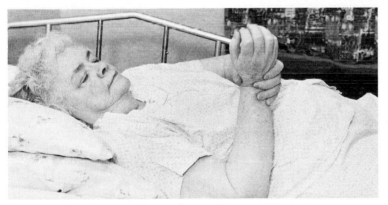

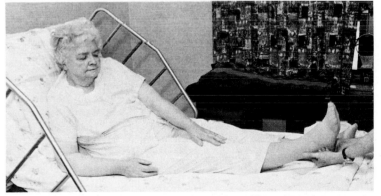

Proper positioning and frequent repositioning will go a long way toward preventing contractures. However, to gain maximum use of body parts affected by paralysis, your patient also needs exercise. Follow these guidelines:
• Perform passive range-of-motion exercises on each affected joint four times a day to help form new motor pathways to the brain.
• Have your patient *actively* put affected joints through full range of motion four times each day (see left photo).
• Have your patient perform gluteal-setting exercises while lying supine. Ask her to contract her buttocks muscles for a count of five, and then relax them for a count of five. Instruct her to perform this exercise five times, twice each day.
• Place your patient in a sitting position, and have her perform quadriceps-setting exercises by contracting her unaffected leg's thigh muscles and raising her heel. Ask her to concentrate on trying to push her popliteal space into the bed. Encourage her to hold this position for a count of five, and then to relax for a count of

five. Have her perform this exercise five times. Then, have her repeat it twice with her affected leg. If necessary, support her affected heel with your hand, and have her push on her affected knee with her *unaffected* hand (see right photo).

If your patient's affected leg is very weak or flaccid, you may have to provide additional help. To do so, support her affected heel with one hand, and place your other hand *under* the affected knee. Supporting her knee with your hand provides resistance and prevents possible knee injury. Then, ask her to push on her affected knee with her unaffected hand.
• Help your patient achieve a sitting and standing balance and early ambulation, following instructions given on pages 88 and 89.
• Encourage self-care in feeding, hygiene, and dressing, as a form of exercise.
• Work out a schedule to coordinate your patient's exercises with her other daily activities.
• Document all exercises and your patient's tolerance of them.

Stroke rehabilitation

Achieving a sitting and standing balance

After suffering a stroke and lying in bed for several days, your patient probably has an impaired sense of balance. She'll need time to recover it. *Note:* She'll find regaining her balance particularly difficult if she has a lesion affecting the cerebellum.

For your patient's first effort toward regaining balance, help her sit up in bed, as ordered. To do so, simply raise the head of the bed slowly until she's in a sitting position, rather than having her try to sit up independently. For safety, be sure to keep the bed's side rails up. She'll probably find this precaution reassuring. The rails also provide sensory feedback for a patient with proprioceptive (sensory) impairment on her affected side. And, by holding one rail with her good hand, she can balance more easily.

As your patient grows stronger, she'll be able to raise herself to a sitting position with little help from you. She'll use her functioning body parts to maneuver into this position. She can use an overhead trapeze or the bed's side rails to help, as shown in the photo below. Be ready to assist her, if needed.

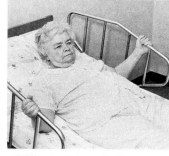

Sitting at the bedside

Your patient's next step in regaining her balance will be to sit on the edge of the bed. First, lower the bed to its lowest position, and lock the bed wheels. Then, help her put her legs over the bedside. Make sure her feet rest solidly on the floor. Or use a footstool, if necessary. Have her place her unaffected hand

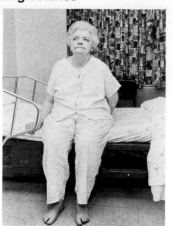

behind her, to help her maintain her balance, as shown above. Tell her to look straight ahead and deep breathe. Stand at her affected side and observe her for any changes in skin color or respiration, or for any signs of dizziness.

Initially, have your patient sit for 3 to 5 minutes. Increase sitting time gradually for each sitting period. Schedule three to four sitting periods each day—preferably at mealtimes—to help her feel more independent.

If your patient can sit on the side of the bed, she can also sit up in a chair or in a wheelchair. Her self-esteem will probably increase dramatically when she can move around in a wheelchair.

Be sure to obtain the right size wheelchair, with a seat low enough so your patient's feet touch the floor but high enough so she can transfer easily. For safe transfer, always place the wheelchair on your patient's unaffected side. Also, make sure that the wheelchair has a good brake. *Important:* Familiarize yourself with proper transfer technique before trying to help her into a chair or wheelchair. For detailed information on transfers, see the NURSING PHOTOBOOK PROVIDING EARLY MOBILITY.

Standing by the bed

Can your patient maintain her balance while sitting? Then, with doctor's orders, help her

try to stand. Ask a co-worker to be ready to assist.

First, lower the bed into its lowest position, and lock the bed wheels. Or, brace the bed against the wall for added support. Place nonskid, supportive, lace-tied shoes on her feet. Rest her feet firmly on the floor.

Now, place a straight-backed chair on her unaffected side, and position yourself on her affected side. Have her grasp the chair with her unaffected hand. Support her affected arm at the elbow and encourage a grasp reflex by clasping her hand with yours. Reassure your patient and help her come to a standing position, supporting her affected leg with your leg. As she stands, encourage her to look straight ahead and breathe deeply (see photo below).

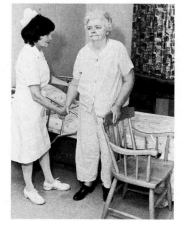

Document each procedure in your nurses' notes. Repeat the appropriate procedure several times each day.

Note: To promote the patient's independence in achieving a sitting and standing balance, consider using an electric bed equipped with half side rails. This allows the patient to independently raise or lower the head of the bed. With half side rails she can more easily maneuver herself into a sitting position on the edge of the bed. From there she can stand and pivot into a chair.

Is your patient ready for ambulation?

Of course, you want to ambulate your patient as early as possible. The doctor will ask you or the physical therapist to help her ambulate when she seems to have adequate locomotor power in one side of her body and sufficient stability in the other. But proceed with caution. Don't assume she's ready to walk just because she can stand. For her safety, follow these guidelines to assess her readiness to begin walking.

First, determine whether she can stand on the affected leg long enough to move her other leg forward. To test this, have her stand at the bedside and steady herself by grasping the bed rail or a chair. Or, you may support her around the waist. If she stands easily on both legs, ask her to shift her weight from one leg to the other (as shown in the photo). Then, note whether she can temporarily balance her weight on her affected leg.

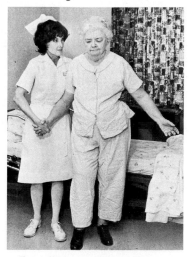

Even if she performs this test with ease, she may not be ready to walk. Keep in mind that sensory or spatial perceptual impairment can hamper balance too. The doctor may ask you to assess possible perceptual impairment in these two ways:

• Have your patient hold her affected hand up with her index finger pointed. Then, move her finger in space. Ask her to close her eyes and pinch her

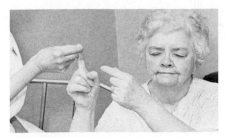

index finger with her unaffected hand (see photo). If she can't find her finger, and gropes in the wrong direction, she probably has a significant perceptual problem.
• Now, have your patient make a pistol shape with her unaffected hand. Ask her to pretend that her index finger is a gun barrel, and her thumb is a sight. Tell her to aim her index finger at her great toe on her affected side, and say "Bang!" when she feels she's pointing directly at her toe. Then, have her repeat the test with her eyes closed (see photo). If her aim isn't accurate when her eyes are closed, she probably has a significant perceptual problem.

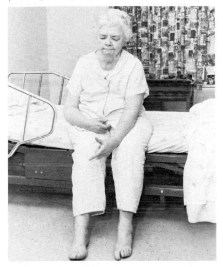

Other impediments to your patient's walking ability include being unaware of paralysis, as well as neglecting an affected extremity. This neglect phenomenon ranges from complete denial of the extremity's existence (total neglect), to paying little attention to objects and space on the affected side.

Total neglect is very common in the first few days following a stroke, but most patients quickly recover at least some awareness of the affected side. The less severe forms of neglect,

however, may persist for months and remain indefinitely.

To determine whether your patient's neglecting her affected side, conduct a visual confrontation test. Simultaneously present objects on both sides of her visual field (see photo). If she fails to react to the object on her affected side, she's neglecting it. *Note:* Don't consider this test conclusive unless you're sure the patient has adequate peripheral vision in both eyes.

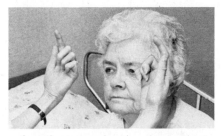

A patient experiencing the neglect phenomenon may bump into objects, leave food on the side of the plate nearest her affected side, or seem unaware of your presence when you stand on her affected side. In general, always try to approach such a patient from her *unaffected* side, and encourage family and staff members to do the same. Also, try to engage several of her senses at once by talking to her as you begin to approach her and touching her when you're near enough.
☎ *Nursing tip:* You may try occasionally approaching her from the affected side, to stimulate her awareness of this side.

Suppose the doctor decides your patient has adequate strength, balance, and perceptual ability for ambulation. Assist her in ambulating with the ordered ambulation aid. For safety, use a transfer belt and have a co-worker stand by. Also, be sure to position yourself on your patient's affected side. Encourage her to look straight ahead and breathe deeply.

Gradually increase her periods of ambulation. Begin by having her take a few steps to a chair. Then, perhaps, she could walk to the bathroom. Next, have her walk around the room. Finally, encourage short, and then longer trips down the hallway. Document your patient's progress, including how well she tolerated each walk, in your nurses' notes.

Coping with emotional problems

Up to this point, we've emphasized the physical changes associated with a stroke. But, your patient may experience emotional problems as well. These problems can be either *organic* or *psychological.* That is, they may have physiologic causes, or they may be primarily emotional in nature.

Lability is one organic problem associated with stroke. A patient with this disorder changes moods rapidly and inappropriately, moving readily from laughter, to anger, to crying.

Perhaps you're wondering how to distinguish lability from other emotional problems. Can you easily distract your patient from crying or laughing by having him perform some simple activity? Does he seem to be aware of and embarrassed by his behavior? Do you have a strong sense that he'd like to control it? If the answer to these questions is yes, he's probably labile.

Explain to your patient that his uncontrolled emotions result directly from physical changes induced by stroke. Whenever you witness an inappropriate emotional display, intervene by engaging his attention in other activities. *Remember:* He'll find excess emotional activity exhausting and frustrating.

Also, make sure his family understands that his behavior bears little relation to his real feelings. This will help them view it more objectively. Encourage them to avoid reacting negatively to his behavior. Instead, teach them to interrupt it with other activities.

What sort of psychological problems is your stroke patient likely to develop? Depression is one common problem. But, your patient's emotional response to stroke depends very much on his personality before the stroke. How well was he able to cope with difficulty previously? To help assess his emotional status, find out as much as you can about him from his family.

Help your patient cope with his organic *or* psychological problems by accentuating the positive. For example, emphasize the body functions he's retained, rather than those he's lost. Be generous with encouragement, support, and reassurance.

Also, attempt to keep your patient stimulated mentally and physically. He may find that watching television, visiting with his family, or performing self-care helps him avoid dwelling on problems. *Important:* In assigning your patient self-care tasks, try to break them down into small, easily completed components. Successfully achieving small goals will give your patient a sense of accomplishment.

Encourage close interaction with the family. Your patient will need a strong support group to sustain him. Remind him and his family to take each day at a time. Reassure them that setbacks are a natural part of the recovery process. Arrange for psychological counseling for both the patient *and* his family, as necessary.

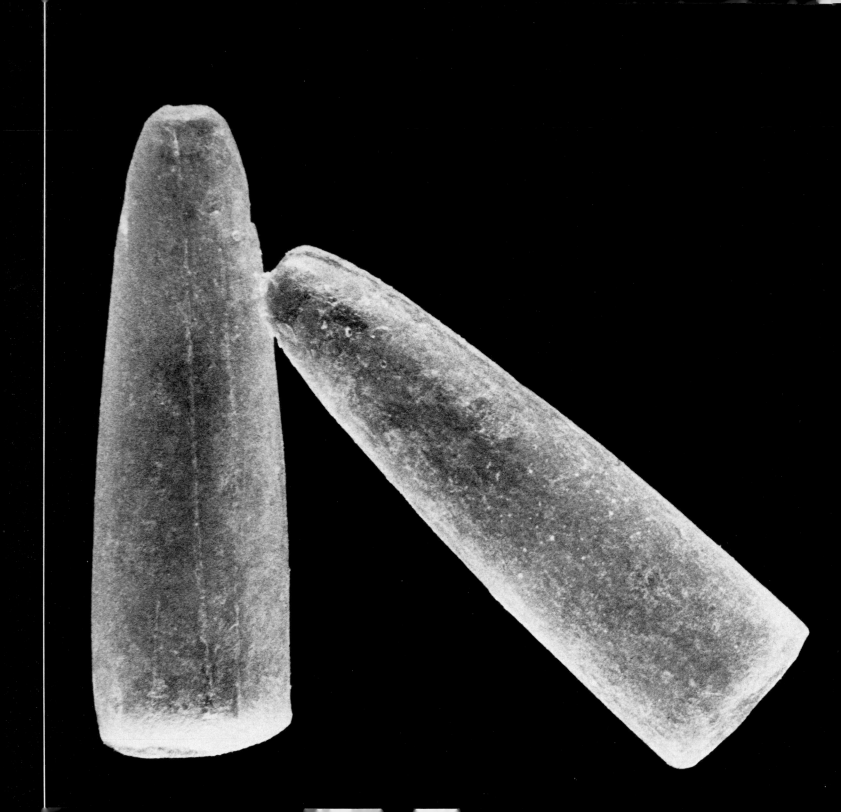

Dealing with
Digestion
and Elimination

Nutrition
Bowel training
Urinary tract care

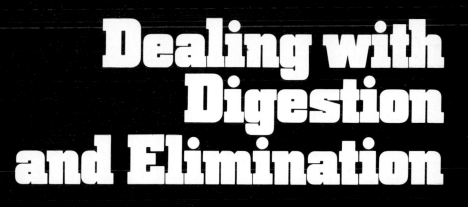

Nutrition

Finding ways to provide your geriatric patient with adequate nutrition should be part of each patient-care plan. But helping your patient develop a diet—and follow it—isn't always easy. Before beginning, you'll have to consider his physical condition, as well as his cultural background, previous eating habits, environment, and available finances.

Do you know how to recognize some of the signs and symptoms of overnourishment? Why an obese patient may be malnourished? Or how vitamins and minerals affect your patient's body?

Your first step is to learn as much about your patient as possible. Then, review your knowledge of nutrition. To prepare yourself for these tasks, study the information on the next few pages.

Understanding nutrition

Before we discuss good nutrition, we have to consider essential nutrients. What exactly is an essential nutrient? Simply speaking, it's a carbohydrate, fat, protein, mineral, or vitamin necessary to maintain life, allow normal body function, and promote growth.

With this in mind, then, consider foods containing essential nutrients (for example, dairy products, fruit, vegetables, meat, whole-grain bread, and cereal) necessary for good nutrition.

Of course, good nutrition is important no matter what your patient's age. But, because of a variety of interrelated factors—inactivity, low income, lack of transportation, special diets, and the disappearance of the corner grocery store—an older adult is more likely to suffer from some type of malnutrition.

As you probably know, malnutrition is the lack of essential nutrients, but not necessarily food. It can take one of three forms:

Overnutrition

Usually a geriatric patient suffering from overnutrition consumes foods that lack essential nutrients but contain large amounts of sugar, saturated fat, salt, cholesterol, phosphates, and calories; for example potato chips, french fries, and butter. Experts say an overnourished patient is more likely to develop such conditions as obesity, heart disease, high blood pressure, hardening of the arteries, stroke, arthritis, osteoporosis, cancer, diverticulitis, colitis, and cirrhosis of the liver.

Subclinical malnutrition

This subtle form of malnutrition is hard to detect. Because the patient consumes somewhat less than the required amounts of essential nutrients, he usually has a low resistance to infection and is in less than perfect health.

Undernutrition

In most cases, a geriatric patient suffering from undernutrition consumes far less than adequate amounts of foods containing nutrients. This essential nutrient deficiency may predispose him to anemia, weakness, brittle bones, infection, gum disease, loss of teeth, and depression.

How to assess your patient's nutritional status

Although diet-planning may strike you as a rather routine task, it's the foundation of adequate nutrition. It requires skilled assessment, careful planning, and systematic implementation, including follow-up. Keep in mind that a well-balanced diet will help your geriatric patient by:
• maintaining normal weight.
• improving the body's resistance to infection.
• keeping arteries and blood fat-free.
• protecting vital organs from degeneration.

Wondering how to plan a diet that meets your patient's nutritional needs as well as his food likes and dislikes? Begin by assessing his present nutritional status. Consider using the following format.

Physical examination/ medical history

• *Note his physical condition.* If all's well, you'll see: shiny hair; healthy scalp; normal-sized neck glands; pink, moist lips; pink tongue with surface papillae present; straight, uncrowded teeth; pink, firm gums; well-shaped jaw with no discoloration; smooth, slightly moist skin with pink mucous membranes; well-developed, firm physique with well-toned arms and legs that aren't tender, weak, or swollen.

Check to see if your patient's in pain. How well does he see, hear, smell, and respond to touch? Does he have weakness or paralysis? How mobile is your patient? For example, he may be physically unable to obtain and prepare his own food. Does he have any physical limitations that may affect his ability to eat? For example, he may have difficulty swallowing or chewing (possibly from dentures).

• *Check body measurements and lab results.* Compare his height, weight, and body frame with the physical standards for his age and body type. *Note:* Find out whether taking anthropometric measurements (such as skin fold measurements) is

your responsibility or the nutritionist's.

Of course, laboratory urine and blood tests can help you immediately detect nutritional deficiencies. Check your patient's urine for protein, glucose, albumin, and acetone levels; and his blood for hemoglobin, hematocrit, total protein, and albumin levels.

• *Check his medical history.* Has your patient recently gained or lost weight? If so, how much? Has he been dieting to lose or gain weight? Does he have a medical condition, such as high blood pressure, diverticulitis, or diabetes, that may require a special diet? If so, is he on a special diet? If not, why? Is he taking any medications that may suppress or stimulate his appetite? Does he have any medication allergies?

If your assessment data reveals that your patient's recently lost more than 10% of his total body weight; has anthropometric measurements less than 85% of standard; a diminished serum-albumin and lymphocyte level; or any serious clinical signs or symptoms; refer him to a nutritionist or metabolic specialist for further evaluation.

Social/psychological assessment

• *Evaluate your patient's mental and emotional status.* How's his memory? Is he alert and oriented? Does he appear anxious, confused, or uninterested? How does he react to you, other staff members, and his family or friends?

• *Assess your patient's lifestyle.* What are his daily activities? Does he work or spend a lot of time watching television?

An active person's nutritional needs will differ from those of a patient who is sedentary. Remember, the recommended daily allowance of nutrients varies from patient to patient, depending on activity level.

• *Determine your patient's financial status.* Is he living on a fixed income? Does he avoid eating meat, poultry, and fish because of the expense? If so, you may want to suggest he substitute other high-protein foods in his diet; for example, beans, nuts, and cheese.

• *Ask your patient about his living situation.* Does he live alone? If so, does he know how to store and prepare food properly? Does he have food storage space and cooking facilities? With whom, if anyone, does he eat?

• *Talk to your patient's family and friends.* Can they provide you with additional information about your patient; for example, details on his home environment, financial status, and eating habits? Do they seem motivated to help him plan and maintain a healthy diet?

Diet history
Find out where, when, and what your patient eats. What's his largest meal? Does he eat junk food (such as potato chips) heavily? How's his appetite? Has it changed recently? Estimate your patient's caloric needs based on how active his lifestyle is. What does he know about nutrition and proper diet? Does he have a clear understanding of the foods he should eat—and those to avoid? Is he willing and motivated to plan and implement a diet?

Goals and interventions
Suppose you learn that your patient's unable to obtain, store, or prepare his food. Recommend he participate in a community nutrition program, if your area has one. These programs offer nutritious meals as well as beneficial human contact. Some communities offer meals at local outreach centers, such as churches or senior citizen centers. If your patient's unable to get to an outreach center, suggest that he enroll in *Meals On Wheels* (if offered in your area). Tell him that for a small weekly fee, this program will entitle him to one hot meal, delivered once a day, five days a week. Keep in mind this program does not include weekends or holidays.

Let's say that on completion of your nutrition assessment,

you feel your patient's willing to talk about improving his nutrition. In that case, establish a time to talk to him about food and vitamins and how they relate to his health. Explain what foods he should eat and how much. Also, advise him

about what foods to avoid. Then, encourage him to let you know how the diet's going. Remind him to write down what he eats and drinks each day for at least 2 to 4 weeks. That way, you'll be able to assess additional nutritional needs. If

necessary, you can adapt the diet to better meet his needs. Remember, call on your patient to find out his physical and mental reaction to the diet.

Finally, document your findings in your nurses' notes. (See the assessment form below.)

NUTRITION ASSESSMENT

Name: *Ellen Johnson*   Age: *67*   Sex: *F*   Date: *7/10/82*
Diagnosis: *Cancer of large bowel, 6 months postcolostomy*
Patient profile: *Returned home 2 weeks ago after 5 month nursing home stay.*

PHYSICAL EXAMINATION/MEDICAL HISTORY:

Weight: *96 lbs.*   Height: *5'1"*   Ideal weight: *110*   Significant weight change: *8 lb. loss*
Body frame: Small _____   Medium *X*   Large _____   (time span) *3 months*
Clinical signs and symptoms: *Tires easily, poor skin turgor, poor control of colostomy.*

Major illnesses (including surgery)   *Right radical mastectomy, 1961   Transverse colostomy, 1982*

Medications (including allergies)   *Librium 10 mg B.I.D.   1 multivitamin daily   Allergic to sulfa drugs*

Laboratory results
Blood: Hemoglobin *9.6 g/dl*
        Hematocrit *27.8 %*
        Total protein *5.0 g/dl*
        Albumin *2.8 g/dl*

Urinalysis: Protein *Negative*
             Acetone *Negative*
             Sugar *Negative*
             Albumin *Negative*

SOCIAL/PSYCHOLOGICAL ASSESSMENT:

Mental and emotional status (alertness, orientation level, memory, motivation) *Alert, oriented to time, place, and person; extremely depressed since death of husband 4 years ago.*

Socioeconomic factors (cultural background, financial status, lifestyle, employment) *Retired telephone operator, has small pension and social security benefits from husband. Lives with divorced son.*

Support systems (family interview; social services) *Son would like to spend more time with mother but holds two jobs. Daughter occasionally visits but lives 1 hour away.*

DIET HISTORY

Describe appetite: Good _____   Fair _____   Poor *X*
Recent change in appetite: *yes*   If yes, describe: *Food intake decreased*
Diet: Regular *X*   Special (describe) _____
Food preferences: *Soft foods, tomatoes, bread, milk*
Food dislikes: *Steak ("too tough"), lima beans*
Food allergies: *Strawberries*
Usual mealtimes (time and place of largest daily meal, food eaten and amount; other meals and snacks) *No breakfast, tea and toast for lunch at noon; makes son's dinner at 6 p.m.; eats only small portion herself.*

Nutritional problem: *Poor protein, fluid, and caloric intake.*
Goal: *Increase weight by 3 lbs. every month up to ideal weight.*
Intervention: *Frequent small, high-calorie, high-protein meals.*

Nutrition

Diet planning: Some general guidelines

After you assess your geriatric patient's nutritional status, your next step is to assist him in planning well-balanced meals and snacks. You'll want to help your patient develop a nutritious, as well as realistic, diet. Be sure he understands that he's the only one able to make his diet work effectively.

Emphasize the importance of eating at least three well-balanced meals each day. Explain that because lunch takes place during the most physically active part of the day, it should be his heaviest meal. Also, suggest that your patient work into his diet nutritious snacks, such as raisins, fresh fruit, cottage cheese, celery, and cheese and crackers.

Recommend that your patient keep a daily food diary. Suggest he record what he eats, what time he eats, and how he feels when he eats and shortly after eating. That way he'll know how various foods affect him physically and emotionally. Now, review the following general dietary goals with your patient.

• *Reducing fat intake*. Advise your patient to trim visible fat off meat and drain fat off food during cooking. Also remind your patient never to use meat fat, such as lard or salt pork, for cooking. Tell him to cut back on fried foods and substitute low-fat milk for whole milk. Recommend he use margarine instead of butter.
• *Avoiding higher cholesterol foods*. Tell your patient to cut down on eggs; organ meats; shellfish, such as shrimp, lobster, and crab; dark-meat fish, such as mackerel and sardines; and non-dairy creamer.
• *Increasing fruit intake*. Encourage your patient to eat fresh bananas, apples, grapes, peaches, pears, and plums. Explain that these fruits supply vitamins A, C, and E as well as potassium. In addition, stress that fresh fruits help satisfy a craving for sweets. Remind your patient to buy seasonal fruits; they're usually ripe and inexpensive. Fruits packed in heavy syrup, on the other hand, contain excess sugar and calories.

Identifying nutrient sources

We've explained how the proper balance of nutritious foods helps keep your geriatric patient healthy. But, how familiar are you with specific nutrients and their sources? Do you know how vitamins and minerals affect your patient's body? If you're uncertain, read the chart that follows.

VITAMIN A
Action
• Maintains healthy skin and lining of mouth, nose, throat, and digestive tract
• Helps build resistance to infection
• Functions in rhodopsin (retinal rod pigment) formation and prevention of night blindness
Sources
Carrots and sweet potatoes; dark-green leafy vegetables, such as endive and collard; fish liver oil; egg yolks; cantaloupe; animal fats, such as butter, cream, and lard
Recommended daily allowance
4,500 to 5,000 IU
Considerations
• Encourage patient to have at least one ½ cup serving (0.12 l) or one piece of fruit per day.
• Warn that excessive amounts of vitamin A may cause patient's skin to appear yellow (carotenemia).

VITAMIN B COMPLEX
Action
• Functions in normal metabolism, cell growth, and blood formation
Sources
Whole-grain cereal, seeds, yogurt, buttermilk, cottage cheese, lean meat, fresh liver, kidney, dark-green leafy vegetables
Recommended daily allowance
B₁ (thiamine), males: 1.3 to 1.5 mg; females: 1.0 to 1.1 mg
B₂ (riboflavin), males: 1.3 to 1.7 mg; females: 1.3 to 1.5 mg
Niacin, males: 14 to 20 mg; females: 12 to 16 mg
B₆, males and females: 1.4 to 2 mg
B₁₂, males and females: 5 to 6 mcg
Biotin, males and females: 0.1 to 0.2 mg
Folic acid, males and females: 0.4 mg
Pantothenic acid, males and females: 4 to 7 mg
Considerations
• Consider increasing vitamin B complex intake for a patient taking hypotensive drugs (as ordered).

VITAMIN K
Action
• Influences formation of prothrombin and other clotting factors in the liver
Sources
Dark-green leafy vegetables, citrus fruits, bananas
Recommended daily allowance
Because it's synthesized by intestinal flora and also abundant in most normal diets, no daily recommended allowance has been determined. Adults are believed to require 0.3 to 15.0 mg/kg body weight.
Considerations
• If patient uses cathartics, anticoagulants such as dicumarol, or antibiotics, be alert for vitamin K deficiency. Keep in mind that a vitamin K deficiency rarely results from insufficient dietary intake of this vitamin.

IODINE
Action
• Increases circulation and boosts energy
Sources
Iodized table salt, seafood, dark-green leafy vegetables
Recommended daily allowance
1 mcg/kg body weight
Considerations
• If deficiency exists, problem may be failure to retain iodine in thyroid gland, decrease in anterior pituitary function, or failure to convert inorganic iodine to organic iodine.

ZINC
Action
• Promotes synthesis of DNA, RNA, and ultimately, protein
• Maintains normal blood concentrations of vitamin A by mobilizing it from the liver
Sources
Seafood, oatmeal, wheat bran, meat, eggs
Recommended daily allowance
15 mg/day
Considerations
• Advise patient that alcohol and corticosteroid medications increase renal excretion of zinc. If he uses either of these substances, have him increase his zinc intake.
• Vegetarians risk zinc deficiency.

- *Increasing vegetable intake.* Emphasize that vegetables contain fiber which helps prevent constipation and keeps blood cholesterol at a low level. To get maximum nutrients from vegetables, your patient should eat them raw or steam them and drink the broth. He can save the broth for use in soups and sauces, if he prefers.
- *Increasing intake of whole grain cereals and bread.* Tell your patient that these foods, like vegetables, contain fiber, which helps prevent constipation.
- *Eliminating sugar.* Recommend that your patient substitute fresh fruits, honey, nuts, seeds, and raisins, for sugar. Tell him sugar can cause headaches, nervousness, anxiety and apprehension. Explain that he'll get enough natural sugars from fresh fruits.
- *Decreasing salt intake.* Explain to your patient that processed food contains large quantities of salt, which can cause water retention and irritability. Recommend he read labels on products he uses. Suggest he sprinkle herbs on vegetables and meat for added flavor. Recommend that he use lemon juice in cooking. And, tell him to ask the doctor if he can use a salt substitute.
- *Increasing intake of minerals, such as calcium and fluoride.* Encourage your patient to eat more low-fat dairy products, whole grains, nuts, and dark, leafy vegetables. Also tell him to drink fluoridated water. Explain that minerals are vital to healthy bones and gums and also help maintain mental equilibrium.
- *Ensuring adequate fluid intake.* Tell your patient to drink plenty of fluids—at least 30 ounces (1,000 ml) a day, unless contraindicated.
- *Stopping smoking.* Tell your patient that smoking—whether a cigarette, cigar, or pipe—interferes with the absorption of nutrients.
- *Decreasing alcohol consumption to under five drinks per week.* Emphasize that more than five drinks per week will prevent proper absorption of minerals and vitamins. However, if your patient's used to having a glass of wine with his meals, or the doctor's prescribed wine to stimulate his appetite, he should continue this pattern.

VITAMIN C
Action
- Holds body cells together and strengthens blood vessel walls; helps keep bones strong
- Helps heal wounds and bone fractures
- Helps build resistance to infection
- Prevents scurvy
Sources
Cantaloupe, citrus fruits, strawberries, broccoli, brussels sprouts, peppers, tomatoes
Recommended daily allowance
Males: 40 to 60 mg; females: 40 to 55 mg
Considerations
- Advise patient that vitamin C in foods can be destroyed by overexposure to air or overcooking.
- Provide larger amounts of vitamin C during periods of physiologic stress: for example, infection.
- Supply patient with vitamin C foods daily because the body can't store large amounts of this vitamin.

VITAMIN D
Action
- Promotes absorption and regulates metabolism of calcium and phosphorus
Sources
Fortified foods (especially milk), butter, egg yolks, fish liver oil
Recommended daily allowance
Males and females: 400 IU daily
Considerations
- Be alert for a vitamin D deficiency if your patient has chronic pancreatitis, celiac disease, Crohn's disease, gastric or small bowel resection, fistulas, colitis, hepatic or renal disease, or biliary obstruction. These conditions lower vitamin D absorption.

VITAMIN E
Action
- Necessary for reproductive function
- Functions in development of smooth muscle, skeletal muscle, and vascular tissue; protects erythrocytes from hemolysis
Sources
Vegetable oils (corn, safflower, soybean, and cottonseed), margarine, whole grains, dark-green leafy vegetables, nuts
Recommended daily allowance
Males: 20 to 30 IU; females: 20 to 25 IU
Considerations
- If patient consumes large amounts of polyunsaturated fatty acids, you may want to increase his vitamin E intake.

IRON
Action
- Functions in erythropoiesis and prevents anemia
Sources
Red meats, green vegetables, eggs, whole-wheat bread, iron-fortified bread, milk
Recommended daily allowance
1 to 2 mg
Considerations
- Assess your patient's medication history. Keep in mind that some drugs (for example, pancreatic enzymes and vitamins) may interfere with iron metabolism.

CALCIUM
Action
- Essential for blood clotting, heart and muscle function, and development of healthy bones and teeth
Sources
Milk, cheese, sardines, turnip greens, broccoli, kale, citrus fruits
Recommended daily allowance
800 mg
Considerations
- For effective absorption of calcium, the patient must also receive adequate amounts of vitamin D.

MAGNESIUM
Action
- Regulates body temperature
- Activates enzymes necessary for carbohydrate metabolism
Sources
- Milk, cheese, poultry, whole-grain breads and cereals, vegetables
Recommended daily allowance
350 mg
Considerations
- Four servings of vegetables per day will guarantee adequate magnesium intake.
- Low magnesium concentration in blood causes irritability of nervous system, peripheral vasodilation, and cardiac arrhythmias.

Nutrition

Home care

Adapting a diet to your needs

Dear Patient:
The nurse has shown you how to plan a diet that meets your nutritional needs. But sometimes physical problems—such as ill-fitting dentures, sore gums, constipation, gas, diarrhea, or a special diet—can make eating unpleasant. We've included some tips to help you deal with these problems. But remember, if you feel pain, or for any reason you can't eat the foods included in your diet, notify your doctor.

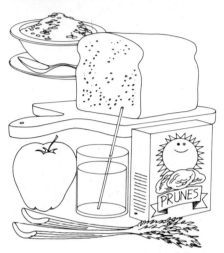

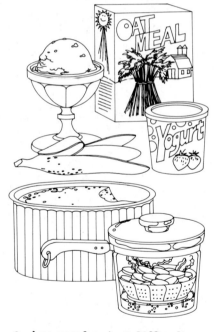

• Are you having difficulty chewing? If so, try including softer foods in your diet; for example, such dairy products as cottage cheese or yogurt; casseroles made with finely ground meat or cheese; canned or very soft fruits, such as bananas and mangoes; steamed fruits and vegetables that can be chopped or mashed; and cooked cereals, such as oatmeal.

• To help prevent constipation, be sure to include high-fiber foods in your diet. Select from whole-grain breads and cereals; cooked or raw fruits or vegetables; prunes in any form; or juice. Also, drink plenty of water. Avoid using laxatives, unless ordered by your doctor. And, if you take mineral oil, take it upon rising or 1 hour before bedtime. Mineral oil hinders absorption of some vitamins and medications.

• Gas is usually caused by swallowing air while eating rapidly, gulping liquids, chewing gum, or sucking hard candy. If you seem prone to gas, try to eat and drink slowly and avoid chewing gum and eating hard candy. Remember to sit up straight when eating, and try eating small meals frequently. Also, avoid eating gas-producing foods and beverages, such as onions, beans, cabbage, and beer.

• Do you experience painful cramps when you drink milk or eat other milk products? If you do, your body may not be producing enough of the digestive enzyme lactase. This enzyme breaks the milk sugar lactose into smaller products during digestion. Notify the doctor of your problem. He may want you to reduce your milk and milk-product consumption. Keep in mind that people who can't drink milk for this reason may find they can consume milk in small amounts or use such fermented milk products as buttermilk and cheese.

• Do you find you don't have much interest in food? Try using herbs, spices, and lemon juice to flavor your foods. Take a cooking class to learn new food preparation techniques. Also, dish out small portions of food for yourself on a small-sized plate rather than heaping your plate with food you don't really want. Garnish your plate attractively with parsley or lemon slices. Make a special effort to make your place setting appealing, using attractive placemats, napkins, and tableware. You may find a glass of wine will increase your appetite.

• If you eat alone and don't enjoy it, try eating while you watch television or listen to music. Or, eat outside in good weather.

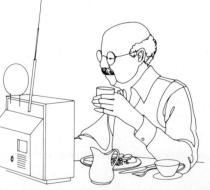

Bowel training

A person faces many changes in his daily routine when he's admitted to the hospital. For starters, being away from his normal environment will probably decrease his appetite and activity and may disorient him. These changes can affect his normal bowel pattern.

In the following pages, we'll explain how you can plan a bowel program that best suits your patient's individual needs. We'll tell you how to alleviate any bowel problems he's experiencing; for instance, how to assess and remove a fecal impaction. To promote perineal cleanliness and comfort, we've included a photostory on how to give your patient a sitz bath. We'll also identify the common types of enemas and laxatives you can give your patient to relieve his bowel problems.

Are you ready to learn more? Then read the next few pages carefully.

Promoting proper bowel function

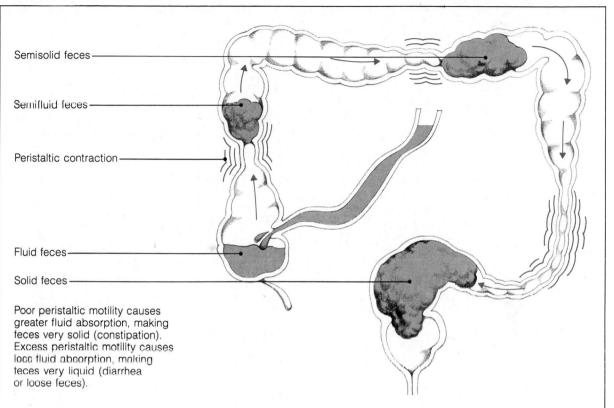

Semisolid feces

Semifluid feces

Peristaltic contraction

Fluid feces

Solid feces

Poor peristaltic motility causes greater fluid absorption, making feces very solid (constipation). Excess peristaltic motility causes loss fluid absorption, making feces very liquid (diarrhea or loose feces).

Catherine Gilbin, a 66-year-old schoolteacher, has been admitted to your hospital with a respiratory infection.

You'll want to help maintain or restore proper bowel function during her stay. First, quickly review bowel function by studying the illustration above. This shows how feces move through the large intestine and how bowel problems might develop.

Now, as part of your assessment, you'll want to take a bowel-function history. This will alert you to any problems, so you can prepare a schedule that best suits her needs. For guidelines, see page 13.

Usually, the geriatric patient is very conscious of bowel habits and takes laxatives to promote regularity. Teach your patient that a *daily* movement isn't necessary. A bowel movement every 1 to 3 days may be normal for a geriatric patient, who usually has diminished muscle tone, decreased activity, and reduced food intake. Establish a program that helps your patient achieve bowel control *without* using laxatives or enemas.

If your patient has a daily bowel-movement pattern already established, have her maintain that pattern, if possible. If her regular time for a bowel movement doesn't fit into her hospital schedule, or she's never been on an established schedule, set up a time after a meal, when the urge to move the bowels may be the strongest. Drinking 4 to 6 ounces (120 to 180 ml) of warm prune juice

before the meal may help establish this pattern regularly. Hot coffee, if permitted, may also help.

Have the patient attempt to move her bowels each day within 15 minutes of the scheduled time. If she can't, abandon the effort for that day, and try again the following day. Inserting a glycerine suppository 30 minutes before the scheduled bowel movement time (as ordered) may help stimulate the anorectal reflex. Positioning can also help. Assist your patient to a sitting position (if possible), the most beneficial posture for achieving a bowel movement. Then, ask her to contract her abdominal muscles and gently bear down. *Caution:* Because bearing down can elicit a vagal response, make sure your patient doesn't have a cardiac disorder. You may find that applying gentle pressure to her abdomen helps such a patient avoid Valsalva's maneuver. Or, have her lean forward to increase intra-abdominal pressure.

Provide as much privacy as possible when your patient defecates. This will give her a sense of control over her own body functions.

Finally, help design a diet for your patient that both contributes to proper bowel function and meets her nutritional needs and appetite. Encourage her to drink 2 to 3 quarts (1.9 to 2.9 l) of fluid daily, unless contraindicated, and make sure she gets a generous amount of fresh fruit, fresh vegetables, and roughage. Prunes, apricots, and bran may also help promote regularity.

Bowel training

Assessing for a fecal impaction

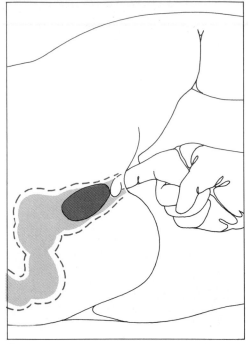

Do you know how to assess your patient for a fecal impaction? Suspect an impacted bowel if your patient has one or more of the following:
• diarrhea
• liquid bowel contents continuously oozing from his rectum
• abdominal cramping and rectal pain
• urge to defecate without being able to do so
• constipation
• abdominal distention
• hard palpable mass in his lower abdominal area
• urinary retention
• no recent bowel movement recorded.

If you think your patient has an impaction, confirm its presence by manually checking his rectum. You'll need an examining glove and lubricating jelly for this procedure. First explain to him what you'll be doing. Then, position your patient on his left side with knees flexed, as shown in photostory at right. Drape him, and provide privacy.

Now, put a glove on your dominant hand, and thoroughly lubricate the index finger of that hand. Next, insert your lubricated finger into his rectum. In normal cases, the rectum feels pliable and soft. It may contain soft stool or no stool. But, you'll know your patient has an impaction if you can't insert your finger into his rectum at all. Also, impaction is likely if you encounter a large, solid mass or many small, hard formations.

Document your findings in your nurses' notes.

PATIENT PREPARATION

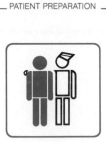

Preparing your patient for a fecal impaction removal

Will you be removing a fecal impaction from your patient's rectum? If so, first determine whether your patient can tolerate manual removal. Note any conditions in his history that would contraindicate the procedure, such as a myocardial infarction or a spinal injury. (If you're unsure whether your patient can tolerate the procedure, check with the doctor first.)

Also, remember to evaluate the medications your patient's receiving. You may need to suggest a prescription change to the doctor if, for example, your patient's receiving a drug that causes constipation.

Before starting the procedure, the doctor may order an oil retention enema given to soften the stool and promote evacuation.

If you can't insert your finger into the patient's rectum during the assessment, instill 30 to 60 ml of hydrogen peroxide solution into the rectum (as ordered). The solution's foaming action will help break up the mass into smaller pieces.

Removing a fecal impaction

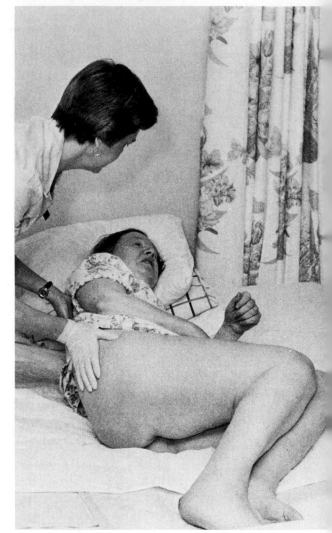

1 You've determined that 72-year-old Margaret Cowling has a fecal impaction. The doctor's ordered you to remove the impaction as soon as possible. Remember, the longer a stool remains in the colon, the firmer it becomes, because the bowel continually absorbs the stool's water content.

First, gather the following equipment: a non-sterile examining glove, lubricating jelly, bed-saver pads or plastic sheets, and a bedpan.

Now, wash your hands thoroughly, and put on your glove. Explain to your patient the procedure and the position you'll be placing her in. Then, turn and position her on her left side, with her knees flexed, as shown. *Note:* If your patient can't tolerate a side-lying position, obtain a fracture pan, and position her supine with the pan under her buttocks and her knees flexed.

After positioning your patient, spread the bed-saver pads or plastic sheets beneath her, tucking the ends under her hips. Then, cover her with a bath blanket to provide privacy.

2 Before you begin, instruct your patient to take slow, deep breaths during the procedure. Doing so will minimize her discomfort and reduce the risk of Valsalva's maneuver occurring.

Then, lubricate your gloved index finger generously, as shown.

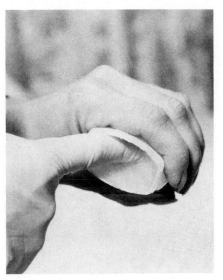

3 Insert your finger into your patient's rectum, and swirl it in a circular motion as you assess for any small fecal masses. This procedure may induce a spontaneous bowel movement of soft stool trapped behind the blockage.

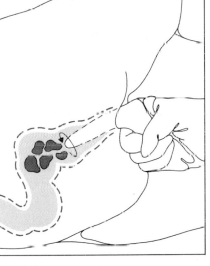

4 Remove any small masses that you encounter in the rectum, as the nurse is doing here.

Important: Give your patient rest periods throughout the procedure. Monitor her tolerance, watching for signs of pain and bleeding. Continuously observe her respiratory rate and consciousness level. If she has any problems, you may need to stop the procedure and resume it the following day.

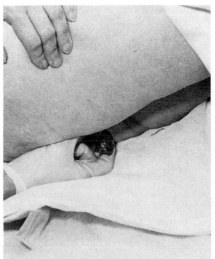

5 Suppose the fecal mass is too large for you to remove through your patient's anus. Then, break the mass into smaller pieces. To do this, lubricate your gloved middle and index fingers, insert them both into your patient's rectum, and move them in a scissors-like motion to divide the mass. Remove the smaller pieces with your fingers, and place them in the bedpan.

☎ *Nursing tip:* Conversing with your patient at this point in the procedure will help relax her.

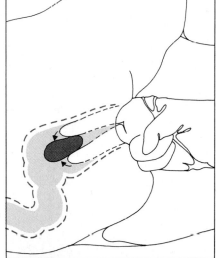

6 Once you've removed the impaction, withdraw your fingers. If no spontaneous bowel movement follows, ask your patient to gently bear down. At the same time, insert your index finger as far as possible into the rectum, as shown, to remove any additional masses or soft stool.

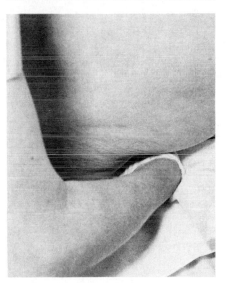

7 After you've finished removing any additional stool, give her a tap water enema, unless contraindicated.

Observe the form and contents of the stool, before disposing of it in the toilet.

Finally, wash and dry your patient's perineal area, as the nurse is doing here. Then, place her in a comfortable position. Document the procedure, noting if the impaction was removed or relieved, the appearance of the stool, your patient's tolerance, and any abnormal findings, such as bleeding or continual pain.

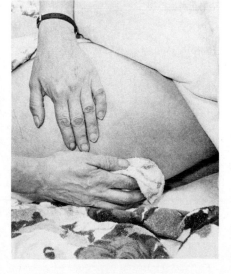

Bowel training

Reviewing enemas

Let's say your patient is constipated. To help him move his bowels, you've obtained a doctor's order to give him an enema. *Caution:* Enemas are contraindicated in patients with undiagnosed abdominal pain.

Although you'll be using only one of many enema types, follow the general guidelines below, whichever type you administer.
• Provide for your patient's privacy.
• Tuck bed-saver pads under the patient to protect the bed linens.
• Position your patient on his left side with his knees flexed.
• Instruct the patient to take slow, deep breaths throughout the enema procedure.
• Generously lubricate the nozzle tip with water-soluble lubricating jelly.
• Gently insert the nozzle 4″ to 6″ (10.2 to 15.2 cm) into your patient's rectum. Proceed cautiously when inserting the nozzle, to avoid damaging the mucous membrane that lines the rectum. Also, keep in mind that if he has external hemorrhoids, he may also have internal hemorrhoids.
• Periodically interrupt enema infusion to avoid overloading your patient with solution.
• Inspect the nozzle tip for new or old blood after removing it from your patient's rectum. Also, inspect expelled fluid and feces for blood. Document any bleeding in your nurses' notes.
• Clean the perineal area thoroughly after the patient's expelled the enema.
• Ventilate the patient's room to keep offensive odors from accumulating.
• Document the time the enema was given, amount of solution given, amount expelled, and the color and consistency of feces.

Now, review the major types of enemas by studying the chart at right.

OIL

Purpose
• Lubricates the rectum and softens fecal material to ease evacuation

Nursing considerations
• Warm solution to 105° F. (40.6° C.).
• Tell patient to lie quietly and retain enema solution for as long as possible (at least 30 minutes).
• This type of enema may be followed by a cleansing enema, after the patient rests.
• Enema is available in disposable form (Fleet Mineral Oil Enema*), which can be self-administered.

CLEANSING

Purpose
• Softens feces, stimulates peristalsis, relieves flatulence and distention, and produces immediate bowel evacuation

Nursing considerations
• Use tap water or normal saline solution as cleansing agents. Use soapsuds with caution, as ordered.
• Warm solution to 105° F. (40.6° C.).
• Elevate the enema bag no higher than 18″ (46 cm) above the patient's rectum during administration.
• Administer enema solution slowly, using well-lubricated rectal tubing.
• Give minimum amount of enema solution—only as much as is necessary to expel feces.
• A cleansing enema is available in disposable form (Fleet Enema*), which can be self-administered.

CARMINATIVE

Purpose
• Relieves gas pain and abdominal distention

Nursing considerations
• Milk and molasses is the most commonly used solution for this type of retention enema.
• Add milk to molasses slowly. Stir to blend thoroughly.
• Warm the milk and molasses together until they combine well. Then allow them to cool to 105° F. (40.6° C.).

*Available in both the United States and in Canada

Using laxatives

As you know, laxatives prompt bowel emptying by facilitating the passage of feces through the gastrointestinal tract. They may do so in one or more of the following ways:
• softening the feces
• adding to the bulk of the feces
• lubricating the feces
• stimulating peristalsis.

Your geriatric patient may occasionally need laxatives to compensate for abdominal and rectal muscle laxity, which slows fecal expulsion. This difficulty in maintaining good muscle control is compounded by an older person's lack of activity.

Use laxatives only when other measures, such as increasing your patient's fluid and fiber intake, have failed. Obtain a doctor's order before giving this medication.

Caution: Never give a laxative to a patient with undiagnosed abdominal pain.

You may be asked to administer one of several types of laxatives, depending on the condition causing the bowel problem. But, whichever the doctor prescribes, follow these guidelines:
• Note in your patient's bowel-function history whether he routinely takes a laxative and how often he takes it. Also, note the brand he finds most effective.
• Select a laxative that will cause the least amount of dehydration.
• Give a laxative only when needed, and use the mildest type that's still effective.
• Administer the smallest effective dose.
• Discourage chronic use of laxatives because they foster dependence and can cause excessive fluid and electrolyte losses.

You'll give your patient one of these five types of laxatives, depending on his needs.

Managing incontinence

Loss of bowel control can cause great concern and embarrassment for your geriatric patient. He'll worry about his lack of control and may fear that the condition will continue indefinitely. Bowel incontinence may occur from:
• a fecal impaction, causing liquid bowel contents to leak around the impaction and ooze from the rectum.
• inability to control the anal sphincter muscle against the defecation reflex.
• long-term dependence on laxatives.
• lack of sufficient bulk or fluid in the diet.
• serious illness or disorder; for example, bowel cancer or a stroke.
• stressful situations.
• medications that reduce cerebral awareness and control over the anal sphincter response.

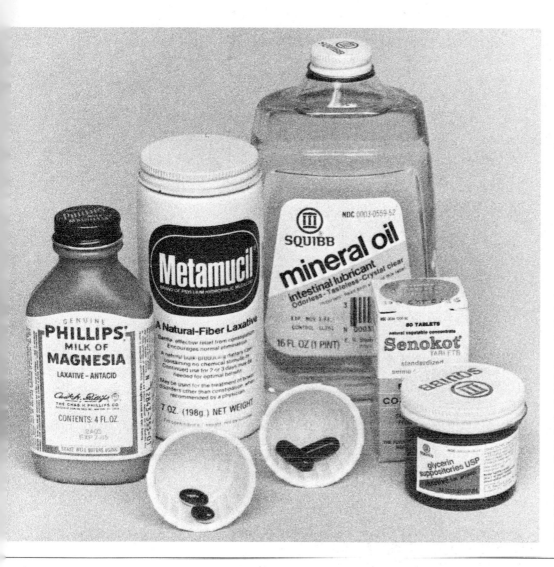

Bulk-forming laxatives, such as psyllium, stimulate bowel evacuation by increasing the bulk of the feces. These are natural or synthetic long-chain polysaccharides which expand in water, forming a gelatinous mass. Bulk-forming laxatives are probably the safest medications for promoting stool evacuation, because they act slowly and more gently than the other types of laxatives.

Emollient laxatives soften the stool by allowing water to enter the fecal mass, which also increases its bulk. Two examples of emollient laxatives include docusate calcium and docusate sodium. These are useful for patients who must avoid straining during defecation; for example, those with hemorrhoids or myocardial infarction.

Lubricant laxatives, such as heavy mineral oil and glycerin suppositories, soften the feces and reduce friction between the feces and the intestinal wall. These are also useful for patients who must avoid straining during defecation.

Saline laxatives include magnesium salts, sodium phosphate, and sodium biphosphate. These produce an osmotic effect in the small intestine by drawing water into the intestinal lumen. This action increases the bulk of the feces, which then encourages peristalsis and bowel movement. These medications work rapidly, usually within 3 hours after administration.

Stimulants, such as senna and cascara sagrada, act directly on intestinal smooth muscle, increasing peristaltic movements and intraluminal fluid. Cramping and passage of semisolid stool usually occur within 6 to 8 hours after drug is given.

● excessive doses of iron, antibiotics, or digitalis preparations.

Your thorough bowel assessment, including a bowel-function history, will help determine what's causing your patient's lack of control. As you investigate his bowel habits, consider the following:
● How much fluid and bulk food does he get in his diet?
● Is he taking any medications that would influence peristaltic action, fluid balance, or mental awareness?
● Can he use the toilet or commode when he needs to? Is he able to walk?
● How long does it take him to reach the bathroom? Once he's in the bathroom, can he manage by himself?
● Is the nurse call button within his reach in the bathroom and at his bedside?

Any program you develop to reestablish your patient's bowel control will require time and patience to be effective. Also, you'll have to be tactful and considerate to relieve his embarrassment. For example, preserve his self-esteem by allowing him to help in his own cleanup, if he can do so adequately. If your patient has limited mobility, you may want to position a commode at his bedside or offer him a bedpan at about the time he usually defecates. To eliminate offensive odors, ventilate the room.

As you work toward helping him regain continence, try to follow these guidelines:
● Establish regular bowel evacuation times.
● Provide meticulous skin care to lower the risk of decubitus ulcers and excoriation.
● Thoroughly cleanse your patient with soap and warm water, as necessary.

● Prevent constipation and impaction.
● Include adequate fiber in his diet, if possible, which adds bulk, weight, and form to the stool and improves evacuation of the sigmoid colon and rectum.
● Provide a daily fluid intake of at least 1,000 ml, unless contraindicated.
● Increase his activity level, if possible.
● Evaluate your patient's medications. Discuss with the doctor whether they may be causing diarrhea or impaction.

To reduce the likelihood of an unscheduled bowel movement, you may need to obtain an order for suppositories or a sodium biphosphate enema (Fleet Enema*). Suggest that your patient wear specially designed underwear with disposable liners, which will provide him with some security when he's mobile (see page 108).

*Available in both the United States and in Canada

Bowel training

Giving your patient a sitz bath

1 *Let's assume you've removed a fecal impaction. Now, to soothe and cleanse the perineal area, you're going to give your patient a sitz bath. Are you familiar with the procedure? If you're unsure, read this photostory.*

First, obtain the sitz-bath pan and tubing, and wash your hands thoroughly. Then, explain to your patient what you're going to do.

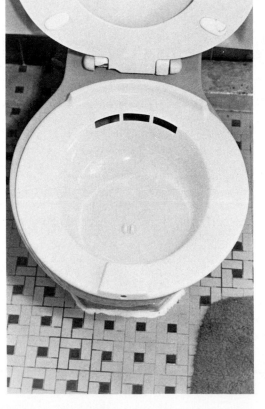

3 Next, insert the end of the tubing through the middle rear slot in the pan (see upper photo). Now, clamp the tubing in the notch on the bottom of the pan (see lower photo).

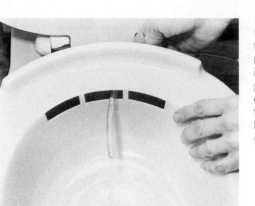

2 Now, raise the toilet seat and place the sitz-bath pan on the toilet bowl. Align the pan so its drainage slots are in the rear of the bowl, as shown here.

Note: The pan may have the word *front* marked on it. If so, follow this guide to place the pan in the correct position on the bowl.

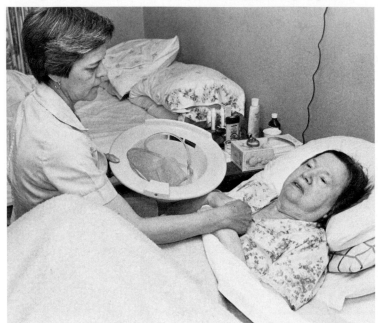

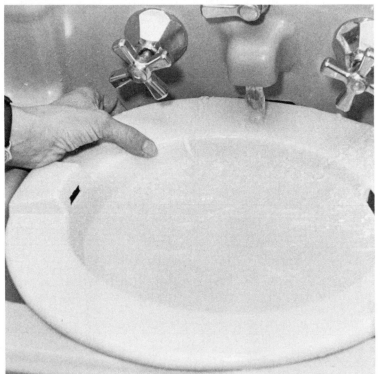

4 Fill the pan two-thirds full with water that's been warmed to between 100° F. and 110° F. (37.8° C. and 43.3° C.).

5 Next, tightly clamp the tubing above the pan, using the flow-control clip. Fill the plastic bag with water warmed to between 115° F. and 120° F. (46.1° C. and 48.9° C.). Place this filled bag on a small hook or nail, no more than 18″ (45.7 cm) above your patient's shoulders.

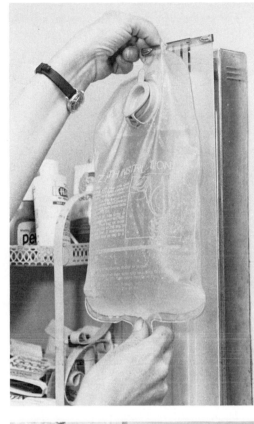

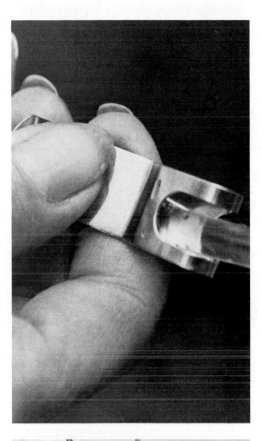

7 To keep the water temperature warm, intermittently release the flow-control clip and allow a small amount of water to flow into the pan. Any excess will empty into the toilet bowl through the rear slots.

6 Have your patient sit on the pan, assisting her if she needs help. Instruct her to sit on the pan for the prescribed length of time (which is usually 15 to 30 minutes), or until the water begins to cool.
Remember: If you must leave your patient during that time, provide her with a means to summon help.

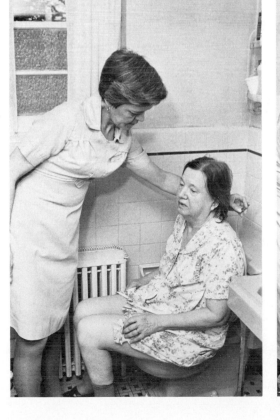

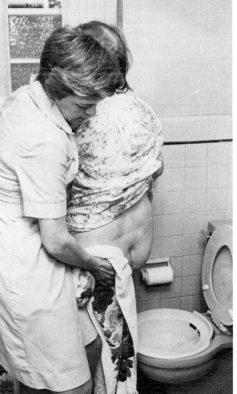

8 After your patient's completed her sitz bath, assist her off the pan, if necessary, and dry her perineal area. Then, tell her to apply any prescribed ointment or dressing to her perineal area. Assist her, if necessary. Finally, prepare the pan for its next use by emptying, cleaning, rinsing, and drying it. Store the pan in a plastic bag or box. Document your observations, the procedure, and any patient teaching, in your nurses' notes.

Urinary tract care

Although urinary incontinence is not a typical aging change, it is one of the more common—and upsetting—conditions that can accompany aging. By one estimate, up to 40% of all people older than age 62 suffer urinary incontinence.

In this section, you'll learn more about urinary incontinence—what may cause it, how to assess it, and how to help your patient cope with it. You'll also learn about external incontinence aids.

Of course, indwelling (Foley) catheterization should be avoided, if possible. But if your patient does go home with a Foley catheter in place, you must teach him how to prevent and cope with any problems.

For all the information you need to manage urinary incontinence, read the text, charts, and home care aids on the next few pages.

Understanding urinary incontinence

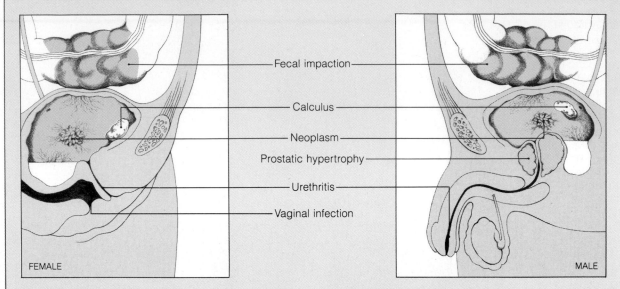

Fecal impaction
Calculus
Neoplasm
Prostatic hypertrophy
Urethritis
Vaginal infection

FEMALE

MALE

For you, dealing with an elderly patient's urinary incontinence may be little more than an inconvenience. But consider the problem from *his* point of view. For him, incontinence signals a profound loss of control that threatens his independence. Shame, loss of self-esteem, social withdrawal—all can contribute to his increasing dependence and isolation. More than ever, he needs your sensitivity, understanding, and reassurance.

Fortunately, incontinence is neither inevitable nor irreversible. Nor is every patient's incontinence problem the same. In order to assess your patient's individual problem, you need the following background information.

What causes incontinence?
As you know, the urge to urinate occurs when the bladder collects enough urine to stretch its smooth muscle walls, sending a message up the spinal cord to the brain stem. Younger adults normally feel an urge to urinate when the bladder's half full.

As an adult ages, his bladder's capacity decreases. In addition, he may not feel the urge to urinate until the bladder's filled almost to capacity.

To complicate matters, an urge to urinate occurs with very little warning and quickly becomes irresistible. If the patient's handicapped by illness or confusion, or if he has difficulty walking or undressing, he may not have time to use a toilet or bedpan before incontinence occurs.

Many underlying causes can contribute to an elderly patient's tendency to be incontinent. They include:
• psychological or emotional factors, such as depression or anxiety from bereavement or a change in lifestyle.
• neurologic disorders or damage (as in neurogenic bladder dysfunction, or after a stroke) that interrupt neural pathways controlling urinary function.
• urinary tract diseases or disorders, such as cysti-

tis, urethritis, lithiasis, or cancer (see illustrations).
• urethral and bladder pressure or obstruction (see illustrations), from fecal impaction; prostatic hypertrophy (in men); and uterine prolapse or trigonitis accompanying atrophic vaginitis (in women). Women who've had many children are especially prone to pelvic musculature weakening or relaxation, which may cause cystocele.
• any condition that tends to raise intra-abdominal pressure, such as chronic obstructive pulmonary disease, obesity, or ascites.
• drug therapy, especially with sedatives, tranquilizers, and hypnotics (which may make the patient drowsy or confused); anticholinergics (which block parasympathetic nerve impulses); and diuretics (which increase urinary output).

Classifying incontinence
Regardless of the underlying cause, incontinence may be divided into these three types:

Stress incontinence is involuntary urination caused by a sudden, transitory rise in intra-abdominal pressure. For example, the patient may experience dribbling when he laughs or coughs.

Urgency is a sudden, intense urge to urinate, followed by incontinence. Urinary tract infection is a common cause of urgency incontinence.

Overflow occurs when the bladder fills to capacity and then releases small amounts of urine to relieve the pressure. The patient may not feel any urge to urinate. Overflow incontinence may be associated with obstruction, drug therapy, or emotional factors. Neither stress nor the patient's usual ability to control the bladder plays a part.

To help your patient correct or cope with incontinence, you must determine both the type of incontinence he's experiencing, and the underlying cause (or causes). Then, you can devise a nursing plan tailored to your patient's specific problem. The following information provides guidelines.

Dealing with incontinence

Never assume that incontinence is a permanent condition that can't be corrected. You may be able to help your patient regain control of urinary function. Here, we suggest some ways to do so. *Remember:* Consider catheterization only as a last resort.

The first step is finding out as much as possible about your patient's incontinence. Ask yourself:
• Do any underlying diseases or conditions contribute to his incontinence? For example, does he have a urinary tract infection, an enlarged prostate, or a fecal impaction?
• Does he suffer from fecal incontinence?
• Is he taking any medication that contributes to the problem?
• When is his incontinence most likely to occur? Is it occasional or continual? Does it occur only at night? Do any particular settings or situations trigger it?
• Is the patient aware of incontinence when it occurs? Does he have the sensation of a full bladder before incontinence occurs? After urinating, does his bladder feel completely empty?
• How much liquid does he drink each day? Does he usually drink something in the evening, before bed?
• Does he have easy access to the toilet? Can he use the toilet without difficulty? If he uses a bedpan, can he do so easily?
• Does he have adequate privacy?
• What's your patient's reaction to incontinence? Is he ashamed? Aggressive? Manipulative? Seemingly unaware of the incident?

Taking action
After gathering all the relevant information about your patient's incontinence, devise a nursing plan. First, try to alleviate any diseases, disorders, or therapies you suspect may contribute to his problem. For instance, if you believe it's related to drug therapy, ask the doctor to consider changing the drug or dosage.

Do you suspect that weakened pelvic musculature plays a part in your female patient's incontinence? Teach her the pelvic-floor exercises described on the next page.

Next, try to reestablish regular urination patterns through bladder retraining. To devise a training program that suits your patient's needs, first establish his typical urination pattern. Carefully record how much fluid the patient drinks, when he urinates, whether urination is continent or incontinent, and the type of toilet he uses. Maintain this record for several days, if possible. *Note:* To estimate urine volume excreted, based on stain size, use the guidelines in the box below.

After you learn when the patient's most likely to become incontinent (for example, after meals, during the night, or every 3 hours), you can help him establish a regular schedule for using the toilet. You may use a time-oriented schedule (for example, taking the patient to the toilet every 2 to 4 hours), or a schedule based on his daily living habits (for example, taking him to the toilet before

and after each meal, and before bedtime). If your patient lives alone, he may appreciate an alarm clock or timer set for the times he should use the toilet. *Important:* If possible, help the patient assume his customary position for urination (standing for a man, sitting for a woman). He may have difficulty urinating in any other position.

No matter what type of schedule you use, remember these important points:
• Make sure the toilet's easily accessible to the patient. Consider using an elevated toilet seat. If he has difficulty balancing, make sure the bathroom has adequate hand rails. Supply ambulatory aids, if necessary, or place a commode at his bedside.
• If he's confined to bed, always keep the bedpan or urinal and call bell within easy reach. Answer his call bell promptly.
• Provide night lights for his bedroom and bathroom, especially if he's prone to nocturia. Remember, awakening in a darkened or strange room can be disorienting for your geriatric patient.
• If he's taking sedatives or tranquilizers, consider awakening him every 2 hours and helping him to the bathroom.
• If he's taking diuretics, make sure they're ordered to be given before 10 a.m., to lessen the risk of incontinence at night.

Suppose your patient's incontinence has psychological origins, such as depression or confusion. Attempt bladder retraining anyway, keeping in mind that you'll have to provide extra attention and supervision. Your patient may improve as he begins to regain control over this part of his life.

Regulating fluid consumption
Although restricting the patient's fluid intake may seem like a logical means to deal with incontinence, this step should never be taken. To maintain adequate hydration, your patient needs between 1,000 and 3,000 ml of fluid a day. Less than 1,000 ml/day may lead to constipation, which can contribute to urinary incontinence. Fluid restriction may result in more concentrated urine, which predisposes the patient to urinary tract infection (see the next page).

You may consider limiting your patient's fluid intake before bedtime, especially if he's prone to nocturia. But never permit him to become dehydrated.

Using urine collection devices
External urine collection devices, such as condom catheters and diapers, can help your patient avoid being embarrassed by incontinence, and restore some of his independence. But keep in mind that these devices have some important disadvantages. For example, they may foster infection or promote skin breakdown. In addition, some patients consider them humiliating. Use them in preference to indwelling catheterization, but consider them a last resort or a temporary measure during bladder retraining, so the patient can be more active. *Never* use them as a substitute for nursing measures. For more on these devices, turn to page 107.

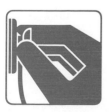

Estimating incontinence volume
Bladder retraining includes keeping accurate records of the amount of urine your patient excretes when he's incontinent. How can you do so? By evaluating the size of the urine stain on his sheet. Use these guidelines:

Stain diameter 9″ (23 cm) **Urine excreted** 50 to 75 ml	**Stain diameter** 12″ (30 cm) **Urine excreted** 100 to 125 ml	**Stain diameter** 18″ (46 cm) **Urine excreted** 150 to 175 ml	**Stain diameter** 24″ (61 cm) **Urine excreted** 200 to 300 ml

Urinary tract care

Teaching pelvic-floor exercises

Barbara Speer, age 68, is troubled by incontinence. Your assessment fails to identify any obvious pathologic or drug-related causes. But you do learn that she's given birth to six children. Chances are, she'll benefit from the pelvic-floor exercises described below.

Begin by telling her why these exercises may help. Explain that she can do them in any position, at any time. They don't require any special preparation on her part.

Then, give her these specific instructions:

• Tighten your anal sphincter, as if to stop a bowel movement or the passage of gas. Keep the sphincter tight for a count of five, and then relax it.

• Now, tighten your urinary and vaginal muscles, as if to stop the flow of urine. Keep the muscles tight for a count of five; then, relax them.

• Repeat each exercise several times. Then, do them again at least four times an hour. Gradually lengthen the time you tighten each group of muscles. As the muscles become stronger, you should have less difficulty with incontinence.

Identifying urinary tract infection

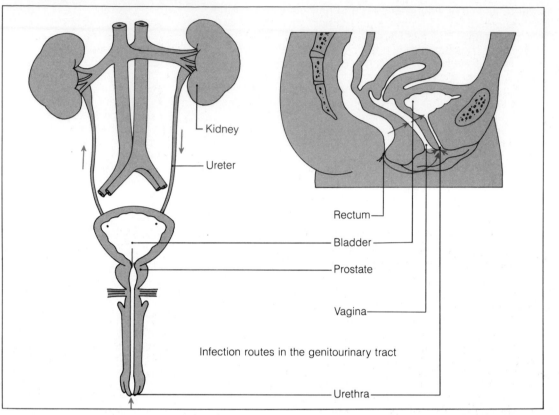

Infection routes in the genitourinary tract

Kidney

Ureter

Rectum

Bladder

Prostate

Vagina

Urethra

If your older patient fails to completely empty his bladder—a common effect of incontinence—he's predisposed to lower urinary tract infection (cystitis or urethritis).

Both men and women may develop such an infection, although women are at greater risk. (See the illustration above for common routes of bacteria entry and infection spread.)

Watch carefully for the following signs and symptoms (which may occur suddenly):
• urgent and frequent desire to urinate, even immediately after urinating
• pain or burning before or during urination
• thick, cloudy, foul-smelling urine
• bloody traces in urine
• possible discharge
• bladder cramps or spasms
• nocturia.

If you suspect an infection, notify the doctor and obtain a urine specimen for culture and sensitivity testing, as ordered. The doctor will prescribe an appropriate urinary tract antiseptic. Reassure the patient that the medication should provide quick relief. If your patient has a history of recurrent urinary tract infections or if he risks recurrence for another reason (for example, because of chronic prostatitis), the doctor may order long-term antibiotic therapy.

Preventing infection
Because bacteria thrive in an alkaline environment, take steps to keep your patient's urine acidic. To do this, make sure he drinks large amounts of cranberry juice each day. Unlike other acidic juices, cranberry juice doesn't lose its acidity in the kidneys. Also, the doctor may order at least 2,000 mg vitamin C administered daily, to help maintain urine acidity.

Remember these additional guidelines:
• Advise the patient to drink plenty of fluids each day (unless contraindicated).
• If possible, avoid using incontinence appliances, such as rubber pants and diapers, since they provide a fertile field for bacterial growth. For the same reason, use an indwelling (Foley) catheter only as a last resort. If a Foley catheter must be used, see the NURSING PHOTOBOOK IMPLEMENTING UROLOGIC PROCEDURES for detailed instructions.
• Encourage your patient to empty his bladder completely during urination, if he can do so. Proper positioning may help.
• Always cleanse a female patient's perineal area from front to back, and teach her to do the same.
• If your female patient's sexually active, advise her to urinate immediately after intercourse. Urination flushes out bacteria that may have been deposited at the urethral opening during intercourse. (Because a man's urethra is longer than a woman's, bacterial migration to the bladder is less likely to occur. As a result, this precaution isn't necessary for a man.)

Nurses' guide to external urine collection devices for males

If your male patient's incontinent, and bladder retraining hasn't yet been successful, you may use one of the devices shown here to manage the problem temporarily.

These collection devices require meticulous nursing care and careful patient teaching. Possible problems include skin irritation, infection, and penile circulatory impairment, as well as disconnection of the collection system. Take care to empty or change the device as often as necessary, following these guidelines:
• Wash and dry your hands before handling the device.
• Each time you change or empty the device, ask the patient to try to urinate.

• After removing the device, carefully wash the penis with mild soap and water, and gently dry it. If possible, expose the penis to the air for a while before reapplying a device.
• When you empty or change a reusable sheath, wash it in mild soap and water. Then, rinse the sheath with 15% white vinegar and water solution to deodorize it. Keep it supple by dusting it with cornstarch.
• Care for a leg bag in the same way. (You needn't dust it with cornstarch.)
• Continually observe the patient for signs and symptoms of impaired penile circulation, skin breakdown, and urinary tract infection.

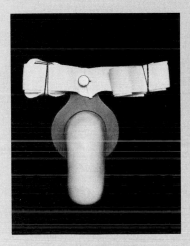

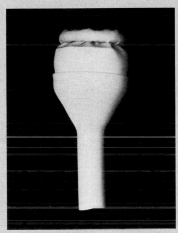

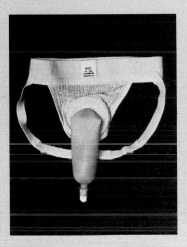

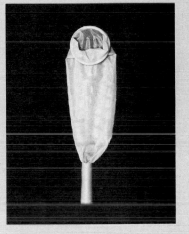

Dribbler sheath (Rusch)

Description
This rubber sheath straps around patient's hips. It has no drainage outlet.

Nursing considerations
• Use for mild incontinence (when patient urinates only a few milliliters at a time).
• Take special care to prevent skin irritation, because the penis soaks in urine until the sheath's emptied.
• Empty sheath every 2 to 3 hours, and perform recommended penile and sheath care.

Single-layer urinary sheath (Chesebrough-Pond Uri-Drain® sheath)

Description
This close-fitting, latex sheath fastens closely around the base of the penis. The sheath adheres to one side of double-sided adhesive tape that's wrapped around the penis. Drain tube at bottom of sheath connects to a leg bag.

Nursing considerations
• Use for moderate to severe incontinence.
• Perform penile care daily.
• Empty leg bag three or four times daily.

Double-layer urinary sheath (McGuire male urinal)

Description
This rubber sheath's held in place by attached athletic supporter. The sheath features an inner, tight-fitting layer that helps prevent urine leakage when patient's sitting or lying and a loose-fitting outer layer for collecting and transferring urine. This design also protects the penis from immersion in urine. The sheath's drainage outlet (with stopper) may be connected to leg bag.

Nursing considerations
• Use without leg bag for mild incontinence; use with leg bag for moderate to severe incontinence.
• Trim inner sheath with scissors to fit individual patient.
• Perform penile and sheath care daily.
• Empty the sheath every 2 to 3 hours, if used without leg bag. If used with a leg bag, empty the bag three or four times each day.
• Hand wash athletic supporter, as necessary.

Condom catheter (Bard® Disposable Uro® sheath)

Description
This soft, condomlike sheath fits closely around the penis. The sheath adheres to one side of double-sided adhesive tape wrapped around penis. The drain tube at bottom of the sheath connects to the leg bag.

Nursing considerations
• Use for moderate to severe incontinence.
• Change catheter daily, using a new one each time; do not reuse catheters.
• Perform penile care daily.
• Empty leg bag three or four times daily.
• Buy commercially made catheters, or make them yourself using condoms and rubber tubing. (For details, see pages 70 and 71 of the NURSING PHOTOBOOK IMPLEMENTING UROLOGIC PROCEDURES.)

Urinary tract care

Learning about incontinent pants

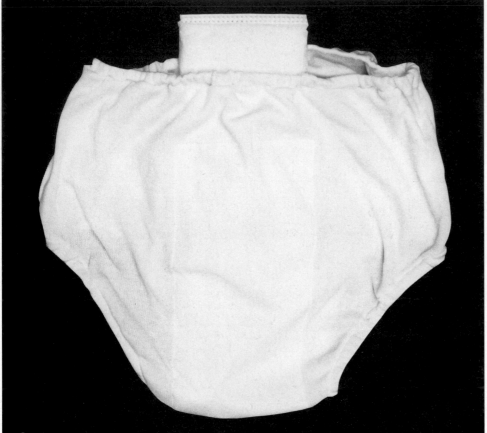

On the preceding pages, you learned about external urine collection devices for men. But what if your patient's a woman? How can you protect her from the embarrassment and discomfort of incontinence, without resorting to catheterization?

If she experiences only intermittent, dribbling incontinence, a sanitary pad designed for menstrual flow may be adequate. To protect her against heavier urine flow, however, consider using a commercially made incontinent pant; for example, the Dignity® pant made by Humanicare International, Inc., shown above.

The pant is made of machine-washable polyester knit, for the patient's comfort and convenience. It's available in six sizes. A disposable liner pad (available in regular or heavy-duty sizes) fits inside the pant's crotch pocket. For a nonambulatory patient, Dignity pants are also available with side openings joined by Velcro® strips.

Of course, the Dignity pant is only one example of the many incontinent pants and diapers on the market.

According to the patient's needs and preference, you may choose, for example, a plasticized incontinent pant with either a disposable or reusable liner pad, or a completely disposable adult diaper.

Note: Like the Dignity pant, all these aids can be used for a male patient, as well as a female.

No matter what type you select, remember these important points:
• Frequently check liner pads and diapers, and change them as necessary. Remember, prolonged skin contact with urine increases the risk of infection and contributes to skin irritation and breakdown.
• Routinely perform perineal and skin care each time you change a pad or diaper. Protect the patient's skin with a skin barrier, such as BARD™ Moisture Barrier Ointment.
• Continually observe for signs of skin breakdown or urinary tract infection. (For details on urinary tract infection, see page 106.)
• Wash reusable pants and liners daily, or as needed.

PATIENT TEACHING

Preparing an incontinent patient for home care

Is your patient going home with an external urine collection device, such as a condom catheter? Carefully inform him of all instructions and precautions for care before his discharge. Then, give him a copy of the home care aid on pages 110 and 111 to help him remember each important step.

But, suppose your patient is going home with an indwelling (Foley) catheter in place. He and his family must care for it themselves, without your help. Be sure to prepare them for this responsibility before discharge. If necessary, contact the local visiting nurse association for help.

First, make sure the patient and his family know what a Foley catheter is, what it's for, and what size he needs. Thoroughly discuss infection precautions and the importance of maintaining aseptic technique when emptying the drainage bag. Also, discuss his fluid requirements and any medication he'll be taking.

Take special care to inform him about possible complications, such as urinary tract infection or catheter blockage. If the patient and his family are willing and able to learn, teach them how to safely remove the catheter in case it becomes blocked. Then, give them a copy of the home care aid on page 109.

Finally, make sure the patient knows when to return to the doctor to have the catheter changed or removed. (A visiting nurse may perform this care instead, with a doctor's order.) In the case of long-term catheter use, the catheter should be replaced only when necessary; for example, when it's blocked or otherwise nonfunctional.

Note: For more information on preparing your patient for home catheter care, see the NURSING PHOTOBOOK IMPLEMENTING UROLOGIC PROCEDURES.

Home care

What to do about catheter problems

Dear Family Member:
Since someone in your family has a Foley catheter in place, you need to know how to tell if it becomes blocked—and what to do about it. Chances are, the catheter is blocked if you notice any of the following:

• the urine level in the drainage bag has stopped rising
• the bed is wet with urine
• the patient's restless or uncomfortable, with pain in his lower abdomen, or he has a strong desire to urinate (but can't).

What should you do? First, look for any obvious reason for a blockage. Is the tubing kinked? Is the patient lying on the catheter or tubing? Is the drainage bag above his bladder level, instead of below it? Correct these problems, if they're present. Also, it may help if the patient changes his position and separates his thighs.

If doing these things doesn't help, try irrigating the catheter. But irrigate *only* if the nurse or doctor has taught you how and you feel confident about it.

Is the catheter still blocked, despite your efforts? Contact your visiting nurse or doctor. But if help isn't immediately available, remove the catheter yourself, as the nurse has taught you. The following illustrations will remind you what steps to take.

As you know, you must first deflate the balloon that's on the end of the catheter inside the patient's bladder. If you don't, you won't be able to remove the catheter—and you'll hurt the patient if you try.

To deflate the balloon, attach a

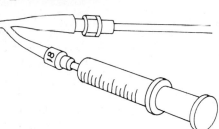

syringe (without a needle) to the unattached end of the tubing's Y-shaped portion (called the inflation port), as shown here. (If the inflation port doesn't have a special tip that the syringe fits into, put a needle on the syringe, and puncture the inflation port.)

Gently pull back on the syringe plunger. The water in the balloon will flow into the syringe, deflating the balloon.

If you have trouble with this method, here's another way to deflate the balloon. (But don't use this way unless the first method doesn't work, because it destroys the catheter.) Place a small basin under the inflation port, to protect the bed. Then, using scissors, cut the catheter in two just above the inflation port, as shown. Now, the water in the

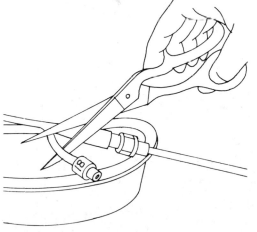

balloon will escape into the basin.

When the balloon's deflated, pull gently on the catheter to remove it. *Important:* If the catheter doesn't come out easily, don't force it. Wait for a nurse or doctor to help you.

Keep the patient dry and comfortable until help arrives. If you can't contact your nurse or doctor, take the patient to a hospital emergency department.

Preventing problems

To prevent catheter blockage and other possible problems, you and the patient must follow these important directions:

• Never pull on the catheter. Disconnect it from the drainage tubing only to clean the bag.
• Always keep the drainage bag below the patient's bladder level.
• Empty the drainage bag every 8 hours.
• Twice a day, use soap and water to wash the patient's skin around the catheter. After washing his skin, dry it gently but thoroughly.
• If the patient's a woman, use a front-to-back motion for washing and drying. This way, you won't contaminate the catheter and her urinary tract with germs from her rectal area.
• Once a day, wash the drainage tubing and bag with soap and water. Rinse it with a solution made from water and white vinegar. (Use one part vinegar to seven parts water.)
• Unless the doctor gives you different directions, the patient should drink at least 1½ quarts (1.4 l) of liquids each day. This simple precaution will help prevent bladder infection.

Urinary tract care

Home care

Caring for your condom catheter

Dear Patient:
When you go home from the hospital, you'll need to care for your condom catheter. Use these illustrations when applying it. In addition, remember these very important points:

• Use a clean condom catheter every day.

• Wash and dry your hands before and after handling your condom catheter, tubing, or leg bag.

• Gently but thoroughly wash, rinse, and dry your penis before putting on the condom catheter. Then, do this again after removing it.

• To keep your urine flowing properly, keep your penis positioned downward.

• Check your penis every 2 hours for swelling or unusual color. If your penis feels uncomfortable or doesn't look normal, take off the condom catheter and call your doctor.

• Also call your doctor if you feel pain or burning when you urinate, feel the urge to urinate very frequently, smell an unpleasant odor from your urine, or see blood or pus in your urine.

• Don't go to bed with your condom catheter in place—you may injure yourself without knowing it. Ask your nurse or doctor to suggest another way to keep urine from wetting your clothing or bed sheets.

• Empty your leg bag every 3 to 4 hours. Never allow it to fill to the top.

• Twice a day, wash your leg bag with soap and water, and rinse it with a solution made from water and vinegar. (Use one part vinegar to seven parts water.) Don't use the same leg bag for longer than 1 month.

1 Do you know what your catheter and leg bag will look like? If not, study this illustration. Then, apply the catheter and leg bag according to the instructions in the following steps.

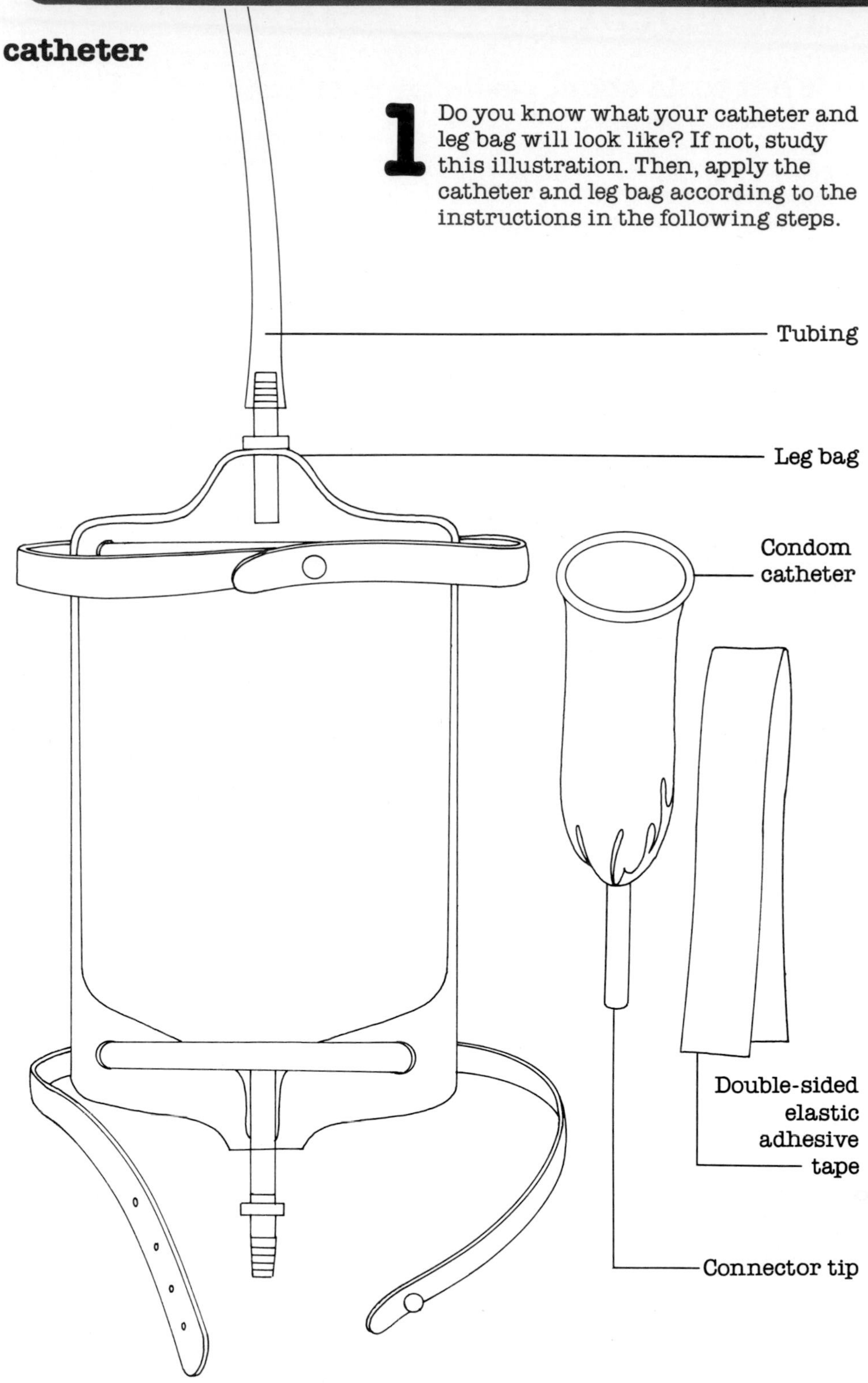

Tubing

Leg bag

Condom catheter

Double-sided elastic adhesive tape

Connector tip

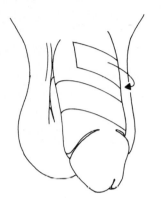

2 After washing, rinsing, and drying your penis, remove the covering from both sides of the double-sided elastic adhesive tape. Starting at the base of the penis, wind the tape in a spiral fashion (see arrow). Don't let the edges of the tape overlap at any point. *Important:* Don't stretch the tape while applying it, or you'll apply it too tightly. Also, never apply tape in a circle around your penis, or you may cut off your blood circulation.

3 Now, you're ready to apply the condom. Make sure the balloon-like part is tightly rolled up to the edge of the connector tip, as shown here.

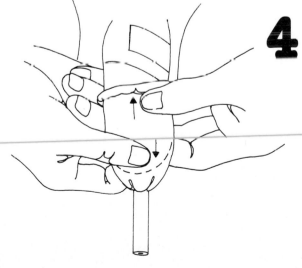

4 Place the sheath on the end of your penis. Leave about ½" (1.3 cm) of space between the tip of your penis and the connector tip.

Unroll the condom along your penis, as shown here. Gently stretch the penis as you do so. Then, when the condom's fully unrolled, gently press it against the penis, so the condom sticks to the adhesive tape.

5 Connect one end of the tubing to the connector tip, and the other end to the leg bag. Finally, strap the leg bag to your thigh.

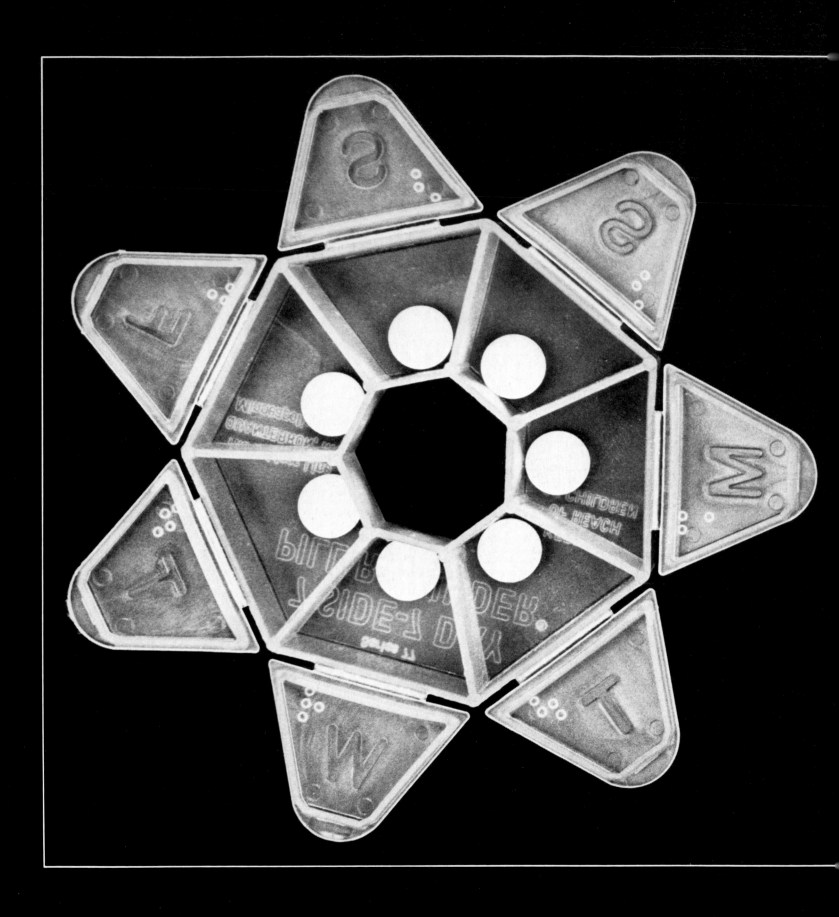

Performing Special Procedures

Eye care

Hearing aids

Medication guidance

Eye care

For your geriatric patient, vision loss can be an important—and devastating—aging change. You can help him by providing the very best patient teaching and nursing care.

In this section, you'll learn about cataracts, their surgical removal, and postsurgical vision correction. You'll also learn how to apply eye ointment, a necessary step in preop patient care. And suppose your patient's lost an eye—or is facing eye loss—for any reason. Can you teach him about the eye implant and prosthesis he'll probably need? Can you provide proper care? In these pages, you'll find the information you need.

Learning about cataracts

As you know, a cataract is an opacity of the eye's normally transparent lens. If you're caring for a geriatric patient with cataracts, he probably has *senile cataracts,* a common result of the aging process. Cataracts may also be caused by a systemic or eye disease (such as diabetes or advanced glaucoma), trauma, or toxicosis. And, of course, some cataracts are congenital.

The extent to which a cataract causes vision impairment depends on the density of opacification. Although opacification is progressive, how *quickly* it develops varies from patient to patient.

Reviewing lens anatomy

A normal lens is biconvex, refractive, avascular, and flexible. It's suspended behind the pupil by zonular fibers attached to the ciliary muscle. Along with the cornea, the lens provides the eye's focusing power; its changeable shape permits the eye to adjust for near and far distances (accommodation).

No one knows exactly what causes senile cataracts, but they probably result from chemical changes that increase the mass and density of lens fibers. Throughout life, the lens' cortical fibers multiply and harden. At first, these fibers are easily contained in the lens' elastic capsule. But as their mass and density increase, the lens loses its elasticity and becomes opaque. If light can no longer reach the retina's macular region, the patient becomes blind in the affected eye.

Understanding cataract surgery

Senile cataracts nearly always develop in both eyes to some degree, but the rate of development is usually unequal. When a cataract significantly impairs the patient's vision, the doctor will probably recommend surgical removal. Although he may remove cataracts from both eyes during the same surgery, he's more likely to first remove only one cataract—the one causing greater vision impairment—and remove the other (if necessary) after a recovery period. He may perform surgery with either local or general anesthetic, depending on his preference and the patient's condition. *Note:* The doctor may not recommend surgical cataract removal if the patient has another condition that makes restoration of good vision unlikely; for example, advanced glaucoma or retinal detachment.

Expect your patient to have questions about his surgery. Prepare yourself to answer them by reviewing these surgical procedures:

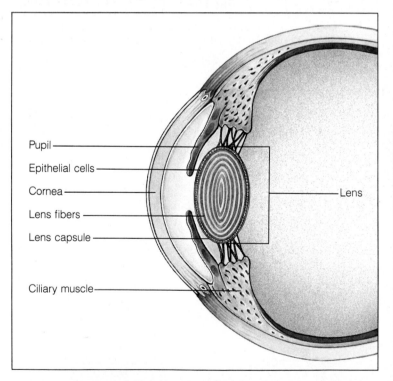

As you see in the illustration above, the lens has three parts:
• a tough but transparent capsule
• a single row of epithelial cells, which produce the capsule and the lens fibers (cortex)
• the lens substance, a clear jelly composed of water, protein, and some minerals. This jelly contains the lens fibers and a nucleus. The nucleus is made of older lens fibers that become compressed in the center as the epithelial cells produce new lens fibers at the lens periphery.

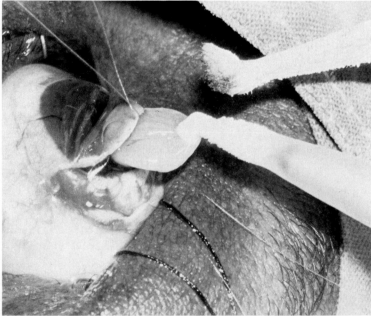

• *Intracapsular extraction.* The more commonly chosen technique for removing senile cataracts, intracapsular extraction results in the complete removal of the intact lens, including its capsule. The doctor may remove the lens with specially designed forceps or with a cryoprobe cooled to −40° F. (−40° C.).

Removal with a cryoprobe is called *cryoextraction*. When the doctor inserts the cryoprobe through a small incision in the eye, the lens sticks to it—in the same way your tongue sticks to a cold ice cube. Then, the doctor can easily pull out the cataractous lens and its capsule (as shown on the opposite page). This technique works so well that it's no longer necessary to wait until the cataract's ripe (fully hardened and opaque) to remove it.

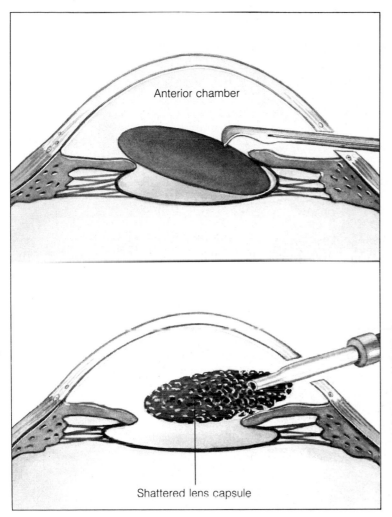

Anterior chamber

Shattered lens capsule

• *Extracapsular extraction*. This procedure removes the lens but leaves the posterior lens capsule in place. It's especially useful if the patient's under age 40 or if he has a traumatic cataract. This technique's also necessary before implantation of some types of intraocular lenses.

To perform extracapsular extraction, the doctor may use a method called *phacoemulsification*. First, he makes a small incision and maneuvers the cataractous lens into the eye's anterior chamber (see upper illustration above). Then, he inserts a probe the size of a pencil tip into the anterior chamber. Ultrasonic waves produced by the probe shatter the lens capsule (see lower illustration above). Lens material is removed through the same incision by irrigation and aspiration. When performed successfully, this method causes less trauma than other methods of cataract removal; the patient may not even need to wear an eye patch during recovery.

Restoring vision

With the lens removed, the eye loses some of its ability to focus and all of its ability to accommodate near and far distances. The solution? An artificial lens, in the form of cataract spectacles, a contact lens, or an intraocular (implanted) lens. Let's consider them one at a time.

• *Cataract spectacles*. The most conservative method of restoring normal vision, cataract spectacles have some disadvantages. They magnify images 20% to 30%; as a result, if the patient has had unilateral cataract surgery, the size of images seen by each eye is considerably different. This situation deprives the patient of normal binocular vision. The patient may have difficulty judging distances, resulting in poor hand-eye coordination.

Cataract spectacles also impair peripheral vision by causing circular blind spots around the edges. As a result, images seen through the edges appear to jump. (Advise the patient to look through the centers of the spectacle lenses and to turn his head to see objects off to the side.)

Although more expensive than glass lenses, plastic cataract spectacle lenses reduce some of these problems. They're significantly lighter than glass spectacle lenses and usually require less adjustment time.

• *Contact lenses*. A wide variety of hard and soft contact lenses exist. They permit normal peripheral vision, and their very slight image-size distortion isn't noticeable. Their disadvantage? An older patient may have difficulty inserting and removing these tiny lenses. Extended-wear lenses, specially made soft lenses that can be left in place for up to 2 months, may provide the solution to this problem for some patients. For more on contact lenses, read the information beginning on page 118.

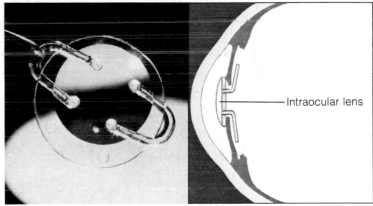

Intraocular lens

• *Intraocular lenses*. For geriatric cataract patients, intraocular lenses provide a promising alternative. An intraocular lens (see photo above left) is made of the same material as hard contact lenses. It's implanted at the time of cataract removal (see illustration above right). It doesn't magnify image size, requires no manual dexterity (because the patient never removes it), and causes no discomfort or inconvenience. It also permits binocular vision, full vision field, and improved depth perception. Of course, the artificial lens can't accommodate distance the way a real lens can. So, the doctor usually prescribes for the patient both an intraocular lens that allows good distance vision and either bifocal or reading spectacles for near vision.

Note: Because intraocular lenses may be dislodged within the eye during strenuous activity, they're considered more desirable for older, less active patients than for younger patients.

Eye care

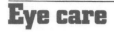

Cataract surgery: Providing total patient care

"I don't mind the surgery so much," says Mrs. Cucci, age 71. "But my sister tells me I'll probably have to stay in bed for 2 weeks afterward. I'm not looking forward to that!"

Mrs. Cucci, who has bilateral senile cataracts, is scheduled for cataract surgery on her left eye the day after tomorrow. Like many patients you care for, she clearly has some misconceptions about cataract surgery. Take recovery time, for example. Not many years ago, patients were confined to strict bed rest for 48 hours and stayed in the hospital 7 to 10 days after cataract surgery. Today, most patients are ambulatory (with help, of course) the day of surgery.

As a nurse, you can give Mrs. Cucci a more accurate picture of her hospital experience. In fact, patient teaching must be one of your top priorities. But of course, you have other nursing responsibilities, too. Use the information on this page for complete guidelines.

Patient teaching

How much does your patient understand about her condition and surgery? Never assume she's completely informed, even if the doctor's given her a thorough explanation. Remember, many patients are too worried to absorb many facts. Carefully assess her level of understanding, as well as her emotional condition, physical limitations, and goals and expectations. Use your assessment to determine her learning needs.

For example, stay alert for any worries and misconceptions she may have. Many patients have a basic misunderstanding about what cataracts really are—they may believe that a cataract is a film over the eye, or that it can be dissolved with drops.

Your patient may think that the doctor will remove her entire eye from its socket during surgery. Or, she may be concerned that her right eye will become strained and deteriorate while her left eye is recovering from surgery.

Address yourself to the patient's foremost concerns. If she's to undergo surgery with local anesthetic, prepare her for what she'll see and hear in the operating room and during the procedure. Also, explain that she'll probably be able to resume some activity, such as walking to the bathroom with your help, the day of surgery. But caution her to avoid any activity that causes bending or straining—even a simple motion like bending down to retrieve slippers may strain the suture line, causing complications. Urge her to call for help as often as necessary. Also, tell her that you'll give her a mild laxative, if necessary, to prevent straining during elimination.

Mrs. Cucci's probably worried about pain. Explain that she may feel some discomfort, such as a dull ache. Encourage her to let you know if she's uncomfortable, so you can give her pain medication and provide other comfort measures.

Important: Don't wait for your patient to ask for pain medication. Try to anticipate her needs, and offer medication before the pain becomes severe.

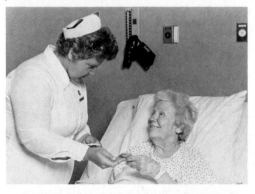

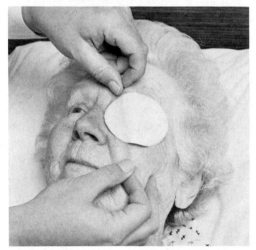

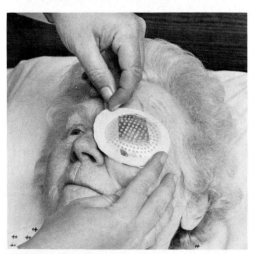

In addition, don't neglect to cover these points:
• Tell her about the postoperative protective measures the doctor plans (see upper left photo). For the first 24 to 48 hours, she'll probably wear an eye patch (see middle left photo). Depending on the type of surgery and the doctor's preference, she may continue to wear the eye patch for up to a week. Or, she may simply wear cycloplegic-style dark glasses during the day and an eye shield at night to protect her eye from injury (see lower left photo).
• Prepare her for the temporary vision reduction or loss she'll experience while her left eye's patched. Familiarize her with her surroundings, to reduce the risk of postoperative disorientation. Explain that for at least 24 hours, her side rails will be raised for her own safety. Place the call bell within her reach, and ask her not to leave her bed without calling for help. At least every 4 hours, check to see if she needs help walking to the bathroom.
• Explain that her vision will be blurry after the patch is removed, but that cataract glasses or a contact lens will eventually correct this. *Note:* If your patient received an intraocular lens during surgery, she'll probably be able to see clearly at once.

Preoperative care

In most respects, preop nursing care for cataract surgery is the same as for any surgery. For complete details, consult the NURSING PHOTOBOOK CARING FOR SURGICAL PATIENTS. In addition, observe these special requirements:
• As part of your preoperative assessment, test and record her visual acuity in each eye, as shown below. Also, document ophthalmoscopic observations.

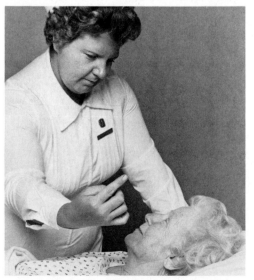

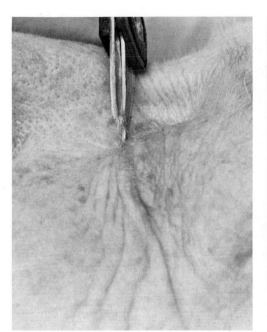

• The day before surgery, trim her left eye's lashes to a length of about 3 mm, if this is a nursing responsibility in your hospital (see photo above). Ask her to hold her eyes closed while you work. Remember to explain why this is necessary, and reassure her that the lashes will quickly grow back.

▣ *Nursing tip:* Prevent clippings from dropping into her eye by applying a dab of vaseline to the scissors.
• Take conjunctival cultures, if ordered, as shown below.

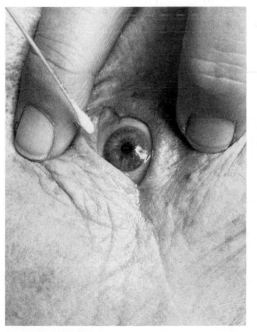

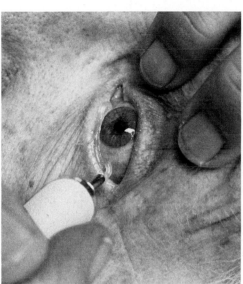

• Apply topical antibiotic drops and ointment to the eye scheduled for surgery (or both eyes), as ordered. Mrs. Cucci's doctor, for example, has ordered chloramphenicol (Chloroptic Ophthalmic*) drops to be instilled four times a day in her left eye, and chloramphenicol ointment applied to the left eye's lower conjunctival sac the evening before surgery (see photo above). See pages 118 and 119 to see exactly how to apply ophthalmic ointment.

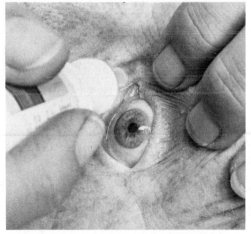

• If ordered, apply mydriatic and cycloplegic drops shortly before surgery (see photo above). If the doctor's using the phacoemulsification technique, for example, the patient's pupil must be completely dilated during surgery.
• Administer preanesthetic medications, as ordered.
• Ask the patient to thoroughly wash her face with a cleansing solution, such as pHisoDerm® the evening and morning before surgery. Caution her to keep the
*Available in both the United States and in Canada

solution out of her eyes, since it will irritate them.

Postoperative care
After your patient returns from surgery, follow these guidelines:
• Position her bed at a 30° angle, as ordered. Lying flat may strain the suture line.
• Closely monitor her vital signs, and watch for sudden, sharp, or excessive pain, excessive bloody or purulent drainage, temperature elevation, and other signs and symptoms of postop complications. Immediately notify the doctor if any occur.
• Try to prevent any activity that may increase intraocular tension, such as bending at the waist, vomiting, sneezing, coughing, straining during bowel movements, and lifting more than 5 pounds (2¼ kg).
• Ask her not to squeeze, scratch, or manipulate her left eye's lids and not to lie on her left side.
• If your patient seems disoriented after surgery, consider having a family member stay with her to help prevent her from touching her left eye. Take steps to reorient the patient (see page 140). Obtain an order for arm restraints only as a last resort.
• Be prepared to help her with even the simplest activities and tasks. Remember, when one eye's patched, she loses depth perception. And if her other eye has a well-developed cataract, or is aphakic (without a lens) from prior cataract surgery, she may have very little vision. *Note:* If she wears glasses, put them on for her.
• Provide extra attention and support. Keep in mind that she may become frightened or disoriented by this temporary vision loss.
• Instill eye drops, as ordered. *Note:* If your patient received an intraocular lens implant, the doctor may order miotic eye drops after surgery, to constrict the pupil and reduce the risk of lens displacement.
• Teach her to instill the ordered eye drops, since she'll continue to need them after discharge. Also, show her how to tape an eye shield in place before she sleeps. If she lives with family or friends, teach them too, so they can help her. *Note:* Determine whether she'll need help from the local visiting nurses' association, and make the necessary arrangements.
• Teach her about activity restrictions after discharge, while healing continues. Also, if she's to receive cataract glasses or hard contact lenses, explain that she'll need several weeks to fully adjust to them. The adjustment period for soft lenses is shorter. (For more on both types of contact lenses, see the information beginning on the following pages.)

Eye care

Administering eye ointment

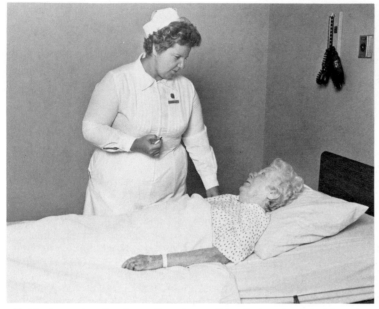

2 Position your patient so she's sitting with her head tilted slightly back, or lying on her back (whichever position's more comfortable for her).

3 Cleanse her eyelids and canthus areas with a moist cotton ball, as the nurse is doing here.

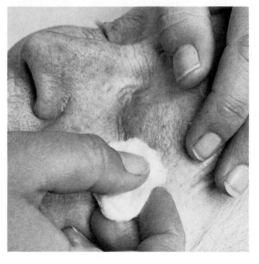

1 *You're caring for Anna Cucci, age 71, who's scheduled for cataract surgery on her left eye. To prepare her eye for surgery, the doctor's ordered chloramphenicol (Chloroptic Ophthalmic*) drops four times a day, and chloramphenicol ointment the evening before surgery. In the following photostory, we'll show you how to instill the ointment. For details on instilling eye drops, see the* NURSING PHOTOBOOK GIVING MEDICATIONS.

First, gather the equipment you'll need: the ordered medication, dry cotton balls or tissue, and cotton balls moistened with sterile normal saline solution, for cleansing Mrs. Cucci's eyelids and lashes. Then, thoroughly wash and dry your hands.

Explain the procedure to Mrs. Cucci and answer her questions. Inform her that the ointment will temporarily blur her vision. Ask her to hold as still as possible while you instill the ointment, to reduce the risk of injuring her eye or contaminating the tube's tip.

Learning about contact lenses

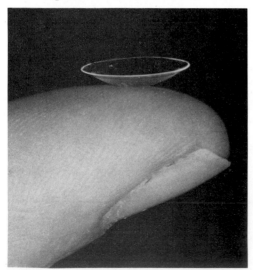

*Available in both the United States and in Canada

Your patient, 67-year-old Robert Collier, underwent cataract surgery on his right eye 6 months ago. Since then, he's been wearing cataract spectacles and is dissatisfied with the results. "Every time I turn my head, I feel like something's jumping at me," he complains. "Sometimes they make me feel dizzy. And I'm always tripping on the stairway. I hear that contact lenses don't cause these problems. What can you tell me about them?"

Today, more and more older patients opt for contact lenses after cataract surgery. Make sure you can knowledgeably discuss the pros and cons of lens wear by reviewing the photos and information here.

As you probably know, contact lenses come in two basic types: hard and soft. The photo at left shows a hard contact lens prescribed for an aphakic patient (a patient whose natural lens has been removed). Look closely at it. Like the cataract spectacle lens this patient wears, the contact lens has a thick center and thin periphery. In a spectacle lens, this design causes considerable vision distortion. But, because a contact lens fits *directly* on the cornea, its thick center causes no noticeable vision distortion. (A *soft* contact lens prescribed for an aphakic patient is designed the same way.)

Before prescribing a contact lens for Mr. Collier (or any patient), the doctor will rule out any contraindications; for example, insufficient lacrimation (tearing). Sometimes called dry eye, this condition affects many older people and makes wearing contact lenses uncomfortable.

Then, the doctor will consider the specific pros and cons for each type of lens avail-

4 Remove the cap from the ointment tube, and lay the cap down on its side on a clean surface. Ask your patient to look up and focus on a specific object. With one hand, place your index finger on her upper eyelid to help keep her eye open. Then, place your little finger on her cheekbone and gently pull down on her skin to expose the conjunctival sac, as shown here.

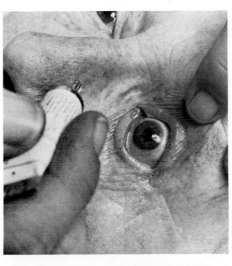

5 Starting at the inner canthus, as shown, squeeze a thin ribbon of ointment along the lower conjunctival sac. As you approach the outer canthus, rotate the tube to detach the ointment. Take care not to touch her eye, eyelid, or lashes with the tube's tip.

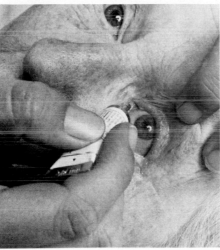

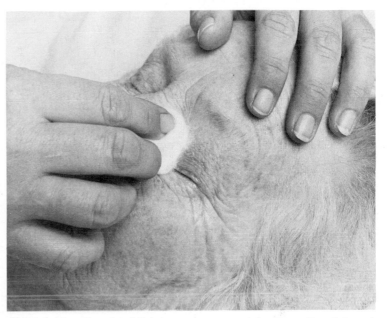

6 Ask Mrs. Cucci to blink her eyes several times, so the ointment can spread and be absorbed. But ask her not to *squeeze* her eyes shut, since this may force out the ointment. Using a clean dry cotton ball or tissue, gently press on her inner canthus, as shown, to prevent possible systemic absorption through the tear duct. Replace the tube's cap, and wash and dry your hands.

Nursing tip: Suppose you're applying ointment to Mrs. Cucci's right eye, too. Depending on her level of awareness, consider waiting a short time to treat the right eye. An older patient may become disoriented if her vision's blurred in both eyes at once.

Properly store the medication. Document the procedure in your patient's medication administration record, and note any observations in your nurses' notes. *Important:* Use this ointment for Mrs. Cucci only. If you contaminated the tube's tip during the procedure, dispose of the tube and use a new one for future applications.

---

able (see the chart on the next page) and decide which suits the patient best. He'll ask himself:
• Is the patient alert enough to provide daily lens care?
• Is he motivated enough to endure some initial discomfort while adjusting to hard lenses?
• Does he have the manual dexterity that's necessary to insert, remove, and clean his lenses?

For an older patient, lack of manual dexterity may be the biggest roadblock to successful adjustment. Conventional lenses (both hard and soft) require daily handling and care. He may have difficulty handling them if he has severe arthritis or if his hands tremble. For such a patient, extended-wear soft lenses may provide a welcome alternative.

Extended-wear lenses
Extended-wear lenses look the same as conventional daily-wear lenses. Unlike daily-wear lenses, however, the patient can wear them continuously for up to 2 months, because they allow more oxygen to reach the cornea. To allow high oxygen permeability, most types of extended wear lenses are very thin and have a very high water content (approximately 71% for one type).

Every 2 months (or as directed), the patient must remove his extended-wear lenses, clean them in a chemical solution or a special low-heat system, and reinsert them. If he can't handle the lenses himself, a family member or visiting nurse can do this procedure for him. To learn how, see the photostory beginning on page 120.
Nursing considerations
An older patient will probably tolerate con-

tact lenses well, in part because his corneas aren't as sensitive as a younger patient's—especially after cataract surgery. But this can cause problems, too. Because his corneas are less sensitive, he's less likely to notice a foreign object under one of his lenses, or to feel the first signs of a corneal abrasion. That's why continuing professional care's important. Urge the patient to have periodic checkups with his eye care specialist. If his eyes look red or irritated, or he complains of discomfort, blurred vision, or pain, ask him to immediately remove his lenses (or remove them for him), and notify the doctor.

Periodically reassess your patient's ability to wear lenses. Any changes in his alertness, orientation, or manual dexterity might mean that wearing glasses is the more practical alternative.

Eye care

Contact lenses: Hard or soft?

Do you know why the doctor's selected a particular type of lens for your geriatric patient? If not, study this chart. It will help you perform follow-up assessments of your patient's contact lens use. *Note:* Here we cover only a few general types. Special types of lenses (for example, gas-permeable hard lenses) may have different advantages and disadvantages. Whatever type of lens your patient wears, familiarize yourself with the manufacturer's and doctor's instructions.

Hard lenses
Hard plastic lenses shaped to fit the corneal contour. They float over the cornea on tears and are held in place by capillary tension between the tears and lenses.
Pros
• May be prescribed for glaucoma patients and for other patients requiring frequent application of eyedrops, because the lenses won't absorb medication
• Are less expensive and more durable than soft lenses
• May be tinted, for easier visibility if dropped
Cons
• Require daily handling and cleaning. Lens insertion, handling, and care may be difficult for a geriatric patient with impaired manual dexterity.
• May cause temporary blurred vision when the lenses are removed and replaced with glasses (spectacle blur)
• Must be removed for sleeping, including naps
• More likely to cause painful corneal abrasions than soft lenses, especially if the patient falls asleep with them in place

Daily-wear soft lenses
Larger, close-fitting flexible lenses made of a hydrophilic (water-absorbent) polymer (or a similar compound)
Pros
• Require little adjustment time; are usually immediately comfortable. Patient may attain maximum wearing time (about 14 hours, or as recommended by the doctor) within a few days. Because of this easy adjustment, patient may wear lenses infrequently, if he wishes. Also, he may be able to wear them for longer periods at a time than hard lenses.
• Less likely than hard lenses to damage patient's eyes if he naps with them in place; however, this is *not* recommended
• Don't cause blur when removed and replaced with glasses
Cons
• May be more difficult than hard lenses for patient to insert and remove, because they're flexible and close-fitting
• Require scrupulous daily care, including sterilization (by boiling, electrical heating, or treatment with special chemicals). Care instructions may be difficult for geriatric patient to follow.
• Must be removed for sleeping, including naps
• Most types aren't recommended for patients requiring frequent applications of eye medication, since the lenses absorb substances in the eye
• Are more expensive and less durable than hard lenses. Require replacement every 1 to 2 years.
• Can't be tinted

Extended-wear soft lenses
Most types are made of hydrophilic compounds similar to those used for daily-wear soft lenses
Pros
• May be worn continuously, including during sleep, for up to 2 months
• Don't require daily sterilization (but must be cleaned and sterilized periodically)
Cons
• Are the most expensive type of lenses
• Are very fragile and easily damaged
• Require replacement every 6 to 8 months, because of protein buildup

---

Inserting and removing a soft contact lens

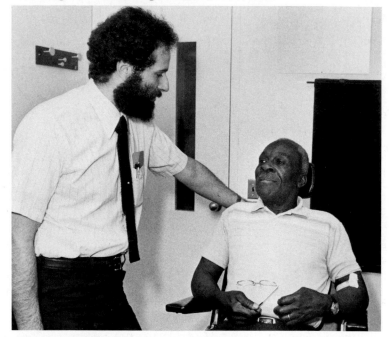

1 *Let's say that Robert Collier's been fitted with a soft contact lens for his aphakic right eye. Do you know how to insert and remove it? Read the following photostory for guidelines. Note: Your patient's eye care professional may use a procedure that differs slightly from this one.*

Begin by positioning Mr. Collier comfortably, either sitting or lying down. Explain what you're going to do. If necessary, assure him that lens insertion and removal is quick and painless. Then, obtain the lens and the wetting and cleaning solutions approved for his type of lens.

Important: Whether Mr. Collier has a daily-wear or extended-wear soft lens, the insertion and removal procedures remain the same. But remember, you'll need to use wetting and cleaning solutions recommended or approved by the manufacturer. Carefully read the manufacturer's instructions, and scrupulously follow all directions.

2 Thoroughly wash and rinse your hands. Dry them on a paper towel, because it's less likely to leave lint on your fingers. To minimize the risk of injuring the patient's eye or damaging the lens, make sure the nails on your thumb and index fingers are short.

Now, remove the lens from its container of sterile solution, and examine it closely. As you see, the lens shown here is torn. Never put such a lens in your patient's eye. Also, don't insert a lens if it looks cloudy, or has specks of lint or other debris on it. If necessary, rinse debris from the lens using approved wetting solution. If it still looks dirty after rinsing, or if it's cloudy or damaged in any way, don't insert it. Instead, notify the patient's eye care professional.

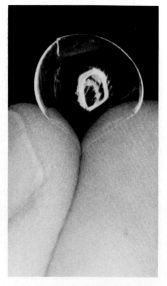

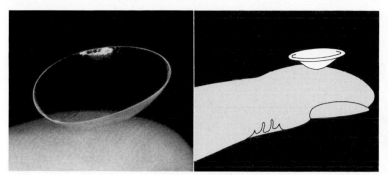

3 If the lens looks okay, place it on the tip of your finger, and make sure it's not inverted. The lens shown in the photo at left is positioned correctly. The lens shown in the illustration is inverted. As you see, its edges point slightly outward and downward.

☎ *Nursing tip:* Here's an alternate way to check. Gently squeeze the lens between two fingers. If it's positioned correctly, its edges will point inward. If not, its edges will turn slightly outward.

If the lens is inside out, gently return it to its correct position. Now, get ready to insert it. *Important:* Before proceeding, make sure the lens is fully wet. Remember, it dries quickly after you remove it from solution. If necessary, rewet it with approved wetting solution.

4 To insert the lens, position it on the index finger of your dominant hand. Use your other index finger to raise Mr. Collier's upper eyelid, and instruct him to look straight ahead. While gently applying downward pressure on the lower lid, move the lens toward his cornea, as shown here. Place the lens directly on the cornea, and remove your finger.

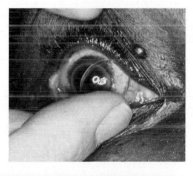

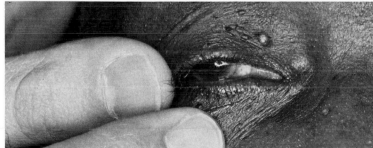

5 To expel any air bubbles that may be trapped under the lens, release the patient's upper eyelid and gently massage it, as shown. Then, ask him if he can see clearly and if he feels any discomfort. If he can't see clearly, look closely to see if the lens is positioned properly on the cornea. (If not, hold his eyelids apart, ask him to look straight ahead, and gently push the lens onto the cornea with your finger.) If the lens feels uncomfortable, it may have a speck of dust or lint trapped beneath it. You'll have to remove the lens, (as explained in steps 6 to 8), rinse it with approved wetting solution, and try again. Never leave a lens in place if the patient complains of discomfort.

Note: If your patient complains of blurred vision, and he wears a lens in each eye, you may have mixed up the lenses.

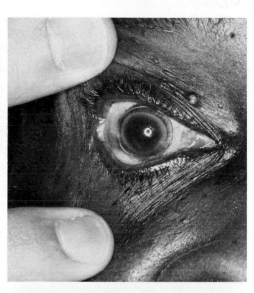

6 Now, suppose you want to remove Mr. Collier's lens. Use two fingers on your nondominant hand to hold his eyelids open, as shown here.

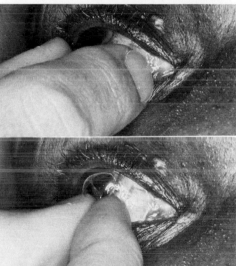

7 Ask Mr. Collier to look up and to the right. (If the lens was in his left eye, you'd have him look to the left.) Then, using your index finger and thumb, lightly grasp the lens's lower edge, as shown in the upper photo.

As you can see in the lower photo, the lens folds up between your fingers.

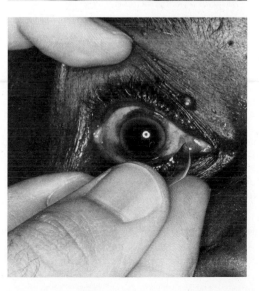

8 Remove the lens, as shown. Clean and sterilize it, according to the manufacturer's instructions.

☎ *Nursing tip:* If your patient wears contact lenses in both eyes, get into the habit of handling the right lens first, and teach your patient to do the same. This lessens the possibility of mixing them up.

Eye care

Learning about eye implants and prostheses

Your patient, Ralph Lundgren, is a 78-year-old retired cook. Like other elderly people, he's already coping with many normal aging changes affecting his body image. But Mr. Lundgren faces another significant body image change, too—the loss of an eye.

An older patient like Mr. Lundgren may lose an eye for one of many reasons—for example, uncontrolled glaucoma, a ruptured cataract, or trauma. Whatever the reason, its loss is emotionally traumatic. Be prepared to give him special support.

Expect him to be concerned about his appearance. He's probably wondering if he'll ever look normal again. Fortunately, you can reassure him that he'll be fitted with a prosthetic eye that looks almost completely natural. To gain information for patient teaching, study the following information and illustrations.

Understanding implants and prostheses

The type of prosthesis your patient needs depends on many factors, including whether he underwent *enucleation* (surgical removal of the entire eyeball from its socket) or *evisceration* (surgical removal of the eyeball's contents, leaving the sclera, and sometimes the cornea, intact). We'll discuss the type of prosthesis appropriate after enucleation.

This type consists of two parts: an implant permanently sewn into the eye socket at the time of enucleation and the visible, removable, shell-shaped prosthesis painted to resemble the patient's other eye.

An implant reduces socket retraction after enucleation. Most implants used today are plastic spheres, like the one shown here. During enucleation, the doctor inserts the implant into the back of the eye socket, and sews the conjunctiva over it. As a result, the implant isn't visible in the socket.

Within 2 to 4 weeks after enucleation (when healing's

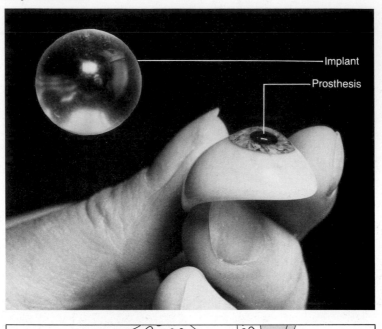

Implant
Prosthesis

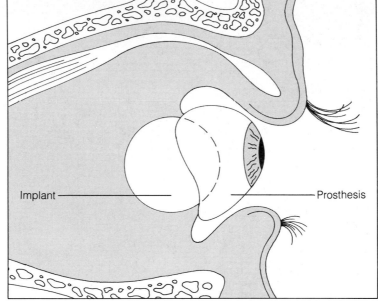

Implant
Prosthesis

complete), the patient can be fitted with a prosthesis. (Under some circumstances, fitting may occur even sooner.) Contemporary prostheses are made of plastic or glass. Changes in the socket's shape, erosion by mucous secretions (in the case of a plastic prosthesis), and daily wear and tear make replacement necessary every 3 years or so. Although glass and plastic prostheses are equally comfortable for the patient, plastic ones have the

advantage of being virtually unbreakable.

Providing support

Teaching your patient about his prosthetic eye is only one part of helping him adjust. Remain sensitive to his special fears and anxieties, even if he doesn't verbalize them. For example, he's probably afraid that he might lose vision in his remaining eye.

Tell him that, to protect the remaining eye, the ocularist (a skilled professional who makes

and fits the prosthesis) may recommend safety glasses. Of course, if the patient has a glass prosthesis, the safety glasses will protect it, too.

Provide additional support and reassurance by following these guidelines:

• If appropriate, reassure him about the health of his remaining eye. Urge him to safeguard it with periodic eye examinations—at least one a year.

• Emphasize that after a period of adjustment, during which he'll learn to compensate for his vision loss, he'll be able to resume a nearly normal life. By learning to turn his head appropriately, he can learn to compensate for lost peripheral vision. Then, he'll be able to drive a vehicle specially equipped with mirrors. He can swim too, although his ocularist may advise him against diving.

• To relieve anxiety about his appearance, explain that he can wear his prosthesis day and night. Removal for cleaning may be necessary only once every few months, or as directed by the ocularist.

• Assure him that a properly fitted prosthesis will be comfortable. Under some circumstances, however, the ocularist may recommend silicone base drops to alleviate possible dryness.

• Warn him not to touch his prosthesis or eyelids any more than necessary, to minimize the risk of infection.

Caring for a prosthesis

If you're caring for a patient who already has a prosthesis, he's probably skilled at caring for it. Allow him to do so, if possible. But you need to know how to properly insert and remove it, too. For example, you'll have to remove the prosthesis before any kind of surgery performed under a general anesthetic, if your patient's too debilitated to do so himself. After surgery, he'll appreciate your replacing it as soon as possible. Review the procedure by reading the photostory that follows.

Performing prosthetic eye care

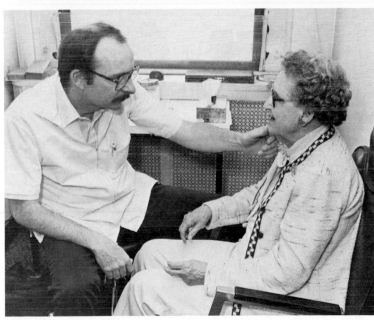

1 Do you know how to care for a patient with a prosthetic eye? If necessary, can you remove and clean the prosthesis, irrigate the patient's eye socket, and replace the prosthesis? This photostory shows you how. (If your patient's had her prosthesis for long, she's probably skilled at caring for it. Give her the choice of doing so, whenever possible.)

Begin by gathering this equipment: suction device, tissues, sterile eye irrigation solution (such as Dacriose or normal saline solution), a basin filled with sterile cleaning solution (for example, Dacriose, normal saline solution, or boric acid), and cotton balls (not shown).

☎ *Nursing tip:* To protect the prosthesis from scratches during cleaning, line the basin with a 4"x4" gauze pad, as shown here.

Also, obtain a plastic bag for disposal of used equipment and a gooseneck lamp, if necessary. Thoroughly wash your hands, and observe clean technique throughout the procedure.

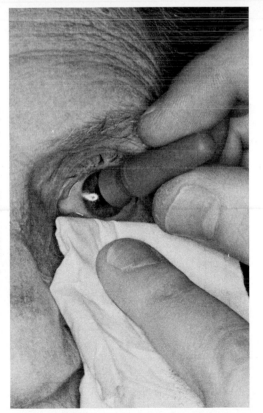

3 To catch any fluid that appears when you remove the prosthesis, place folded tissue against her lower eyelid, as shown. Then, gently raise her upper eyelid and place the suction cup against the iris of the prosthesis, as the nurse has done here.

2 Tell the patient what you're going to do, and answer her questions. Then, position her comfortably, either sitting up or lying on her back. *Note:* If your patient's prosthesis is glass, ask her to lie on a soft surface, such as a bed. This way, if you accidentally drop the prosthesis, it won't break.

If you're using a gooseneck lamp, position it so it lights the patient's face. But don't shine the light directly into her eye.

Eye care

Performing prosthetic eye care continued

4 Then, pull the prosthesis toward you and slightly away from the lower lid. After breaking the eye socket's suction, you can easily remove the prosthesis, as shown here.

Immediately place the prosthesis in the bowl of cleaning solution. If incrustations are present, gently remove them by rubbing with a cotton ball. *Important: Never* use alcohol to clean a prosthetic eye. Also, avoid using extremely hot or cold solutions.

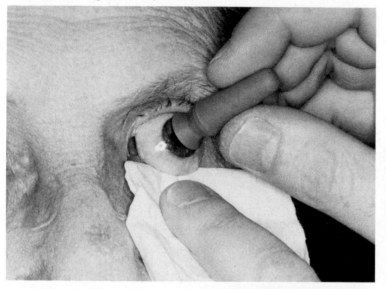

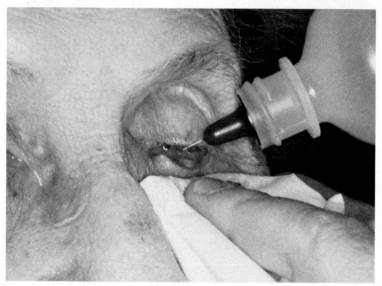

5 While the prosthesis is soaking, prepare to irrigate the patient's eye socket. Fold a clean tissue and place it under her lower eyelid, as shown, to catch the irrigating solution. (If your patient's lying down, protect her clothing by draping a towel over the shoulder nearest the eye socket. Then, ask her to incline her head toward this shoulder and hold the empty basin next to her face.)

Next, lift her upper eyelid, and gently irrigate the eye socket with about 30 ml of irrigating solution, as shown here. Remember to irrigate from the inner canthus toward the outer canthus. (If your patient's lying down, allow the solution to wash around the socket and flow into the basin.)

Dry her eyelids and cheek with tissue.

6 Now, you're ready to reinsert the prosthesis. Remove it from the basin, but don't dry it—the cleaning solution will lubricate it, making insertion easier.

Using your thumb, raise her upper eyelid. Hold the prosthesis so its narrow side points toward the patient's nose, and ask her to look down or straight ahead. Then, gently insert the prosthesis, as shown here.

When it's about halfway in, pull the patient's lower lid downward, toward her cheek. The prosthesis will slip all the way in. Ask the patient to gently move it in her socket, until it fits comfortably.

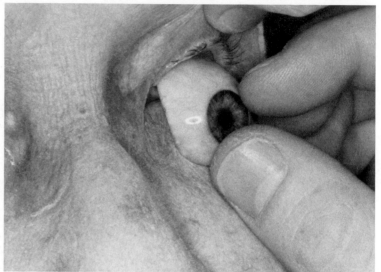

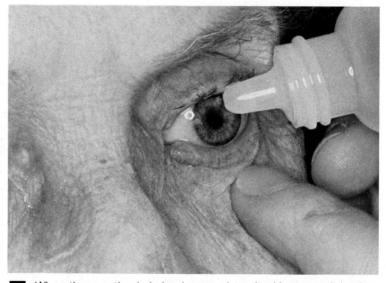

7 When the prosthesis is in place, moisten it with an eye irrigation solution.

Note: If you don't reinsert the prosthesis, store it in water.

Wash your hands and document the procedure and your observations. Notify the doctor if your patient felt any pain during the procedure or if you observed any discharge from the socket. (For the first few weeks after surgery to remove an eye, expect to see moderate serosanguinous drainage. But, notify the doctor if you notice a foul odor or if the amount of drainage increases or changes in color or consistency.)

Hearing aids

When a person's hearing deteriorates, he loses one major channel for interpersonal communication. Sometimes an obstruction such as cerumen creates the hearing loss. But the primary cause is degenerative aging changes, which gradually diminish the ears' ability to interpret the spoken word.

In this chapter, we'll explain how you can assess your patient for signs of hearing loss and what to look for in his history that could indicate or lead to a hearing deficit or loss. Does your patient have cerumen buildup? We'll give you several suggestions for coping with this problem.

Suppose he needs a hearing aid. You can use the information on the following pages to teach your patient how to adjust to and care for it. We also tell you how to troubleshoot a hearing aid problem. And, we'll provide tips on communicating with a hearing-impaired patient.

Remember, in many cases, hearing loss from aging can be corrected—with your assistance. Read the following pages to find out how.

Understanding hearing loss

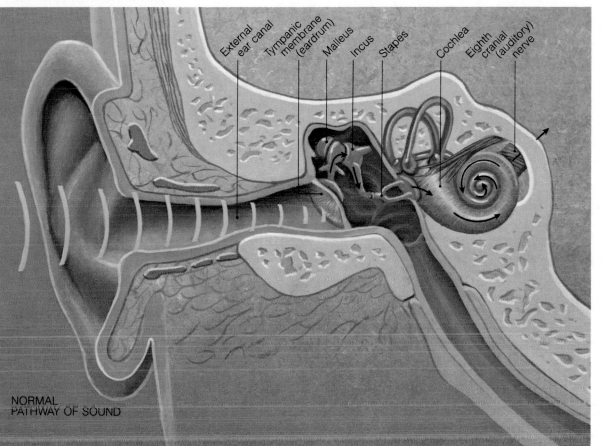

External ear canal · Tympanic membrane (eardrum) · Malleus · Incus · Stapes · Cochlea · Eighth cranial (auditory) nerve

NORMAL
PATHWAY OF SOUND

By the time a person reaches age 65, he's likely to experience some degree of hearing loss. The degenerative process begins in childhood and progresses gradually as a person ages.

Since the process occurs slowly, the geriatric patient unknowingly compensates for hearing loss and in many cases doesn't realize that subtle changes are taking place. These changes can affect his family relationships, his social interactions, and his everyday activities. And, as the condition worsens, he risks not hearing important warning sounds, such as an automobile horn or siren.

Hearing loss can be perceptive (sensorineural) or conductive. Perceptive loss occurs from a natural deterioration of cochlear hair cells, which commonly affects the older adult. This deterioration—known as presbycusis—muffles sounds and impairs ability to interpret those in the high-frequency speech range (such as f, s, th, ch, and sh). Additionally, the person's own speech loses quality and tone because he can't hear properly. Many hearing loss problems are alleviated by aural rehabilitation; for instance, amplification by a hearing aid or speech training.

Conductive hearing loss is a blockage of sound transmission in the passage from the external

ear, through the ear canal and middle ear, into the cochlea. The obstruction may simply be an accumulation of cerumen in the ear canal, which the doctor can remove by irrigating the ear or using an ear spoon.

Other common conductive hearing problems include otitis media, cholesteatoma, and otosclerosis, which may be treated conservatively or may require surgery.

Corrective measures exist for hearing loss, but the major way to combat its effects is by early detection through routine screening for hearing and communication problems. This screening requires a thorough assessment and keen observation. Often, the geriatric patient won't admit that he has a hearing loss and instead claims his family and friends don't speak loudly or clearly enough. They, in turn, may feel that he hears only what he wants to hear or is deliberately being uncooperative.

Your patient's lack of awareness about his condition may cause inappropriate behavior and responses. Don't misconstrue these actions as signs of aging. Instead, increase your sensitivity about the impact hearing loss has on your geriatric patient, so you can improve your interactions with him.

Hearing aids

Detecting hearing loss

By observing your geriatric patient closely, you can probably determine more about his ability to hear and communicate than he'll tell you himself. Why? Because many geriatric patients won't admit they don't hear clearly. So, you'll need to watch carefully for signs and symptoms of perceptive or conductive hearing loss. These include:
• inattentiveness to others
• inappropriate response when he's addressed
• irrelevant comments during verbal interactions
• frequently asking to have something repeated
• turning one ear toward the speaker
• difficulty in following directions
• poor response to environmental sounds
• tendency to withdraw from activities requiring verbal communication
• unusual voice quality or unusually loud speech.

If your patient has *perceptive* hearing loss, he'll probably also have these particular signs and symptoms:
• diminished ability to hear high-pitched voices, such as women's and children's voices
• exaggerated sensitivity to loud sounds
• tinnitus (a ringing or buzzing in his ears)
• dizziness
• difficulty in understanding speech, especially when there's background noise
• inability to follow or participate adequately in a conversation.

Assessing for a hearing problem

Let's say you're assessing your geriatric patient for a hearing or communication problem. First, obtain his medical history and that of his family. Note if any of them have a hearing loss. Also, find out if he's experienced any conditions that might lead to a hearing problem. These include:
• head trauma
• exposure to loud noises, especially over a prolonged period; for instance, a job history of construction work
• frequent ear or upper respiratory tract infections
• drugs with ototoxic effects, such as aspirin
• tinnitus
• frequent ear drainage problems
• tendency to build up cerumen
• previous ear surgery.

Using an otoscope, inspect the external ear canal for any obstruction, such as cerumen or a foreign body. Also, look for redness, swelling, drainage, lesions, or scales. Be gentle. This procedure can be very painful if your patient's ear is inflamed. As you proceed, examine his internal canal and eardrum for signs of inflammation, drainage, or accumulated blood. For more information on examining the ear, see the NURSING PHOTOBOOK ASSESSING YOUR PATIENTS.

Other ways to assess your patient's hearing include testing whether he can hear a ticking watch or your whisper. This indicates whether he's lost some ability to hear high-frequency sounds. To differentiate between perceptive and conductive hearing loss, perform the Rinne and Weber's tests (see page 19).

If you suspect your patient has a hearing loss, be tactful about suggesting further tests. If further tests indicate he needs a hearing aid, help by:
• motivating him and his family to establish and meet goals for the hearing rehabilitation program.
• providing the opportunity for them to discuss their feelings about the value of the program developed for the patient.

Learning about cerumen

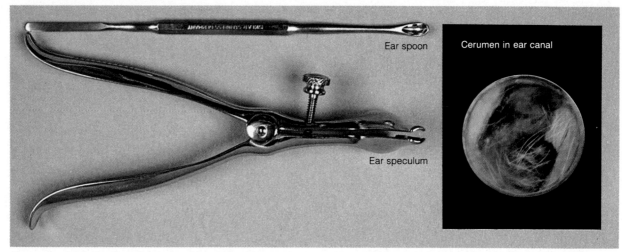

Ear spoon

Cerumen in ear canal

Ear speculum

If your geriatric patient has a hearing loss, his ears may be obstructed by a natural protective secretion called cerumen (see illustration). This brownish substance is created by the wax and oil glands located in the ear canal. The amount and consistency of the cerumen varies in each person, depending on heredity as well as exposure to the environment. For instance, a person with oily skin and a dark complexion usually has more cerumen. Also, excessive cerumen formation may result from irritating dust or from fungal or bacterial infection in the inner ear.

When inspecting your patient's ears, make sure you ask him about any ear disease he has now or had previously. What appears to be cerumen may actually be hardened discharge from a perforated eardrum or a disorder such as chronic suppurative or secretory otitis media. For patients with these conditions, the doctor will remove the cerumen or discharge.

However, if it's *your* responsibility to remove the cerumen (in cases where no contraindications exist), you may do so by irrigating the ear canal.

Caution: Irrigation's contraindicated in patients with a history of ear drainage or a perforated eardrum. Also, whenever you irrigate a patient's ear, make sure the solution's at body temperature, to avoid provoking extreme dizziness.

Before trying to remove cerumen, first soften it with a ceruminolytic agent, such as carbamide peroxide (Debrox*). Then, you may irrigate the ear with a bulb syringe or (very gently) with a water jet-spray appliance, such as a WaterPik®. Continue irrigating until you've thoroughly cleansed the ear. After removing cerumen, you'll want to reassess the ear for cerumen buildup periodically, using an otoscope.

If the cerumen can't be removed by irrigation, the doctor may use an ear spoon (see photo). This spoon is smooth edged and used only with an ear speculum (see photo), for direct viewing of the ear canal.

He'll insert the spoon into the ear canal through the speculum and gently pull out the cerumen. During this procedure, he'll take special care to avoid injuring the epithelium and the eardrum.

*Available in both the United States and in Canada

Learning about hearing aids

Do you know how a patient's fitted with the proper hearing aid? After a hearing loss has been confirmed, he'll undergo further tests to determine his specific needs. The doctor or audiologist will evaluate his ability to recognize pure tones and speech, his hearing in a normal environment, and his tolerance of loud noises. With this information, the doctor can try various hearing aids to find the most suitable amplification—and most comfortable aid—for his patient.

Encourage your patient to have a qualified person fit him, especially if he's had one of the following conditions:
• active drainage from the ear in the past 90 days
• sudden or progressive hearing loss within the past 90 days
• acute or chronic dizziness
• unilateral hearing loss of sudden or recent onset
• visible evidence of significant cerumen accumulation or a foreign body in the ear canal
• pain or discomfort in the ear
• visible congenital or traumatic deformity of the ear.

All hearing aids contain three basic parts: microphone, amplifier, and receiver. The microphone converts sound waves into electrical energy, which is then fed into an amplifier to increase the signal's energy. This amplified electric signal activates a receiver, which changes the energy back into amplified sound waves. A battery usually provides the hearing aid's power.

Also, all aids have an on/off switch and a volume-control switch. (In some aids, the volume-control switch serves both purposes.) Many newer models feature external tone control, which can amplify or mask certain sound frequencies, depending on the patient's needs. Other models have a switch setting that specifically amplifies telephone conversations.

Your patient will wear one of four types of hearing aids: a behind-the-ear aid, an in-the-ear aid, a body aid, or an eyeglass aid. Each of these is used with an earmold which is specially fitted to match the anatomical shape of the individual's ear. Read the following chart to find out more about each type.

BEHIND-THE-EAR AID

Description
This small curved case, housing all the components (including the battery), fits neatly behind the ear. The amplified sound feeds into the ear through a plastic tube attached to an earmold.

Advantages
• Easy to conceal
• Used for mild to moderate hearing losses
• Comfortable to wear
• No long wires required
• Durable
• Some models are equipped with a telephone pickup device

Disadvantages
• Close proximity of microphone and receiver causes feedback, which limits the amount of amplification possible

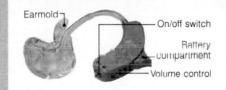

Earmold
On/off switch
Battery compartment
Volume control

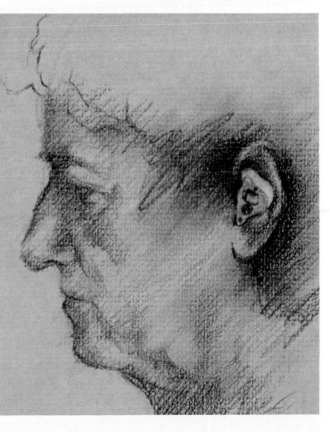

IN-THE-EAR AID

Description
This aid, housing all components, fits directly into the ear canal and is supported by the outer ear.

Advantages
• Lack of external wires or tubes make the aid more attractive than other models
• Easy to conceal
• Lightweight

Disadvantages
• Suitable only for mild hearing loss
• Provides less amplification than others
• Allows some sound distortion
• Small controls may make unit difficult for geriatric patient to operate
• Less durable than others

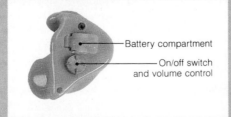

Battery compartment
On/off switch and volume control

Hearing aids

Learning about hearing aids continued

BODY AID

Description
The microphone, amplifier, and battery are located in a single case, which the patient attaches to clothing or carries in his pocket. The external receiver attaches directly to the ear mold and connects to the amplifier by a long wire.

Advantages
• Most powerful aid; allows patient to hear wide amplification ranges
• Can be used in serious hearing loss
• Controls are more easily adjusted than in other aids
• Separation of receiver and microphone prevents acoustic feedback
• Some models contain variable tone control
• Usually the least expensive model of hearing aid

Disadvantages
• Requires external wiring
• Large size may make it look unattractive
• Doesn't allow full hearing in high-frequency ranges

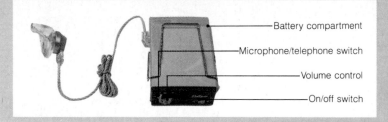
— Battery compartment
— Microphone/telephone switch
— Volume control
— On/off switch

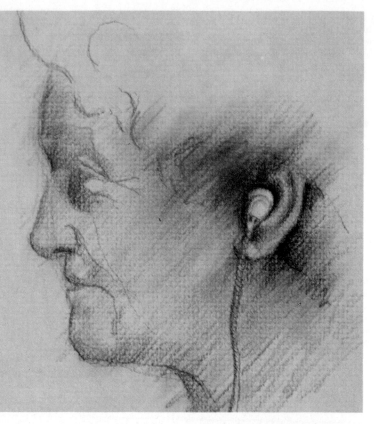

EYEGLASS AID

Description
Similar to behind-the-ear model, except that the unit is built into the arm of the eyeglass frame. A short length of tubing connects the hearing aid to the earmold.

Advantages
• Frame can carry signal from one ear to the other; good for binaural amplification
• Used for mild to moderate hearing losses
• Eyeglass frame largely conceals aid; hides wires connecting microphone and receiver within the frame
• Bone-conduction hearing aids are also available in the eyeglass style

Disadvantages
• Requires wearing eyeglasses
• Eyeglass frame is bulky and unattractive
• If aid or frame breaks, patient must do without both or find substitute

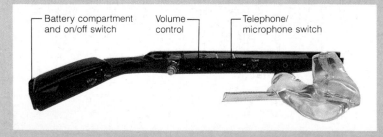
┌ Battery compartment   Volume ─   ┌ Telephone/
  and on/off switch   control   microphone switch

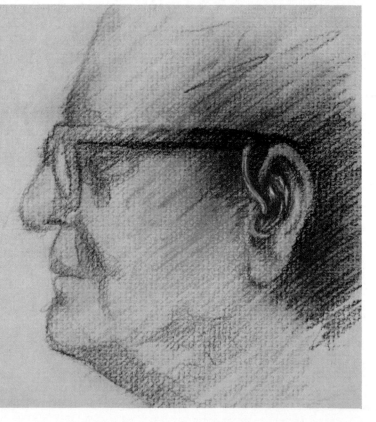

Applying a hearing aid

Your patient with moderate loss has just returned from having reconstructive surgery on both her hands. In order to communicate with her, you'll have to put her hearing aid in her affected left ear. Do you know the correct procedure?

First, familiarize yourself with her hearing aid, which is a Beltone® behind-the-ear model. Observe the location of each marking and control. Then, place your patient in a comfortable position.

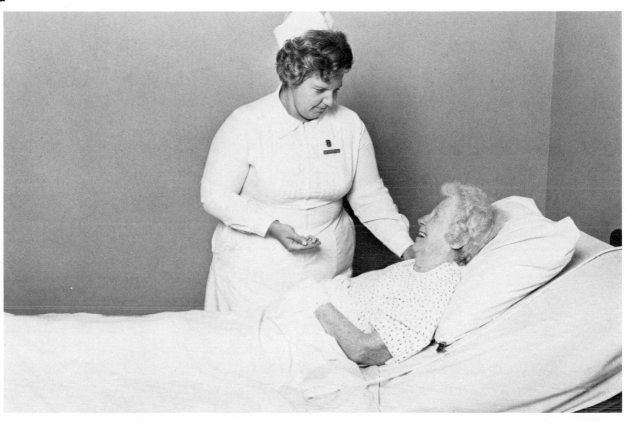

2 Now, test the battery. To do this, turn the control switch to the M (microphone) setting (see left photo). Then increase the volume by pushing the dial upward (see right photo).

3 Cup your hand over the earmold, as the nurse is doing here. If you don't hear a constant whistle, replace the battery with a fresh one.

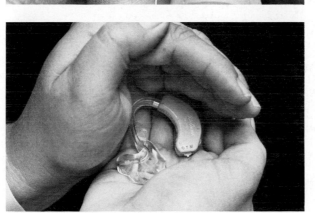

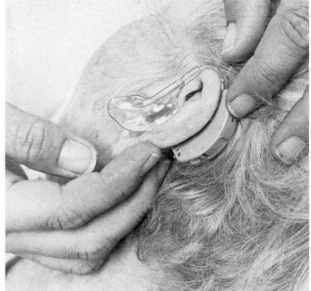

4 Next, check the control switch at the base of the hearing aid. Make sure the switch is positioned under the O, which means OFF. Also, turn the volume control to its lowest level. Then, place the aid over your patient's ear, allowing the earmold to hang free, as the nurse is doing here. Check the tubing, to make sure no kinks or twists can obstruct sound transmittal.

Hearing aids

Applying a hearing aid continued

5 Now, grasp the earmold, and gently insert the tapered end into your patient's ear canal, as shown. Then, lightly twist the earmold into the cradle of her ear. Using your other hand, pull on her earlobe as you push gently upward and inward on the bottom of the earmold.

Eliminating hearing aid problems

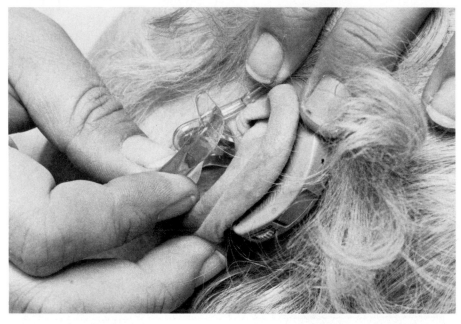

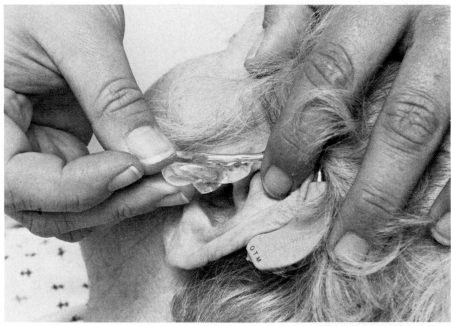

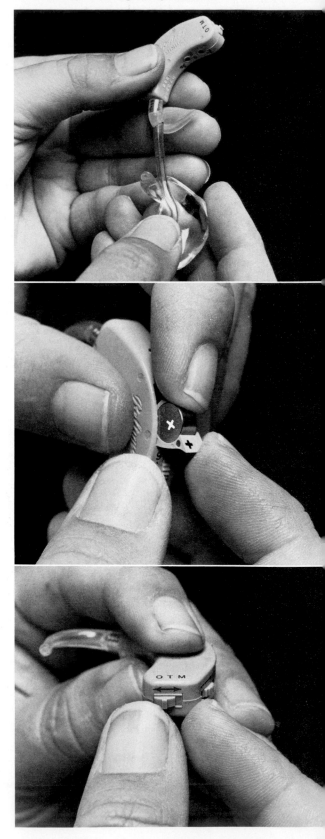

6 Next, turn on the hearing aid by moving the control switch to the position marked M. Then, adjust the volume to the setting most comfortable for your patient. Note the desired setting on her nursing care chart.

Suppose you want to remove the hearing aid. First turn it off. Then, gently loosen the upper portion of the earmold, and simultaneously lift it up and outward, as the nurse is doing here.

Important: Never remove the earmold by gripping the aid or the plastic sound tube.

Finally, document the application—or removal—in your nurses' notes.

Problem
Whistling or howling noise

Possible cause
- Excessively high volume
- Improper seal between ear canal and earmold
- Crack in the plastic tubing
- Bad connection between earmold and amplifier
- Improperly selected aid

Nursing intervention
- Turn down the volume, if needed.
- Make sure the earmold fits well and seals the ear canal completely.
- Check the tubing for cracks or faulty connections, as shown.
- Refer the patient for evaluation, if you can't identify his problem.

Problem
Inadequate amplification

Possible cause
- Aid turned off or volume set too low
- Weak or dead battery
- Cerumen or other material in earmold
- Cerumen in ear canal
- Improperly fitted earmold
- Wire or tubing disconnected from aid
- Improperly selected aid

Nursing intervention
- Make sure the aid is turned on.
- Check volume setting.
- Check tube connections.
- Check battery alignment.
- Replace battery with a fresh one, if needed. To do so, hold the hearing aid over a soft surface. Be sure to match the positive mark on the battery with the positive mark on the battery contact (as shown).
- Remove any obstruction from the earmold, or cerumen from the ear, using the proper procedure.

Problem
Intermittent loss of sound

Possible cause
- Dirt lodged in the switch
- Loose connection between amplifier and tubing
- Poor battery contact
- Cracked hearing aid case

Nursing intervention
- Work the switch back and forth to loosen any dirt, as shown.
- Check battery alignment.
- Check the battery contact. You'll know there's poor contact if the aid works when you press its sides together. On some models you can remove the battery and clean the metal contact pieces with a small emery board. Also, gently push them closer to the battery, for better contact.
- Instruct patient to return a cracked case to his dealer for repair.

How to clean an earmold

1 *Every hearing aid has a specially fitted earmold that channels amplified sound into the ear. An earmold is made of a clear or flesh-colored synthetic material that is molded to the ear's anatomy. Most models seal the ear canal tightly, to prevent acoustic feedback between the microphone and receiver.*

With daily use, an earmold usually needs replacing every 2 to 3 years. When caring for a patient with a hearing aid, instruct him to check the earmold daily for cracked or rough edges that may irritate his ear. *Important:* If the earmold is causing your patient pain, he should contact a doctor immediately. Remind him to clean the tip weekly to remove cerumen, which can impair the aid's effectiveness.

To clean an earmold, disconnect it from the hearing aid. Then, carefully rotate a pin, needle, or pipe cleaner in the opening of the earmold, as the nurse is doing here.

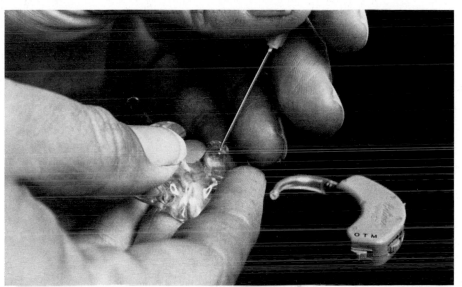

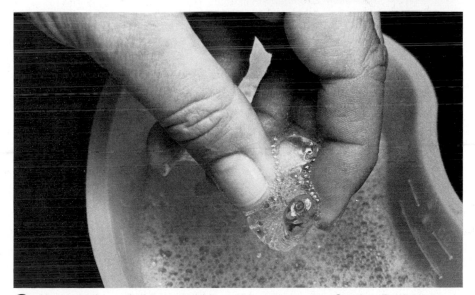

2 Next, gently wash the earmold in warm, soapy water. *Caution:* Don't use alcohol to clean it; alcohol causes dryness and cracking.

Rinse the earmold, and allow it to dry thoroughly before reconnecting it to the aid. Water droplets left in the connecting tube can enter the hearing aid and damage it.

Finally, document the cleaning in your nurses' notes.

Hearing aids

Caring for a hearing aid

Let's assume your patient, 68-year-old Harry Pauls, has just been fitted with a hearing aid. He's received instructions on how to care for it. But you'll also want to give him these important guidelines:
• Turn off the aid when you're not using it, and remove the battery. Leave the battery case open, storing your hearing aid in a properly identified container.
• Take care not to drop the aid on a hard surface. Work over a bed or a similar soft area when changing batteries or removing the aid from your ear.
• Turn off the hearing aid before replacing or inserting a new battery.
• Clean the battery by gently rubbing it with a sharpened pencil eraser. This procedure removes corrosion. If the battery becomes damp, dry the contacts with a cotton swab.

• Store extra batteries in the freezer to lengthen shelf life. *Note:* If you use your hearing aid 10 to 12 hours daily, you'll probably need to replace the battery weekly.
• Avoid getting moisture inside the hearing aid; for example, by wearing it in the rain, in the bathtub, or during activities that cause excessive perspiration. Steam from a vaporizer can also damage the hearing aid. Store the aid in an airtight container with a silica-gel packet, particularly in humid climates.
• Avoid applying any sprays on or near your head while wearing the aid, to prevent clogging the microphone.
• Keep the hearing aid away from excessive heat or cold. Never place it near a stove, heater, or on a sunny windowsill, and don't wear it when using a hair dryer. Also, try not to wear it for long periods outside in extremely hot or cold weather.

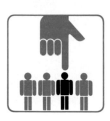

Helping your patient adjust to his aid

Has your geriatric patient recently been fitted with a hearing aid? His orientation period will critically affect the success of his hearing rehabilitation program and could determine whether he wears the aid or hides it away in a drawer. Stress to your patient that he won't adapt to the aid overnight. Getting accustomed to it will require many hours of wear and much patience.
    Follow these guidelines to help him adjust:
• Encourage your patient to use his hearing aid as much as possible.
• However, advise him to wear the aid for only short periods of time during the adjustment period; for instance, have him wear it for 15 to 20 minutes the first 2 days, and then for a half hour more each day until he's completely comfortable with it. Tell him to turn off the aid and rest for awhile if it makes him nervous or tired.
• Warn him not to turn the volume too high. Doing so will distort the sound and may cause a whistling or squealing sound.
    Note: These sounds may also indicate a loose-fitting

earmold.
• Instruct him to ignore background noises when listening to conversations. Blocking out those distractions will require patience. If the background noise gets too annoying, tell your patient to turn down the volume on his hearing aid and to closely watch the speaker's face.
• Tell your patient to get accustomed to his aid by conversing with only one person at a time at first. Have him experiment with the aid in difficult situations; for example, when listening to a stereo or television set or with loud background noise.
• Suggest that he sit as close as possible to the speaker when in a large group.
• Make sure he understands and continues to follow his instructions on wearing and caring for his aid. If he can't maintain it, teach a family member how to assist him.
• Stress that he should immediately contact the doctor if he has pain or drainage in his ear, which could be caused by skin or cartilage infection, a middle-ear infection, an ear tumor, or an improperly fitted earmold.

Communicating with a hearing-impaired patient

Does your geriatric patient have hearing loss? If so, you'll need to adopt special techniques to communicate effectively, even if he's wearing a hearing aid. Keep in mind that a hearing aid doesn't restore normal hearing. It simply amplifies sound, including background noise. Because of this, your patient may still have difficulty hearing what you're saying.
    Because your geriatric patient may take longer to perceive and interpret what you

say, allow extra time when you talk to him. Call him by name to attract his attention.
    When speaking to him, make sure that you face him, that your face is visible, and that you're speaking into his less impaired ear (if he has one). Speak slowly and clearly, and avoid shouting, which distorts sound and can upset your patient.
    Enhance your conversation with facial expressions, gestures, and body language. But, avoid exaggerated lip movements,

which may confuse him or make him feel more self-conscious about his problem.
    Use short phrases rather than long sentences, to help your patient understand you. If he doesn't know what you've said, rephrase your statement using different words. Encourage him to frankly inform his family and friends when he doesn't understand them. *Note:* Teach the family members to use the techniques described above to improve communication with the patient.

Medication guidance

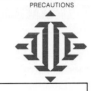

As you know, administering medications to a geriatric patient—and teaching him self-administration—takes special care. Depending on his age, specific health problems, and mental alertness, he may face one or more of the following problems:
• decreased, increased, incomplete, or erratic medication absorption, because of the debilitating effects of aging and disease processes
• adverse medication interactions among several prescribed medications, or among prescribed and over-the-counter medications
• difficulty complying with medication regimens, from lack of manual dexterity or other problems associated with aging.

Fortunately, your thoughtful nursing care can reduce these risks. Read the following pages for medication administration guidelines, as well as some practical suggestions that will help your patient safely give himself medications at home.

Spotting drug misuse

"Dad's really gone downhill these last 6 months," Mrs. Minelli tells you. "He's forgetful and confused most of the time. But I guess that's just part of getting old."

When you hear something like this, do you just nod agreement? If so, you may be overlooking your geriatric patient's real problem—drug misuse.

If you make this mistake, you're not alone. Although widespread, drug misuse affecting geriatric patients is frequently overlooked by health-care professionals. Why? Because the patient's signs and symptoms may mimic the following stereotypical aging changes: weakness, fatigue, confusion, tremors, anorexia, and anxiety.

Don't fall into the trap of assuming that these signs and symptoms are inevitable and irreversible aging changes. In fact, they may be caused by any number of factors related to drug therapy.

First of all, drug action in the elderly is a complicated matter. Decreased gastrointestinal absorption and reduced systemic circulation may reduce a drug's immediate effects. But an increase in fat (which stores chemical substances), combined with impaired liver and kidney function, can allow a drug to quickly accumulate to toxic levels—even when it's given in moderate dosages.

Each patient's response depends on how aging has affected each body system and on the specific drug administered. As a rule, an elderly patient requires smaller than average dosages of most drugs. But if his ability to absorb drugs is impaired while his ability to metabolize and excrete them is unimpaired, he may require *larger* than average dosages.

Throughout drug therapy, continually assess your patient's response. Consider even a slight change in behavior or alertness to be a possible sign of toxicosis, and notify the doctor.

Protecting your patient
To assess your patient, first take a thorough drug history. Then, ask yourself these questions:
• Are all the drugs he's taking necessary? Be especially alert if he's taking several drugs prescribed by different doctors. Remember, some elderly patients change doctors frequently and neglect to tell a new doctor of previously prescribed drugs.

Also, note whether he's taking two drugs that serve the same purpose. For example, suppose the doctor decided to change the patient's diuretic from chlorothiazide (Diuril*) to furosemide (Lasix*). The patient may mistakenly take *both* drugs, unaware that the doctor intended him to stop the chlorothiazide.
• Is he experiencing adverse effects from drug interactions? This is likely if he takes more than one prescription drug. Find out if he takes over-the-counter drugs. He may not know how potent they can be, especially in combination with other drugs.
• Is he experiencing drug side effects? In addition to specific side effects attributable to drugs he's taking, assess for indirect side effects, such as malnutrition. And, remember, physiologic aging changes, as well as disease processes, mean an older patient is twice as likely to have adverse drug reactions.
• Are drug dosages appropriate? As you know, an elderly patient may require a dosage that's significantly different from that required by a younger adult.
• Is the patient complying with doctor's orders? If he's not properly self-administering his medication, assess the reasons. Then, if necessary, teach your patient how to use a chart or device that can help him comply (see pages 134 to 137).

Providing medication guidelines

"I'm glad to be going home soon," says 73-year-old Anna McKay, who was hospitalized for congestive heart failure. "But I'm a little worried about all the medicine I have to take at home. I'm so forgetful these days—how will I ever manage?"

As a nurse, you can help. On the following pages, you'll find many suggestions that can help Miss McKay properly and safely administer her own medications at home. Prepare Miss McKay *before* her discharge, with thorough patient teaching.

Don't wait until the day of discharge to begin. Instead, plan brief teaching sessions several times a day, for a few days before her discharge (or as soon as she feels well enough to be attentive). Plan plenty of time for each teaching session, so she doesn't feel rushed. To avoid misunderstandings, take care to use simple language.

As she learns, encourage her to begin accepting responsibility for self-medication, with your supervision. This way, you can assess her progress.

To help her remember her medications, write down each medication's name, its purpose (in easy-to-understand words; for example, *water pill* rather than diuretic), its dose, the correct times to take it, how to recognize possible side effects, and when to call the doctor. Remember to write with large, clear letters, so she can easily read the words. Finally, tape a sample tablet or capsule next to the appropriate medication name, so she learns to identify each by sight and touch.

As you assess Miss McKay's progress, stay alert for any potential problems she'll have at home. Ask yourself these questions:
• Does she live with family or friends? Include them in your patient teaching, if possible.
• Does she live alone, or with a debilitated spouse? If so, she'll need continuing support from a visiting nurse or social agency. Keep in mind that inadequate supervision may result in drug misuse. Make appropriate contacts for her.
• Can she open medication bottles easily? If she's handicapped by arthritis or Parkinson's disease,

*Available in both the United States and in Canada

Medication guidance

Providing
medication guidelines continued

or lacks manual dexterity for any reason, make sure she has snap—not childproof—caps. Tell her to ask the pharmacist for snap caps in the future. If her medication doesn't require the protection of an airtight bottle, suggest an envelope system like the one shown on page 135. *Important:* Remind her to keep all medications out of the reach of children and pets.
• Can she see well enough to read medication labels or identify medications? She may be reluctant to admit that she can't see as well as she used to, so observe her closely.
• Does she eat regular meals? Remember, many medications are scheduled with meals. If she regularly skips meals, she may miss one or more doses a day. Or, she may take her medications on an empty stomach, causing nausea. Help her work out a schedule based on her eating habits.

Note: If your patient isn't eating adequately (for example, because she's unable to prepare meals), consider contacting a social service program, such as Meals on Wheels.
• Does she feel financially secure? If not, she may be tempted to save money by not refilling prescriptions. Or, she may try to make her medication last longer by taking less than the prescribed dosage. Refer her to your hospital's social service agency for financial guidance.
• Can she get refills easily? If not, help her find a pharmacy that delivers.

Points to emphasize

Don't let your patient leave the hospital before you've taught her the *do's* and *don'ts* of medication use.
• DO tell the doctor if you've ever had an allergic reaction to anything—including food or a vaccination.
• DO call the doctor if you become sick and can't take your medication.
• DO store your medication properly.
• DO continue to take your medication until the doctor says you should stop.
• DON'T take more or less than the prescribed dosage.
• DON'T take anyone else's medication or give yours to anyone else.
• DON'T drink alcohol when taking medication, without your doctor's permission.
• DON'T take outdated medication or medication that's several years old.

Using a chart system

Does your patient need help remembering when to take several different medications? Make him one of the charts shown here, and teach him how to use it.

The first chart helps him remember the names of his medications, their purpose, what they look like, how to take them, and when to take them. In addition, it reminds him at a glance of any special instructions or precautions; for example, *Take with meals* or *Don't drink alcohol.*

☎ *Nursing tip:* If your patient has trouble

Medication and what it's for	Amount, color, and shape	Instructions	Times
DIGOXIN (HEART)	1 YELLOW, ROUND, SMALL	CHECK PULSE FIRST.	9 A.M. MON., WED., FRI.
LASIX (WATER)	1 WHITE, FOOTBALL-SHAPE	DON'T DRINK ALCOHOL.	9 A.M.
MOTRIN (ARTHRITIS)	1 ORANGE, ROUND, SMOOTH	TAKE WITH MEALS.	9 A.M., 1 P.M., 5 P.M., 9 P.M.

Times	DIGOXIN – 1 EVERY OTHER DAY LASIX – 1 EVERY DAY MOTRIN – 1 FOUR TIMES A DAY	S	M	T	W	Th	F	S
9 A.M.	DIGOXIN, LASIX, MOTRIN	✓✓	✓✓✓	✓✓	✓✓✓	✓✓	✓✓✓	✓✓
1 P.M.	MOTRIN	✓	✓	✓	✓	✓	✓	✓
5 P.M.	MOTRIN	✓	✓	✓	✓	✓	✓	✓
9 P.M.	MOTRIN	✓	✓	✓	✓	✓	✓	✓

Medication, color, and shape	Instructions	Times						
		S	M	T	W	Th	F	S
DIGOXIN – YELLOW, ROUND, SMALL	1 EVERY OTHER DAY. CHECK PULSE FIRST.		9 A.M.		9 A.M.		9 A.M.	
LASIX – WHITE, FOOTBALL-SHAPE	1 EVERY DAY. DON'T DRINK ALCOHOL.	9 A.M.	9 A.M.	9 A.M.	9 A.M.	9 A.M.	9 A.M.	9 A.M.
MOTRIN – ORANGE, ROUND, SMOOTH	1 FOUR TIMES A DAY. TAKE WITH MEALS.	9 A.M. 1 P.M. 5 P.M. 9 P.M.	9 A.M. 1 P.M. 5 P.M. 9 P.M.	9 A.M. 1 P.M. 5 P.M. 9 P.M.	9 A.M. 1 P.M. 5 P.M. 9 P.M.	9 A.M. 1 P.M. 5 P.M. 9 P.M.	9 A.M. 1 P.M. 5 P.M. 9 P.M.	9 A.M. 1 P.M. 5 P.M. 9 P.M.

Medication, what it's for, and amount	Times	S	M	T	W	Th	F	S
○ DIGOXIN (HEART), 1 EVERY OTHER DAY	9 A.M.	◐ ●	○ ◐ ●	◐ ●	○ ◐ ●	◐ ●	○ ◐ ●	◐ ●
● LASIX (WATER), 1 EVERY DAY	1 P.M.	●	●	●	●	●	●	●
● MOTRIN (ARTHRITIS), 1 FOUR TIMES A DAY	5 P.M.	●	●	●	●	●	●	●
	9 P.M.							

remembering whether he's taken his medication, and he takes only one dose a day, suggest that he turn the bottle upside down after taking his daily dose. Or, advise him to move the bottle from one side of his shelf or dresser to the other after taking a dose. Before he goes to bed, he can turn the bottle right side up again or move it back to its original position.

As an alternative for your patient who's taking several medications at the same times each day, try making the second chart. As you see, in addition to columns for the time and medication name, it contains a column for day of the week. By checking off each dose as he takes it, he can keep track of what he's taken. Of course, this chart's reliable only if the patient consistently checks off each dose as he takes it.

Suppose your patient's biggest concern is remembering which medication is which. The third chart emphasizes the appearance of each medication, to help the patient easily identify each one. As you see, this chart combines the features of the two charts immediately preceding.

If your patient has a vision impairment, a color-coded chart with accompanying key (such as the fourth chart) may help him correctly administer his medications. Here's what to do: First, assign each medication a color. *Note:* When you make such a chart for your patient, choose colors that he can easily distinguish. Many elderly patients see reds and yellows best, and blues and greens least well. Also, consider using the color of each medication as its identifier.

Using colored stickers or tape, color-code the top and bottom of each medication bottle.

Then, make a color key, like the one shown on the left side of the chart. As you see, the nurse has identified each drug by assigned color, name, purpose, and the time of day to take it. (As an additional visual aid, consider taping a sample capsule or tablet at an appropriate spot on the chart.) Post the key in a prominent place, such as on the refrigerator door.

Finally, color-code a chart, as shown on the right side of the chart, and post it near the color key. Now, the patient can tell at a glance which medications to take each day and at what times to take them.

The type of chart you choose depends on your patient's individual needs. Take care to make it large enough so that he can easily read it. If you're using the second chart, photocopy a number of blank charts, so he'll have a supply to use as needed.

Premeasuring medications

1 *To help your patient give himself correct doses—no more and no less—you or a family member may premeasure his medications for him. Consider using one of the systems shown below. But remember, before taking a medication out of its original container, make sure it doesn't need the protection of an airtight or tinted container. Also, keep in mind that some medications need refrigeration. Check with the pharmacist.*

Caution: Be particularly careful when using any of these systems if unsupervised

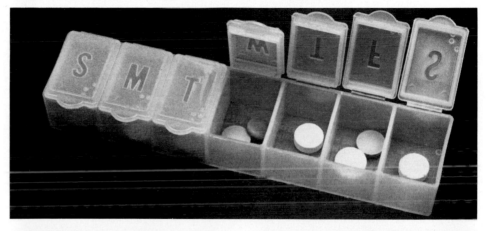

children live with or visit the patient.

Suppose your patient can see well enough to distinguish his medications but lacks the manual dexterity to easily open medication bottles. From his pharmacist, he may be able to purchase a container similar to the one shown here, with one pocket for each day of the week. Once a week, you, a family member, or a visiting nurse can measure the following week's doses. This system's especially useful if the patient takes some medications every other day, rather than daily.

2 Here's a simple alternative. Place each dose of medication in a small envelope, and mark the envelope with the time of day to take it. Then, put the envelopes containing each day's doses into larger envelopes, and label each one with the appropriate day of the week. Put the larger envelopes in order, and place them in an empty shoe box or card file. Instruct the patient to proceed from front to back, according to the day of the week. To avoid confusion, tell him to discard each envelope (or put it in a separate place) after taking the medication from it.

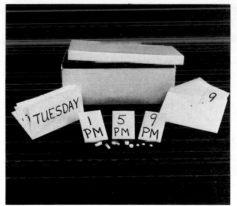

3 Does your patient take more than one capsule or tablet several times a day? Then, he may prefer to use a system such as the one shown here. Using large numbers, label each compartment of an egg carton. Each number represents one of the 12 daytime hours. Instruct a family member to place the prescribed medication in the compartment representing the time of day the patient's scheduled to take it. For example, if he's scheduled to take medication at 9 a.m., 1 p.m., and 6 p.m., he'd find it in the compartments marked 9, 1, and 6.

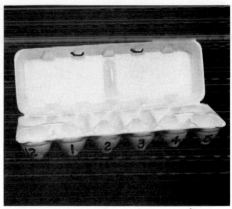

Medication guidance

Learning about medication aids

If your patient can reliably take his medications, he may be able to maintain a more independent lifestyle. Choose one of the aids featured here, depending on his specific needs.

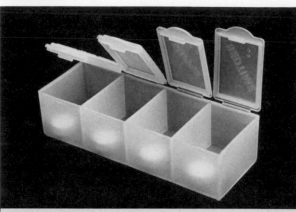

One-day Pill Reminder®

Purpose
To help patient determine if he's taken all the medications prescribed for a single day

Description
Plastic device with four medication compartments marked breakfast, lunch, supper, bedtime. The initial letter of each word is also marked in braille on each compartment.

Special considerations
• Family member or visiting nurse must remember to fill device with ordered medications at the beginning of each day.
• Not appropriate for large numbers of tablets or capsules

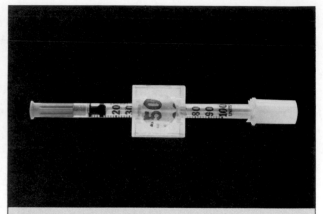

Monoject® Scale Magnifier

Purpose
To help a vision-impaired diabetic patient read syringe markings and independently fill his own syringe

Description
Plastic magnifier snaps onto syringe barrel

Special considerations
• May not be appropriate for an arthritic patient, who may have difficulty attaching the device

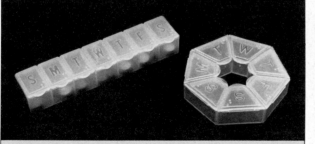

Seven-day Pill Reminder®

Purpose
To help the patient remember if he's taken all the tablets and capsules prescribed for each day of the week

Description
Both plastic devices shown here have seven medication compartments, marked with the initials for each day of the week (in both braille and visible letter characters).

Special considerations
• Family member or visiting nurse must remember to fill device with ordered medications at the beginning of each week.
• Not appropriate for large numbers of tablets and capsules, or tablets and capsules that must be taken at specific times each day
• Useful if patient takes a medication every other day, rather than daily

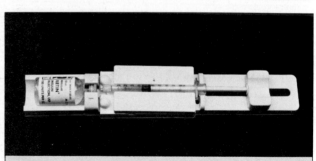

Dos-Aid Syringe Filling Device

Purpose
To precisely measure insulin doses; especially appropriate for a patient with vision impairment

Description
Plastic device designed for use with a disposable U-100 syringe and an insulin bottle. The device is set to accommodate the syringe's width; then the plunger is positioned at the point determined by the dose and the stop tightened. When set, the patient can draw up the precise dose ordered for each injection.

Special considerations
• Not for mixed or variable doses of insulin
• Settings must be checked and adjusted when syringe size or type is changed.
• Screws may become loose after repeated use of device; instruct the patient to regularly check them.
• Needle can be contaminated easily.

Using a bottle adapter and oral medication syringe

1 *If your patient must take daily doses of liquid medication, consider teaching a family member to use a special medication bottle adapter and oral medication syringe. Read the following photostory to learn how. Note:* An older patient will probably find capsules and tablets easier than liquid medications to administer correctly. Ask the doctor to prescribe oral medications in solid form, if possible.

The equipment shown here is made by Quanterron®, Inc. As you see, the medication syringe is marked in both teaspoons and milliliters.

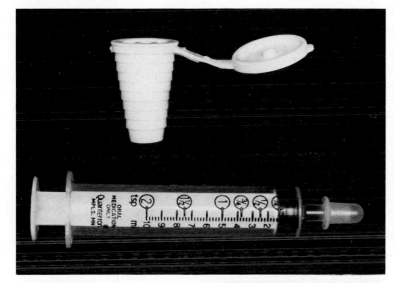

2 To use the adapter, first open the patient's medication bottle, and make sure the outside is clean and dry. Then, press the adapter's narrow end into the bottle with a downward, twisting motion (see arrow). Make sure it fits snugly. If it doesn't, remove it, rinse it with warm water, and try again.

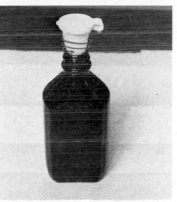

3 Now, remove the syringe cap. Draw back the plunger to the last marking on the syringe barrel.

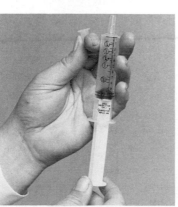

4 Open the adapter's cap, and insert the syringe tip into the adapter, as the nurse is doing here.

Completely depress the plunger, to inject air into the bottle.

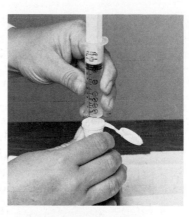

5 Next, invert the entire unit, and withdraw the prescribed amount of medication. *Important:* When teaching the family member this step, explain that he can ensure accurate medication measurement by looking at the top edge of the plunger's stopper from eye level.

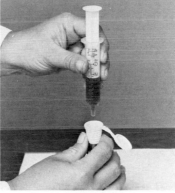

6 Place the bottle right side up and remove the syringe, as shown. Recap the bottle adapter.

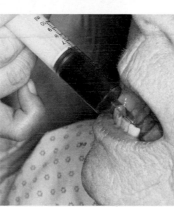

7 Give your patient her medication directly from the syringe, as shown here. Or, if she prefers, squirt the medication into a cup and give it to her. Then, thoroughly rinse the syringe with warm water.

Keep the adapter on the bottle until the bottle's empty. Then, discard the adapter with the empty bottle. Obtain a new adapter for each new bottle of medication.

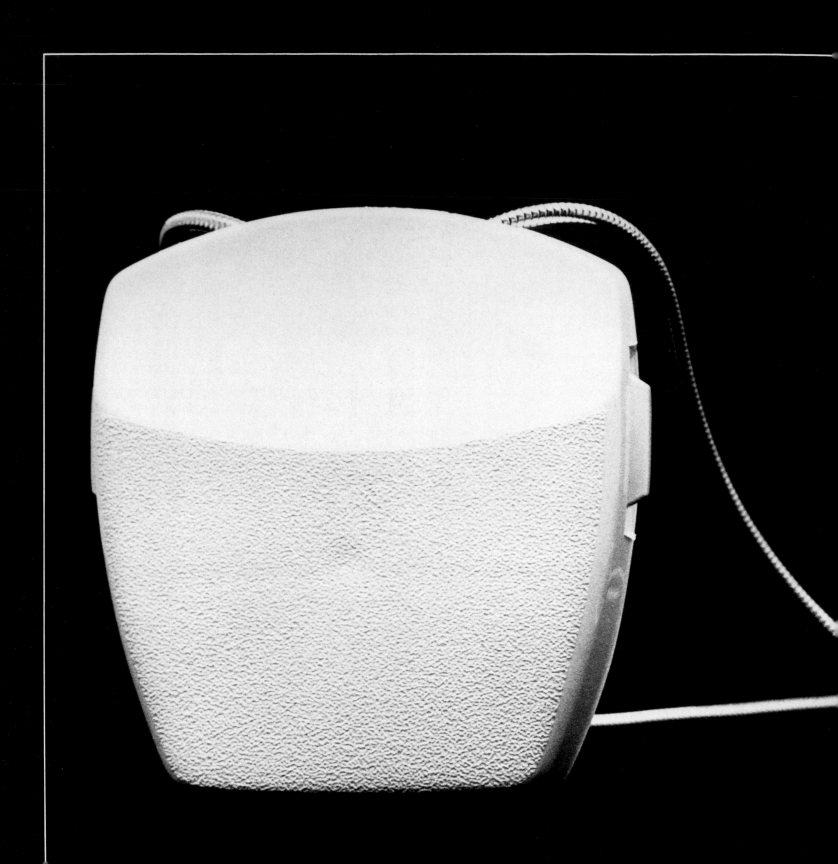

Providing Comfort and Protection

Restraints
Home adaptations
Special services
Nursing homes
Hospice care

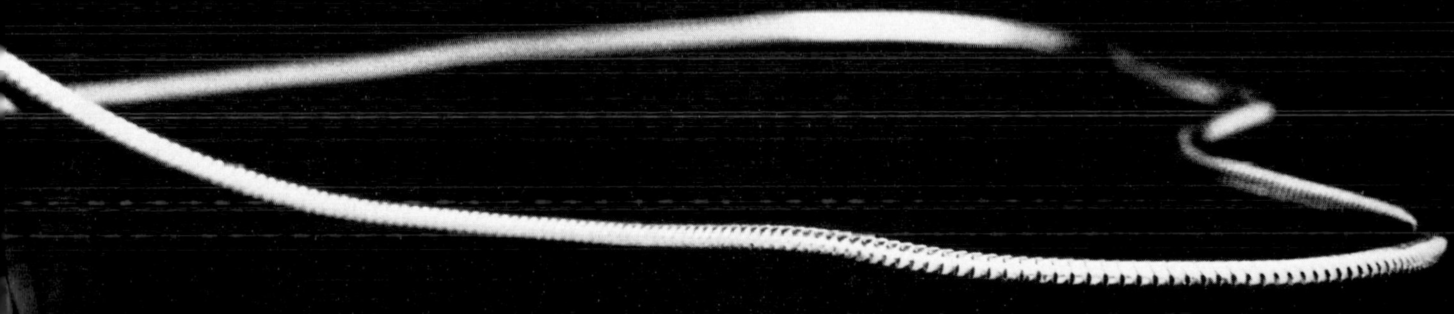

Restraints

Of course, you realize that you should never use restraints routinely. But do you know when to use them— and when not to? In the next few pages, we review some of the ways you can determine whether your patient needs these protective measures. We also outline alternatives to try *before* restraining him. And, we'll give you specific tips on two commonly used protective measures for your geriatric patient: the restraint vest and the geriatric chair.

SPECIAL CONSIDERATIONS

Finding alternatives to restraints

Restraints can never substitute for good nursing measures. Why? Because restraints jeopardize the rights, dignity, and privacy of your patient, and can intensify his anxiety and disorientation. Use protective measures, such as a restraint vest or geriatric chair, only as a last resort. If you must restrain your geriatric patient, apply the restraint properly and release it every 2 hours, to prevent additional problems. Of course, a restrained patient will require close observation and more attentive nursing care, because he'll be dependent on you to fulfill many of his basic needs (see page 142).

A geriatric patient's most likely to need restraints if he's become so disoriented or confused that he could accidentally harm himself. Sources for this disorientation include:
• medication
• environmental changes; for example, being hospitalized or losing a spouse
• acute physiologic problems, such as temperature elevation or electrolyte imbalance
• chronic conditions, such as cerebral arteriosclerosis or impaired renal function
• postoperative stress.

To evaluate your patient's disorientation level, check his orientation to person, time, and place. Ask him simple questions, such as these: Do you know who I am? Where you are? Why you're in the hospital? What day this is? Phrase your questions clearly and try to slant them to his cultural background. Take into account any special commmunication handicaps he has; for instance, lack of fluency in the language you're using, hearing or sight impediment, or preexisting memory problems. Check his hearing aid, if he wears one, to make sure it's turned on and working properly. Also, find out if he's supposed to be wearing glasses. And keep in mind that his speech may sound garbled if his dentures have been removed.

Document this assessment thoroughly with *specific* details about his disorientation. This will help you establish a consistent orientation program so that staff and family members can work together to reorient the patient. *Caution:* An inconsistent approach could disorient the patient even further.

You've completed an assessment and determined that your patient could harm himself. Before restraining him, try to reorient him. Here are some suggestions:
• Introduce and identify yourself each time you speak to him. Talk in a low-key, friendly tone. Make any gestures slowly to avoid frightening or threatening him.
• Explain all procedures to him, in a clear, concise manner, whether or not he appears to understand you.
• Make sure his call bell is always within reach. Answer the call bell as soon as possible. Try to answer him in person rather than over the intercom system.
• Be certain he has some links to the outside world, such as a radio, calendar, newspaper, clock, or watch. Check to see that all appliances and timepieces he has are in good working order.
• Encourage him to move and turn, which will help him reestablish physical reality. If he can't move himself, perform passive range-of-motion exercises.
• Correct your patient gently if he makes a mistake. Never agree with his error, which would only add to his disorientation. For example, if he mistakes you for his daughter, tell him who you actually are.

For a more controlled and consistent environment, consider following these guidelines:
• Involve family members in as many aspects of patient care as possible.
• Try to have the same nurses care for him regularly. Establish a consistent care plan for all nurses.
• Ask his family to bring in some of his belongings, such as personal clothing and toiletry articles. Have them bring in pictures; for example, of his loved ones or favorite pet.
• Use physical reminders to keep him in bed, such as propping a pillow between his body and the side rails.
• Arrange the room so your patient can see out his window or into the hall. If he can safely leave his bed, bring his chair into the doorway of his room, or put him close to the nursing station, where he can be part of the unit's activity.
• Visit his room often to reorient him and relieve his isolation. Encourage visits by friends, relatives, and other familiar staff members and hospital volunteers. Consider asking one family member to remain after the evening visiting hours to help bridge the transition to the late night hours.
• Reduce any disturbing noises, drafts, or shadows in his room. Keep a night-light on so he won't be confused by darkened objects.

If none of these measures work, and you're thoroughly convinced your patient's potentially dangerous to himself, then protect him with a restraint. Use the least amount of restraint necessary. Obtain a doctor's order before you apply any devices.

Familiarize yourself with the policy where you work regarding specific procedures for applying, checking, and removing a restraint. In an emergency, apply it first, and obtain an order as soon as possible afterward.

Applying a restraint vest

1 *Since entering the hospital, your patient has become disoriented at various times during the night. You've observed that she's unsteady on her feet and may fall. To remind her to stay in bed, you're going to apply a Medline® restraint vest and provide her with a call bell. This way, you can make sure you'll be present to help her out of bed.*

A restraint vest secures your patient at her waist, but allows her to sit up and turn on her side. If she's violent, you can also restrain her at the shoulders, using the loops attached to the shoulders of the vest.

Note: Be sure to obtain an order for the restraint. You can probably apply it by yourself. Secure assistance only when your patient's violent.

First, identify yourself to your patient. Then, slowly and carefully explain the restraint vest and why she needs to wear it. Next, seat her on the edge of the bed, unless contra-indicated. This permits easy access for applying the vest and allows her to help you, which should reduce any fear she has.

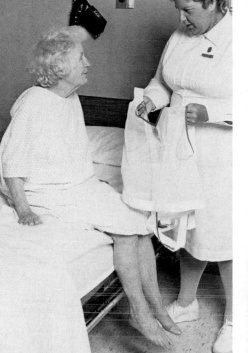

2 Now, make sure the vest is right-side out. Then, carefully slip your patient's arms through the arm holes.

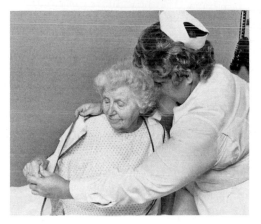

3 Next, pull the strap on the left side of the vest across the front of her body and through the loop at her waist on the right side.

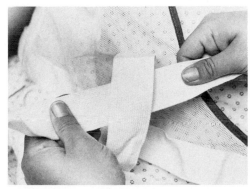

4 Now, help your patient lie down in bed. Then, grasp the strap and thread it through the bed frame. *Note:* Some frames are equipped with a space to loop the strap through. Make sure you secure the strap to the movable portion of the frame, so that when the head of the bed is elevated, the strap moves with it. Otherwise, the strap will pull on your patient, causing dis-comfort and possible injury.

Secure the strap with a knot, as shown here. Then, follow the same procedure on the other side of the bed.

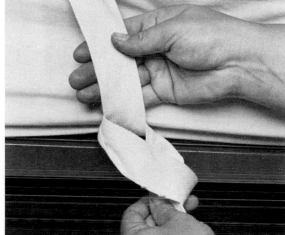

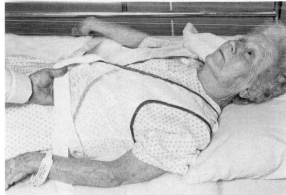

5 Check for tightness by sliding your hand between the vest and your patient's abdomen. Make sure the vest fits well enough to be effec-tive, but doesn't restrict respiration. Either tighten or loosen the straps, as indicated.

Next, elevate the head of the bed slightly and make sure your patient's comfortable. Then, give her the call bell, and remind her to use it whenever she needs assistance. Be sure both side rails are raised. Provide vigilant nursing care, as explained on the following page.

Finally, document the need for the restraint, each application and release, and your patient's tolerance of the restraint.

Restraints

Caring for a restrained patient

Have you put a restraint on your geriatric patient? If so, you must intensify your nursing care. Why? Because restraints take away his independence. You'll have to help him eat, drink, and go to the bathroom, all of which require extra time.

Consider the following as necessary steps in performing care:
• Periodically assess your patient's orientation level, to determine whether he still needs to be restrained.
• Explain to your patient and his family why you've restrained him. Remove the restraint when performing care and when the family's present. But make sure the family members understand that they must observe the patient closely and call you if any problems develop or before they leave him.
• Make sure your patient's bony prominences are padded under the restraint. Every 2 hours, release the restraint. Massage areas subject to pressure, such as the buttocks, heels, and elbows. Reassess your patient, and apply the restraint again only if necessary.
• Check pulses distal to the restraint frequently. Every hour, observe the area under the restraint for signs of abrasion or bruising. If his limbs are restrained, check them for position, alignment, and circulation. Never supplement the restraint by binding the patient with gauze or a sheet, which can constrict circulation when pulled taut.
• If your patient's struggling against his restraints, closely monitor him to make sure he doesn't become entangled or harm himself.
• Don't allow him to remain flat on his back for a long time. Release the restraint and change his position every 2 hours. Gently provide skin care, as needed.
• Ambulate him at least every 2 hours. If he can't ambulate, provide range-of-motion exercises every 2 hours to prevent contractures.
• Assist him to the bathroom every 2 hours or give him a bedpan or urinal. If he's incontinent, remember to wash him and change the linen, as necessary.
• If your patient must remain restrained, you'll have to feed him. If you can remove the restraint, stay with him and allow him to feed himself. Assist if necessary. Also, offer him fluids every 2 hours.

Do you know when to ask the doctor for an order to remove the restraint? As early as possible after your patient regains his self-control and orientation.

Explain to the patient what you'll be doing before removing the restraint. During the procedure, provide him with emotional support and carefully assess his behavior. Document the restraint removal and your patient's reaction to it in your nurses' notes.

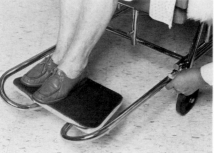

How to use a geriatric chair

1 *Have you ever had to use a geriatric chair? This protective equipment is especially useful for a disoriented geriatric patient who sometimes forgets that she needs assistance to walk.*

Before you place her in the chair, show it to her. Explain how the chair will protect her and how you'll position her in it. Next, lock the chair wheels, to secure it in place.

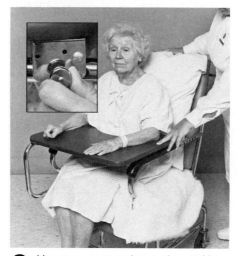

2 You may want to lay a sheepskin or a foam rubber square on the seat to minimize pressure on your patient's buttocks. Then, seat her gently. If she's very thin, place a pillow between her back and the chair for comfort and support.

Next, you'll position the tray. First have your patient raise her arms to avoid pinching them as you adjust the tray. Next, pull it out, and pivot it into position over her lap, as shown. Adjust it far enough away to permit her to move and breathe, but close enough to prevent her from sliding to the floor.

[Inset] Make sure you lock the tray in the appropriate adjustment hole so the tray can't be dislodged when the patient leans on it.

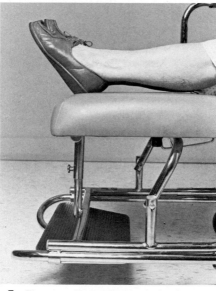

3 At least every 2 hours, change your patient's leg position. Alternate between dangling and elevated leg positions. To elevate her legs, first adjust the footstool outward.

4 Then, pull out and lock the legrest cushion. Next, elevate the legrest cushion to a height that's comfortable for your patient's legs, as shown.

You've positioned your patient comfortably in the chair. But, remember, never let the chair substitute for good nursing measures. Assess your patient frequently for any pressure areas. Assist her at mealtime, if necessary. Take her to the bathroom or provide a commode every 2 hours, or as needed. Also, ambulate her at least once every 2 hours to maintain her muscle strength, promote circulation, and provide an opportunity for her to observe and interact with her environment.

Be sure to document the reason why you're using the geriatric chair, how long she's seated each time, and how well she tolerates it.

Home adaptations

When your geriatric patient leaves the hospital and returns home, he and his family may need to make some household alterations for his safety and convenience. You'll help by assessing your patient's needs and referring him to the appropriate community agency. Then, a visiting nurse or community representative will evaluate his home to determine the adaptations that would best suit him.

On these two pages, we'll show you what a thorough home assessment includes. Study the following information carefully.

Assessing the home

In the blueprints below and on the following page are lists of questions to ask during a thorough home assessment. Areas that warrant special attention include the kitchen, bathroom, bedroom, and the exterior of the home.

Important: To avoid disorienting the patient, any changes made should be introduced gradually.

Interior (throughout)
• Does the home have a functioning phone?
• Does the phone have an enlarged dial (to accommodate the patient with limited vision)?
• Does the phone have an amplifier (to accommodate the patient with a hearing loss)?
• Are emergency phone numbers posted in a convenient location? Are they printed large enough to read easily?
• Are all phone wires located away from household traffic?
• Are the light bulbs bright enough to compensate for any limited vision?
• Are the stairways adequately lighted?

• Are sufficient night-lights installed?
• Are throw rugs anchored securely with rubber backing, or should they be removed completely?
• Are areas that might cause falls marked? For example, are step edges taped with brightly colored tape?
• Does each room have enough uncluttered space to permit easy mobility?
• Do the chairs and stools provide sufficient support for the patient?
• Are handrails securely fastened to walls or fixtures?
• Are pipes and radiators exposed?
• Is the furnace or heater functioning properly and vented adequately?
• Is the inside temperature within the comfortable range of 70° F. to 80° F. (21.1° C. to 26.7° C.)?
• Is the water heater temperature set at the safe level of 115° F. to 120° F. (46.1° C. to 48.9 C.)?
• Are electrical cords in good condition, and located away from household traffic?
• Do any potential firetraps exist?
• Is there a bathroom or portable commode on each floor the patient will use?

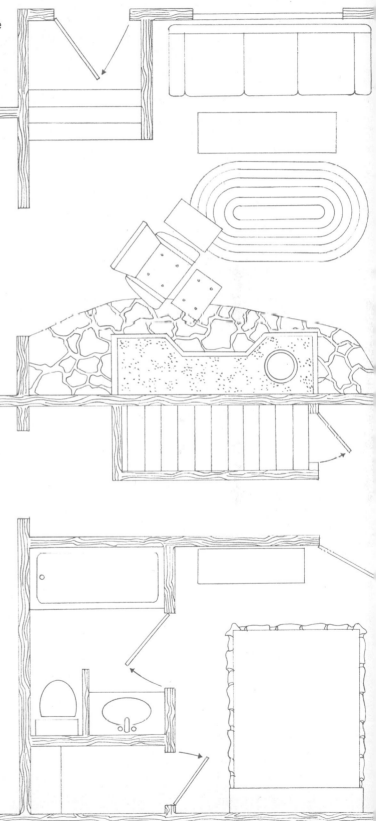

Home adaptations

Assessing the home continued

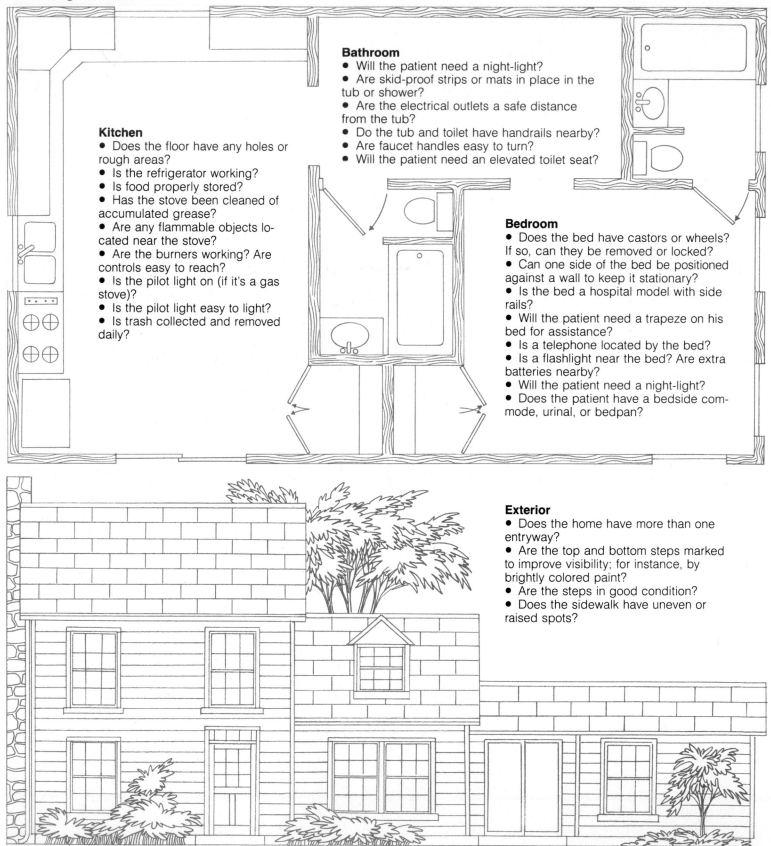

Kitchen
- Does the floor have any holes or rough areas?
- Is the refrigerator working?
- Is food properly stored?
- Has the stove been cleaned of accumulated grease?
- Are any flammable objects located near the stove?
- Are the burners working? Are controls easy to reach?
- Is the pilot light on (if it's a gas stove)?
- Is the pilot light easy to light?
- Is trash collected and removed daily?

Bathroom
- Will the patient need a night-light?
- Are skid-proof strips or mats in place in the tub or shower?
- Are the electrical outlets a safe distance from the tub?
- Do the tub and toilet have handrails nearby?
- Are faucet handles easy to turn?
- Will the patient need an elevated toilet seat?

Bedroom
- Does the bed have castors or wheels? If so, can they be removed or locked?
- Can one side of the bed be positioned against a wall to keep it stationary?
- Is the bed a hospital model with side rails?
- Will the patient need a trapeze on his bed for assistance?
- Is a telephone located by the bed?
- Is a flashlight near the bed? Are extra batteries nearby?
- Will the patient need a night-light?
- Does the patient have a bedside commode, urinal, or bedpan?

Exterior
- Does the home have more than one entryway?
- Are the top and bottom steps marked to improve visibility; for instance, by brightly colored paint?
- Are the steps in good condition?
- Does the sidewalk have uneven or raised spots?

Save $3.00 on each NURSING PHOTOBOOK™

Select your first book and examine it for 10 days FREE.

Subscribe to the NURSING PHOTOBOOK series and save $3.00 on every volume. That's a significant savings on the entire series. And select your own introductory volume from the books shown below.

10-DAY FREE TRIAL

PASS THIS CARD ON TO A COLLEAGUE

Use the card on the right to:

1. Save $3.00 on each book you buy by subscribing to the NURSING PHOTOBOOK series.

or

2. Buy a single selection without joining the series and pay only $18.95 (plus a small charge for shipping and handling).

Send no money with this order card.

Please send me the following volume as my introduction to the NURSING PHOTOBOOK series for a 10-day, free examination.

- ☐ *Caring for Surgical Patients* 76364
- ☐ *Giving Medications* 76406
- ☐ *Managing I.V. Therapy* 76497
- ☐ *Dealing with Emergencies* 76398
- ☐ *Providing Respiratory Care* 76455
- ☐ *Giving Cardiac Care* 76372

If I decide to keep this introductory volume, I agree to pay $15.95, plus shipping and handling. I understand that I will then receive another NURSING PHOTOBOOK approximately every other month, each on the same 10-day, free-examination basis. There is no minimum number of books I must buy, and I may cancel my subscription at any time simply by notifying you.

H1PB

I do not want the series at this time. Just send me:

- ___ *Caring for Surgical Patients* 74575
- ___ *Giving Medications* 74468
- ___ *Managing I.V. Therapy* 74401
- ___ *Dealing with Emergencies* 74476
- ___ *Providing Respiratory Care* 74492
- ___ *Giving Cardiac Care* 74658

I will pay $18.95 for each copy, plus shipping and handling. I've written how many copies of each book I want beside each title.

H1SP

Name _____ (Please print clearly)

Address _____

City _____ State _____ Zip _____

Price subject to change. Offer valid in U.S. only. © 1984 Springhouse Corporation

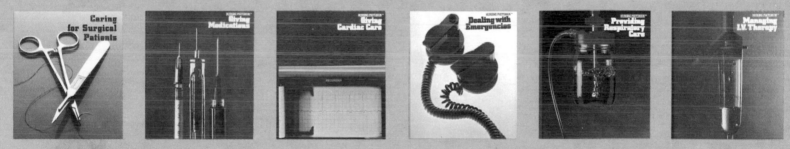

Caring for Surgical Patients · Giving Medications · Giving Cardiac Care · Dealing with Emergencies · Providing Respiratory Care · Managing I.V. Therapy

---

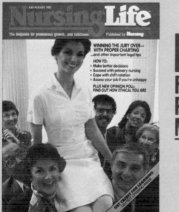

NEW! FROM THE PUBLISHER OF NURSING84®

Mail the postage-paid card at right. ▶

Introducing *NursingLife*®...

RETURN THIS CARD TODAY

the new journal all about "the other side" of nursing.

NursingLife is the new professional journal that gives you practical, workable solutions to the nursing situations you face every day. The legal risks. Getting along with doctors...other nurses...patients...administrators. Supervising others. Handling paperwork. Educational questions. Ethical questions. And more.

And *NursingLife* is published by the same people who bring you *Nursing84,* so you can be sure you'll always get reliable, expert advice you can put to use right away.

Subscribe for 2 years at the special-promotion price of $15.95. Mail the card today and receive an added bonus issue *at no cost!*

☐ Yes! Please send me the next issue of *NursingLife* and enter my 2-year trial subscription. Add the bonus issue to my subscription at no cost for ordering promptly.

Name _____

Address _____

City _____ State _____ Zip _____

NursingLife is published bimonthly. The single-copy price is $3 each, $18 per year.
Tax-deductible for nurses working in the U.S.

RPA3-6

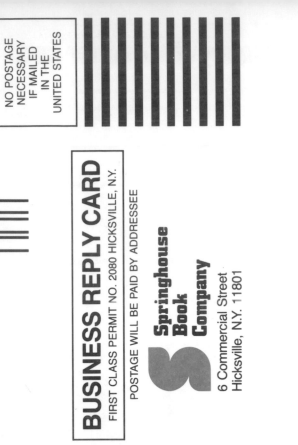
Get acquainted with the incomparable NURSING PHOTOBOOK series and learn important new procedures, step by step.

Hundreds of crystal-clear photographs, diagrams, sketches, and tables give you "how to" instructions quickly. The concise, clearly written text amplifies each highly detailed photostory.

The NURSING PHOTOBOOK series is a remarkable breakthrough in nursing education that can change your career. You actually watch experts at work. You'll learn how to • administer drugs safely • effectively teach your patient about his disorder and its treatment • minimize trauma • understand doctors' diagnoses • increase patient comfort • control pain • and much more.

Each handsomely bound PHOTOBOOK offers you 160 illustrated, fact-filled pages • brilliant, high-contrast photographs • convenient 9"x10½" size • durable hardcover binding • carefully chosen bibliography • complete index.

See for yourself how much you get out of this exciting series and how much your nursing will improve. Return the postage-paid card today.

© 1984 Springhouse Corporation

You can examine each NURSING PHOTOBOOK at your leisure...for 10 days *absolutely free.*

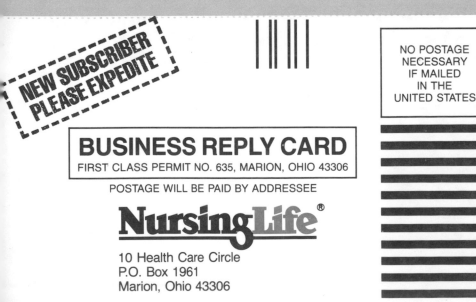
At last! A journal that helps you with "the other side" of nursing. The things they didn't (and couldn't) teach you in nursing school.

NursingLife tells you how to be a better nurse... how to find greater fulfillment in your career... how to grow on the job.

It's all about the skills today's nurses need to round out their professional lives.

Become a subscriber to this exciting new professional journal. Just tear off and mail this card today. There's no need to send money now. This is a no-obligation, free trial offer!

If order card is missing, send your order to:

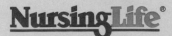

NursingLife ®

10 Health Care Circle
Marion, Ohio 43306

Special services

Mary Ogdin, age 73, was recently widowed. Although she has no debilitating health problems, her son's worried that she can't manage living alone. "Mother doesn't want to move in with me or go to a nursing home—she wants to stay in her own home," he says. "But I don't live close enough to help her every day. Do you have any suggestions?"

If a patient like Mrs. Ogdin wants to continue living independently, you can help. How? By informing her of the many community services available to older people. She and her family may be surprised—and reassured—to learn that considerable community support is available to help her maintain her independence. Of course, specific services vary among communities; here we'll give you an idea of commonly available ones.

You'll also learn about several protective devices your patient can use to make independent living as safe as possible, even if an emergency occurs.

Finally, we'll consider a tragic problem some elderly people face—financial exploitation and physical or emotional abuse by family members or other caretakers. In addition to teaching you how to assess such a problem, we'll provide guidelines for dealing with it.

Using community services
To help Mrs. Ogdin most effectively, you'll have to match her specific needs with the community services locally available.

As always, you must start with a careful assessment.

Assessing your patient
To pinpoint Mrs. Ogdin's needs, ask yourself the following questions:
• Does my patient have special or chronic health problems requiring medical or nursing care?
• Does she have health problems that limit vision, hearing, or mobility?
• Does she live alone?
• Does she live with another elderly person, such as her husband? (If so, consider his needs, too.)
• Has she recently lost a significant family member?
• Is she financially secure? Does she live on a fixed income?
• Does she need help finding or keeping decent housing?
• Does she need help keeping house and making meals?
• Can she easily perform routine chores outside the home, such as shopping and banking?
• Does she need legal help to protect her interests?
• Does she need emotional or psychological counseling?
• Does she have satisfying social and recreational outlets?
• Does she keep a pet for companionship? If so, does she need help caring for it?

Getting help
When you've identified your patient's needs, refer her to the appropriate agency or agencies. In many communities, all services for the aged are administered through one agency, such as an Office on the Aging. If so, that agency may publish a book or pamphlet listing services available. Obtain one, and help your patient select appropriate help.

In other communities, services are administered separately. Investigate local resources by checking the senior citizens listing in the telephone book's guide to human services. Or, contact your local government office or a local senior citizens' center for guidance.

Types of services widely available include:
• *Meal programs.* Meals on Wheels delivers at least one hot meal a day, 5 days a week, to homebound people who can't cook for themselves. Cost depends on each person's ability to pay and how the program's funded. Some programs will make special arrange-

ments to deliver meals throughout the weekend, if needed. Also, some Meals on Wheels programs provide special services, such as kosher meals and meals for diabetic patients. *Note:* Many senior citizens' and day-care centers provide free lunches.
• *Housing assistance.* If a patient on a fixed income is having difficulty finding—or keeping—decent housing, perhaps the local housing authority can help. A patient with a higher income may want to investigate a retirement community. Keep in mind, however, that most retirement communities won't accept residents who can't care for themselves. If your patient's severely disabled, a foster home may be a good alternative to a nursing home.
• *Legal assistance.* If your patient needs any kind of legal help, a variety of agencies, including the American Civil Liberties Union and the local public defender's office, can provide advice at little or no cost.
• *Protective services.* In states with protective service laws, protective service agencies can help an elderly person who's being abused by caretakers. For more information on protective services, see pages 148 and 149.
• *Health services.* You're already familiar with such agencies as visiting nurse associations. If your patient has a specific health problem, such as diabetes, heart and lung disease, cancer, or arthritis, she may also benefit from help available through an organization dealing specifically with her condition (for example, the American Heart Association). Also keep in mind that many hospitals and dental schools provide special low-cost services for older patients. And, if your patient needs emotional counseling, refer her to your community's mental health organization.
• *Transportation.* If your patient needs help getting to her grocery store, bank, or doctor's office, investigate whether low-cost, door-to-door transportation is available in your community.
• *Social and recreational organizations.* Social clubs, senior citizens' centers, and day-care centers can provide daily companionship for an older person who may otherwise be cut off from the community. In addition, most volunteer groups welcome the help of older people, providing them with even more opportunities to be socially active.

These are just a few of the services you may discover in your community. By drawing on these resources, your patient may be able to maintain an independent lifestyle. Now, read the following pages to learn about some protective devices that may also help your patient remain in the community.

Special services

Using an identification bracelet or necklace

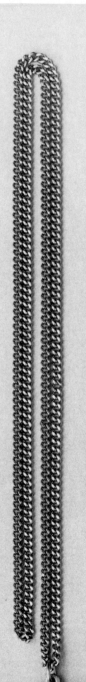

Richard McLeod, 82, hasn't let his age or his diabetes slow him down. Still active, he takes regular bus trips to see his brother, who lives 65 miles away. "My brother worries about me, though," he tells you. "He's afraid that I'll go into insulin shock during one of my bus rides, and no one will know what's wrong or how to help me."

For a patient like Mr. McLeod, independence is precious. But safeguarding his health is equally important. You may be able to help him satisfy both needs with an identification bracelet or necklace, like the Medic Alert™ tags shown here.

You'll probably recognize the Medic Alert emblem on the tag's front. It immediately alerts a rescuer that the patient has a special health problem. Engraved on the tag's back is the patient's health problem (for example, diabetes or hypertension), a 24-hour collect phone number, and the patient's special code number.

Of course, the amount of information that can be engraved on the tag is limited by the tag's small size. That's where the phone number comes in. By calling it and giving the special code number, a rescuer can obtain more detailed information about the patient; for example, his name and address, nearest relative, and personal doctor, as well as additional medical information.

Imagine how this identification tag could help Mr. McLeod. Insulin shock can cause confusion and unconsciousness—conditions commonly associated with senility or drunkenness. Such a mistake could be fatal. By alerting a rescuer to Mr. McLeod's medical problem, the tag may prevent delay of appropriate treatment.

Recommend an identification bracelet or necklace especially for any patient who has a medical problem or condition that may go unrecognized if he loses consciousness or can't speak for himself for any other reason.

Here are a few examples of Medic Alert messages:
- glaucoma
- implanted pacemaker
- heart condition
- allergic to penicillin
- epilepsy
- on hemodialysis
- wears contact lenses.

Note: A patient may also wear a Medic Alert bracelet even though he doesn't have a medical problem himself; for example, if he wants to be an organ donor.

How can your patient get one of these bracelets? Most pharmacists can give him an application. Help him complete it in as much detail as possible. Take care to list all medications he takes. (All information is confidential and divulged by Medic Alert only in an emergency.) Send the form, along with $15 for a lifetime membership, to Medic Alert Foundation International, P.O. Box 1009, Turlock, CA 95381-1009. *Note:* Medic Alert charges a small additional fee for updating the patient's medical file.

In about 1 month, he'll receive his tag and code number, as well as a wallet card containing pertinent medical information. Help him to carefully check his tag and card, to make sure all information is accurate. Then, urge him to wear his tag at all times, and to keep the card in his wallet.

Using a Body Guard® tag
As an alternative, your patient may wear a Body Guard bracelet or necklace. Although similar to Medic Alert jewelry, a Body Guard bracelet or necklace is designed to include the patient's name and address, for instant identification. Another difference is that the Body Guard system doesn't provide a rescuer with any more information than what's on the tag. For more information about this product, write to Body Guard, P.O. Box 747, Brigantine, NJ 08203.

Learning about the Vial of Life
Roberta Schuyler, 74, is a retired store manager who has terminal lung cancer. She lives at home with her husband, Thomas, who is 75. He's able to provide care for his wife, but what if something happened to him? As you can imagine, this couple would find an emergency difficult to cope with.

Think how they would benefit if a rescue crew knew the details of their medical histories, especially Roberta's. This information would help the crew begin appropriate treatment at once, saving precious minutes. Those minutes could make the difference between life and death.

Now, by participating in the Vial of Life program, any patient who lives in the community can place vital medical information—known medical conditions, medications, allergies, and blood type—at the fingertips of a rescue worker. If the Vial of Life program's in practice in your community, recommend this free, easy-to-use service to all your geriatric patients. To help your patients set up the system, follow the steps outlined in the photostory at right.

Using the Vial of Life

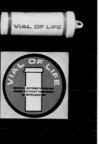

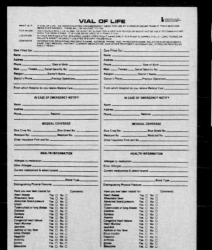

1 How can your patient participate in the Vial of Life program? All that's needed is a kit like the one shown here.

This kit contains a plastic vial, a medical information form (designed to record information about two people), a decal, and an instruction sheet (not shown). Help your patient obtain a kit through his pharmacist, doctor, visiting nurses' association, or a community services group. *Note:* If the program doesn't exist in your community, consider setting it up; then advise emergency personnel of the program. To obtain kits, contact Loral Packaging, Inc., 520 South Avenue, Garwood, NJ 07027.

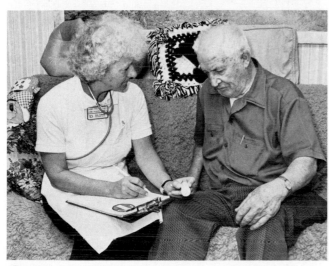

2 First, help the patient or family member fill out the information sheet, as the nurse is helping Mr. Schuyler do here. Be as thorough and detailed as possible. If necessary, write additional information on the back of the form. (Take care to note on the form's front that additional information appears on the back.)

3 Then, roll up the form, and place it inside the plastic vial. Firmly cap the vial.

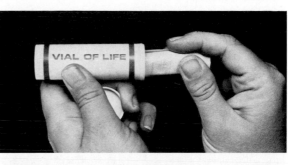

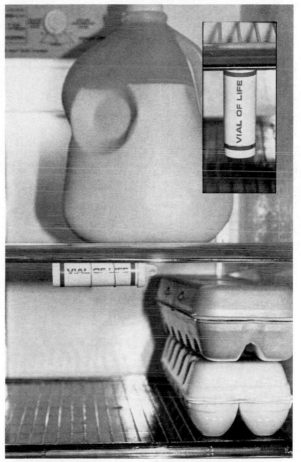

4 Now, using a rubber band, attach the vial to the right side of the refrigerator's top shelf. Or, hang it from the shelf's rung, as shown in the inset photo. To do this, just place the slit in the ring on the cap's top against the rung, and press firmly until the ring snaps in place around the rung.

Why place the vial in the refrigerator? Because nearly everybody has one. And most ambulance crews are trained to automatically check the refrigerator for a Vial of Life.

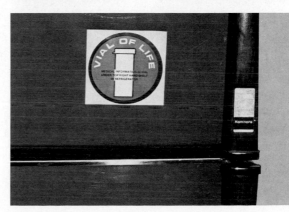

5 Finally, firmly attach the decal to the outside of the refrigerator door. This alerts the ambulance crew that a Vial of Life is inside. Remind the patient to avoid obscuring the decal with a shopping list or note.

Document your patient's use of the Vial of Life.

Special services

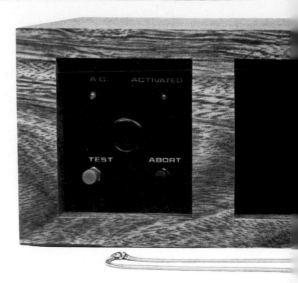

Learning about the Med-Alert system

Imagine this: Your neighbor, 81-year-old Millie Danoff, trips and falls in her living room, breaking her hip. She lives alone, and no one hears her call for help. Although her telephone is only a room away, next to her bed, that short distance seems like miles. Suppose she's unable to drag herself to the phone? She could lie helplessly on the floor for hours—even days.

As a nurse, you know that broken bones and other medical emergencies are a constant threat to the elderly. After imagining a situation like this, you may be tempted to advise Mrs. Danoff against living alone—even if it means giving up her own home.

An independent person like Mrs. Danoff may not even consider such a suggestion. Fortunately, an emergency alert system, like the Med-Alert system shown in the photo at right, provides an alternative.

Med-Alert is designed to electronically summon help in an emergency. To use it, Mrs. Danoff simply wears the plastic pendant around her neck or carries it in a pocket. In an emergency—for example, an accident, heart attack, stroke, or seizure—she squeezes the buttons on both side of the pendant. The pendant transmits a signal to a control console connected to Mrs. Danoff's phone. The console then

Dealing with elderly abuse

You're a visiting nurse. At least once a month, you call on 78-year-old Nell Golding to check her medications and answer any questions her family has about her care. Today, you're disturbed by Mrs. Golding's deteriorating condition. Formerly bright and alert, she's now quiet and apathetic. She seems to have lost weight, and you see signs of dehydration. You also observe that her clothing's damp and smells of urine and her skin's excoriated. Finally, you notice a developing pressure sore on her heel. Could Mrs. Golding's family be neglecting her?

As a nurse, you're familiar with the signs of child abuse, including neglect. But are you equally alert for signs of abuse when your patient's an older adult?

You should be. Although less well-documented, elderly abuse may be almost as prevalent as child abuse. For an elderly patient, as for an abused child, your assessment and intervention can be critical.

Recognizing an abused patient

Although patients in nursing homes and other institutions may suffer abuse, the typical abused adult lives in the community. She's most likely to be a Caucasian woman with at least one physical or mental disability. Her abuser is probably someone responsible for her care. The abuser may be a woman, because women are more likely than men to assume caretaker responsibilities.

An abused patient may suffer from one or more of these types of abuse:
• *Financial exploitation* includes outright theft (for example, of social security checks), fraud, and misuse of the patient's funds and property.
• *Psychological abuse* takes many forms: verbal abuse, coercion, or belittling; threats; and any other behavior that arouses fear and anxiety. Degrading the patient by treating her like a small child (which may include denying her sexuality) may also be a form of psychological abuse.

• *Physical abuse* includes violent assault (beating, shoving, jerking, pushing, burning), overmedication (or withholding necessary medication), sexual abuse, and neglect (for example, leaving a helpless patient unattended for long periods or neglecting to feed her).

Assessing the abused patient

If you suspect that your patient's abused in any way, conduct a thorough assessment that focuses on the signs of abuse. In addition to her physical condition, document your observations of the patient's environment and her interaction with the family. For example, does a caretaker change bed linens as often as necessary? How do family members treat her—with respect? Contempt? Or do they usually ignore her altogether?

Also, interview the patient—in private, so she's not intimidated or embarrassed by anyone. Use tactful, nonthreatening, and open-ended questions; for example, "Can you tell me what a typical day is like for you?" Other questions that may open the door to communication include:
• Has your family experienced any unusual difficulties lately?
• Who cares for you when your caretaker is at work?
• Who manages your finances for you?
• Do you have much contact with others outside your family?
• Do you eat regular meals?
• Do you think that your family has difficulty caring for you?
• If you had a choice, where would you most like to live?

Be prepared for possible resistance or denial of abuse by the patient, especially if you haven't yet established strong rapport with her. She may be reluctant to discuss abuse because of fear ("I'm afraid they'll put me in a nursing home"), guilt ("I know I'm a burden"), or shame ("How could I have raised such a disrepectful child?").

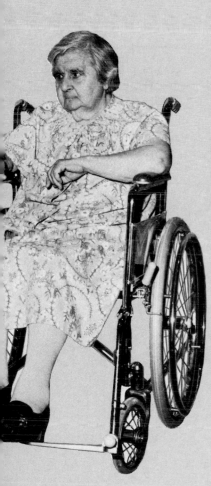

MED-ALERT SYSTEM

emits an audible distress signal; at the same time, it sends a specially coded emergency signal through the telephone lines to a 24-hour monitoring center. There, a computer identifies Mrs. Danoff and the location of her home. An operator immediately sends emergency assistance to Mrs. Danoff. From computer records, the operator can tell rescue workers where to find a house key and give specific information about Mrs. Danoff's particular health problems. The operator also notifies Mrs. Danoff's family members, her doctor, and other designated people. The entire sequence of events takes only moments.

As soon as help's on the way, the audible distress signal ceases. This tells Mrs. Danoff that someone is coming.

The console operates on household current. But, as a precaution against power failure, it also contains a self-recharging battery. The pendant is entirely battery-powered. Tell your patient to check and change the pendant battery as necessary.

Med-Alert can also be adapted for non-medical purposes; for example, it can summon help during a burglary or fire. For information, contact Emergency Life Saving Systems, Inc., Life Call Building, 80 Second Street Pike, Southampton, PA 18966.

She may also attempt to rationalize her treatment to protect her caretaker ("He's been under a lot of pressure lately"). Or, she may be too confused or depressed to accurately report abuse. That's why your thoroughly documented assessment—including your observations—is essential.

Important: Make every attempt to keep your assessment ongoing and up-to-date. If legal intervention is necessary, good documentation on your part is critical.

Identifying causes
If possible, interview your patient's caretaker in private. Remain calm, nonaccusatory, and nonjudgmental. Remember, the caretaker usually doesn't intend to be cruel. Suppose, for example, that you suspect he locks up the patient for hours each day. From his point of view, locking her up may be the only way to keep her from hurting herself while he goes to work.

As you talk with the caretaker, try to identify the reasons for the abuse. Possibilities include:
• Ignorance or disability. Does the caretaker understand what the patient needs? Perhaps he's unaware, for example, that a bedridden patient must be repositioned to prevent decubitus ulcers. Or, he may not realize that a junk food diet, however generous, may lead to malnutrition.

Also consider the caretaker's age and health. If he's caring for an elderly parent, he himself may be elderly and physically unable to provide adequate care.
• Stress. Taking an elderly parent into the home may cause considerable disruption for the parent's child and family. If the child must leave a job to care for a confused or bedridden parent, for example, he must cope with reduced income in addition to physical and emotional stress.
• Resentment. A child may take a parent into his home out of obligation or guilt. If so, resentment can easily grow, especially if the parent is demanding or requires continuous care.

• Poor family communication. Someone who's never been able to communicate well with his parents will probably have even more difficulty as the parent ages.
• Drugs and alcohol. A caretaker who abuses drugs or alcohol may be unable to responsibly care for an elderly patient.
• Revenge. The abuser may have been abused as a child. If so, abusing his parent may be a form of revenge.

Intervention
Base your intervention on your continuing assessment of the patient and his situation. If abuse is caused by ignorance or disability, patient/caretaker teaching or closer supervision by a visiting nurse may help.

If stress and resentment exist, refer caretakers to community resources that can relieve the burden—for example, day-care centers, foster-care programs, Meals on Wheels, and social agencies that offer family counseling. A part-time home-health aide may help, too. If the patient requires constant professional care, and the caretaker can't afford appropriate home care, urge him to consider an institution.

But if abuse is willful or extreme, or if the caretaker refuses your help, seek outside legal assistance. To do so, you first must know your state's laws about elderly abuse. If you live in a state with an Elderly Protective Service Act, begin by contacting a protective service agency for advice. If your state doesn't have such an act, learn what other legal remedies exist. For example, your state may have an Adult Abuse Act; although designed to protect marital abuse victims, its protection extends to the elderly.

Whatever the appropriate remedy, recognize and accept your limitations. If a competent patient refuses help, you can do little. But by recognizing abuse and taking appropriate steps, you can feel confident that you've done your best.

Nursing homes

When an older adult's condition keeps him from caring for himself independently, he may need the special care that a nursing home staff provides. On this page, we present some guidelines to help your patient and his family select the right nursing home for him.

Establishing criteria for choosing a nursing home

Before an older adult and his family discuss nursing-home care, they should first explore other options that may satisfy his needs. Keeping him out of an institution as long as possible by providing care at home can preserve his dignity and independence. As we explained on page 145, many communities have agencies that provide support services for the older adult.

However, he may require nursing home care if he reaches a point where he needs special attention that the family or community can no longer provide. If so, he and his family should perform a thorough search for a nursing home using *his preferences* as a guideline. Doing so will help minimize the impact of the ensuing lifestyle change.

The first step in the process is to identify the older adult's needs. Then, a preliminary list of homes can be investigated by applying these general criteria:
• Is the facility close enough for the family's easy access?
• Can the facility meet the patient's basic physical,

emotional, spiritual, and social requirements?
• Are different levels of care provided (residential, intermediate, skilled nursing) that can accommodate his changing needs?
• What is the ratio of professional to nonprofessional personnel? Is the staff large enough to provide full attention to each resident?
• How expensive is the care? Does the resident pay for all his care? Will the cost increase if he requires additional care?
• What provision is made for medical coverage, especially in an emergency?
• Does a working relationship exist with a local hospital, a mental-health facility, and an ambulance unit to provide services when needed?
• Does a working relationship exist with a home-health agency for discharge planning, if a temporary stay is anticipated?
• Who regulates the quality of the care? Is there a medical director? Is the director responsible for more facilities than this one?

Selecting the right nursing home

You've explained what your patient and his family should look for in a nursing home. But they need help in carrying out their search systematically. Advise them to take these steps:
• Prepare a list of homes that meet the patient's needs, according to criteria listed in the preceding story. To obtain the names of these homes, use these sources: hospital social service departments, visiting nurse associations, senior citizens' groups, social work agencies, churches, the local welfare family assistance office, and the local health department.
• Call the homes on your list and get details about the services and care you're looking for. Then, narrow down your list to those homes you want to visit.
• To arrange a visit, contact the admissions or social service department of each home. Try to schedule the visit during the late morning or midday hours, while

the noon meal is being served. Be sure to take the patient on the visit. Plan to spend at least an hour, and bring along a notepad and pen. During the visit, record your impressions, and ask as many questions as possible, including those suggested in the box below.
• Next, discuss with the patient the advantages and disadvantages of each facility, and narrow the choice to two or three.
• Visit these facilities again, but this time schedule the tour during the evening hours. Doing so will give you the opportunity to determine whether nighttime staffing is adequate. Overall, try to spend several hours at each facility.
• Finally, discuss with the patient the advantages and disadvantages of each facility. Draw up a list of these for use in making the final decision.

MINI-ASSESSMENT

Touring the nursing home

As the older adult and his family tour a nursing home, they'll want to assess the quality of care the facility offers, as well as its suitability for him personally. They can evaluate the nursing home by noting the following:
• What kind of services are offered? For example, does the facility provide occupational therapy, physical therapy, or reality orientation?
• Does each patient have an individual care plan to match his needs?
• What is the quality of the care? Are many residents physically restrained? Do residents appear sedated?

• What type of activities are offered? Do the activities provide opportunities for socializing? Do residents participate in and enjoy these activities?
• Does the food appear appetizing? Are menu choices available?
• Are the building exterior and grounds well-kept? How clean is the interior? Is an odor of feces or urine present?
• Are residents allowed to keep personal belongings, such as a rocking chair, photos, and plants?
• How good is the facility's fire-safety program?

By touring the home personally, the patient and his family can gather enough information to confidently make a good decision.

Hospice care

Undoubtedly, you've confronted death a number of times in your nursing career. But how many times have you helped a patient endure the terminal stages of disease? If you've had this experience, you'll remember his deep apprehension, the importance of pain control, and possibly, the family's or patient's difficulty accepting death.

At the time, you probably wished for a more personal way of dealing with this experience than a hospital setting allows. For some people, the hospice program offers a good alternative. Read the next few pages to find out how a hospice program helps some patients—and their families—live fully and cope successfully in the last stages of the patient's life.

Learning about the hospice program

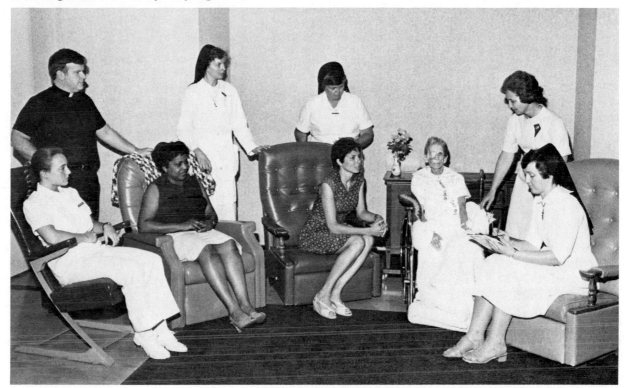

Your geriatric patient may be very healthy, considering the aging changes he's experienced. At age 65, he may well live for another 20 years. But death will eventually occur, and chances of it occurring from a slow chronic process, rather than a communicable disease, infection, or even accident, have been increasing steadily with medical advances.

A person who's aware that he's dying usually experiences three fears: fear of pain, fear of abandonment, and fear that his life has been meaningless. A geriatric patient may have already confronted these fears, as part of his emotional response to aging. Depending on his personality, previous losses (of friends, a close relative, and possibly of his own faculties) may have either strengthened his coping skills, or, conversely, weakened them. Either way, he'll need abundant support and encouragement to help him deal with the ultimate human experience of dying.

What can be done to meet his needs? One recently evolved solution is the hospice program. The avowed goal of such a program is to maintain the dignity of the dying person and his family throughout the dying process, as well as to help the family members through their period of bereavement. When a patient and family work within the hospice setting, they acknowledge that cure is no longer possible. The hospice focuses on improving the patient and family's comfort and well-being until death occurs, *rather than painful, stressful prolonging of life for its own sake.*

To carry out its goals, the hospice employs an interdisciplinary team of professionals and volunteers in a home, hospice institute, or hospice unit of a hospital.

Although a variety of hospice models exist, they all emphasize maintaining continuity of normal daily living by providing a homelike setting. The patient's own home is almost always preferred.

Here's a brief rundown of hospice working principles:
• providing care only at the patient's and family's express request
• caring for the patient and the family as an inseparable unit
• addressing the patient's and family's physical, emotional, and spiritual needs
• preventing distress from chronic signs and symptoms, especially pain
• working with the family as the central component of the hospice care team (or finding individuals who can substitute for the family, if necessary)
• including in the hospice care team (see photo) the patient, primary caregiver (usually a family member), doctor, nurses, social worker, hospice volunteer, clergy, nutritionist, homemaker/home-health aide, any other needed professionals (for example, an occupational therapist or physical therapist), and community agency staff members, as needed
• providing care 24 hours a day, 7 days a week
• extending hospice care into the family's bereavement period
• offering both formal and informal support for the hospice staff.

Of course, accurate assessment is a prerequisite for providing care. To find out more about your assessment responsibilities if you're caring for a patient in a hospice setting, read the text on the following pages.

Hospice care

Assessing the patient and family

Most nursing care requires assessment of the patient only. But, because hospice care addresses the patient and family as a unit, it necessitates an intimate understanding of the entire family—its fundamental values, key individuals, and communication patterns. You'll need to explore these important points: Are any family members especially close? Which members exert authority? Does one member act as the spokesperson? How does the family react to stress? What other stressors is it confronting beside a family member's approaching death? What support systems can it draw on? Are all family members geographically close, and do they have sufficient time and energy to care for a dying patient?

Obtaining the answers to these questions will take time. But the more you know, the more effective you'll be in helping family members help the patient—as well as themselves.

Now, consider your patient's needs. In addition to determining the role he plays in the family, you must assess his physical and emotional status. And remember, the family members' opinions are crucial, since they'll be providing most of his care. Assess him with a family member present. To do so, take a history and perform a physical assessment as outlined on pages 12 to 27. But place special emphasis on the following areas.

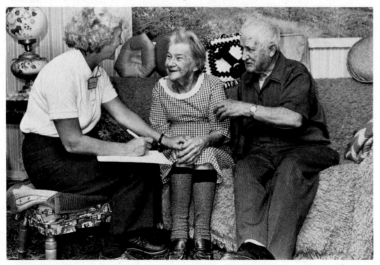

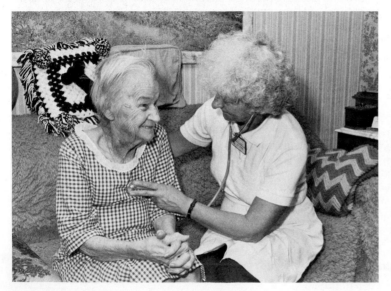

Pain

Most patients and their families request hospice care because they need help coping with the patient's most distressing symptom—pain. If uncontrolled, pain can reduce his existence to the single, all-absorbing experience of physical agony.

First ask your patient to describe his pain in detail. Then ask both patient and his family how pain affects him. Does it limit his activities, social interaction, ability to sleep, or appetite? Also, find out how the patient views his pain. Some patients see it as an unfortunate handicap, while others see it as an unfair burden imposed by fate, or even as a punishment for past offenses.

Finally, ask how the patient's been coping with his pain. Does he use distraction, relaxation, medication, or some combination of these approaches? Get specific information about his medication. Find out the drug name, dose, how often he takes it, and how well it works.

Develop a pain-management plan based on this assessment. (For more information on pain control, see page 154. Also see the NURSING PHOTOBOOK CARING FOR SURGICAL PATIENTS and the references at the end of this book.)

Nutrition

Assess your patient's nutritional status, following the guidelines on pages 92 and 93. But gear your assessment toward your patient's terminal condition. For example, you'll want to know if he can still eat his favorite foods. If not, does he have problems with some foods because his mouth is dry or because he has difficulty swallowing? Does he have a poor appetite? Does he feel nauseated? In addition to such normal aging changes as impaired taste, his disease, therapy, or depression can adversely affect his nutrition.

Also, keep in mind that eating is a family activity. A change in eating habits can disrupt the whole family's routine, and ultimately, their nutritional status.

Work with the family and patient to implement a good nutrition plan. Adequate nutrition will boost your patient's strength and energy and help improve his morale. *Note:* Restrictions imposed by a special diet (for example, a low-cholesterol diet), may become secondary for a dying patient. Curb any tendency on the family's part to be too strict with him, unless deviations from the diet definitely cause him problems. At this stage of his life, experiencing some pleasure from eating is probably more important than long-term dietary consequences.

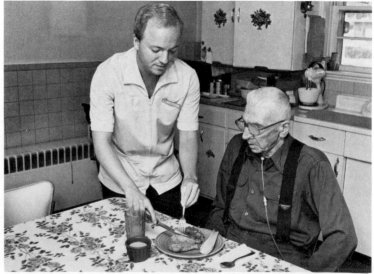

Sleep habits

Sleep habits may change as a person ages. And the pain or depression associated with a terminal illness can compound any existing sleep problems. Obviously, lack of sleep causes fatigue. But it can also contribute to lack of appetite, anxiety, confusion, nausea, and other physical symptoms, which will in turn perpetuate the initial sleeplessness.

Use the sleep assessment on page 14 to find out if your patient's sleep habits have changed. Does he feel he has a problem with insomnia? Does he keep other family members awake at night? What do he and the family think is depriving him of sleep—anxiety, pain, lack of activity, or some other cause?

Be sure to schedule the patient's care around his sleeping pattern. Except where pain management makes awakening him necessary, his sleep requirements should always come first. Keep in mind that very simple measures (as explained on page 14) can sometimes induce the relaxation necessary for sleep.

Elimination

Aging changes, as well as disease and medication, can affect your patient's bowel and urinary function. Use the assessment guidelines on pages 13, 97, and 105 to determine your patient's current elimination pattern. Adapt any bowel training program to allow for the patient's diminished food intake and limited mobility. Evaluate use of catheters and ostomy equipment. Reinforce any patient and family teaching necessary to care for these devices.

Skin condition

Skin breakdown is of particular concern in a terminally ill patient. In addition to reduced mobility, systemic conditions, such as diabetes, can adversely affect his skin. Assess the patient's and family's knowledge of skin care. If the patient's bedridden most of the day, teach family members how to reposition and ambulate him. Perhaps they wash him more vigorously or frequently than his aging skin can tolerate. Conversely, maybe they're neglecting to care for open sores or wounds because they don't know how. Also, sometimes family members avoid touching the patient, from an exaggerated sense of the dying person's fragility.

Activity level

Decreased activity can lead to such physical problems as constipation, insomnia, decreased appetite, skin breakdown, and poor circulation. But it can also compound emotional problems.

Find out how your patient's illness has affected his activity level.

What can he do for himself and what does he need help doing? How does he view his changed activity level? How active does he (and his family) think he should be? Does he remain as active as possible? For example, if he uses oxygen continuously, does he have portable oxygen equipment? *Note:* Sometimes the family overcompensates for a patient's reduced activity level. To be helpful, they perform all tasks for him, without realizing that they're undermining his self-esteem.

Emotional status

Coping with your terminally ill patient's physical problems may seem like a considerable challenge in itself. But, even if he hasn't been an emotionally expressive person in the past, this last phase is likely to elicit intense emotional responses. Anger, hostility, denial, and withdrawal are all typical—and understandable—reactions.

However, although these provide some immediate emotional satisfaction, they may serve to alienate the patient from his family, at a time when he most needs them. You'll have to help both patient and family understand his emotional reaction. First, try to determine how the illness has affected your patient's self-image. Does he feel he's draining the family's emotional and financial resources? Does he think they'll be better off without him? How does the family perceive and respond to his emotional changes? In addition to their concern for him, are they burdened by financial worries? Help the family identify resources they can draw on to meet expenses.

In providing emotional support, be prepared to help your patient and his family confront a series of difficult decisions. These may involve choosing to terminate such life-supporting treatment as chemotherapy. As the patient and family come to terms with these choices, they'll be working through the grieving process. For more information, see page 155.

Goals and intervention

How can you use your assessment findings most productively? By pooling them with information gathered by other members of the hospice team. First, of course, you'll discuss your findings and compare notes to make sure they're valid. Then, you'll formulate a realistic care plan and assign team responsibilities. Remember, both the patient and the family must agree on any goals set.

The level of professional involvement in hospice patient care varies, depending on the patient's needs and the family's receptiveness to outside influence. After all, *family* self-care is a primary goal of the hospice program.

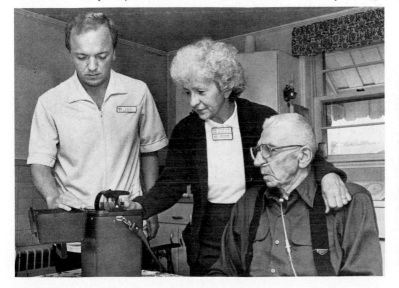

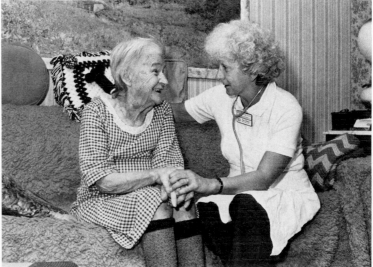

Hospice care

Managing your patient's pain

In managing pain, the goal is to relieve it *without oversedating or disorienting the patient.* A number of measures are available to control pain. For best results, you'll use them in combination, as ordered. *Important:* Be sure to use those your patient feels work best for her.

Consider adopting this three-point approach:
• Reduce the cause of pain.
• Intercept the painful stimulus.
• Influence the perception of pain.

In reducing the *cause of pain,* keep in mind that your patient may have some relatively minor condition (such as constipation, hemorrhoids, pain from poorly fitting dentures, or musculoskeletal aches from poor positioning), which complicates the pain from her primary problem. Thorough assessment will help you detect any such problem, so you can take steps to relieve it.

Also, you may need to administer such medications as antibiotics and anti-inflammatory agents to help reduce painful infection or inflammation. Sometimes surgery or irradiation may be required to relieve the primary cause of pain.

You can reduce or intercept the painful *stimulus* with cutaneous stimulation. For example, transcutaneous electronic nerve stimulation (TENS) overrides the painful stimulus. Warm- or cold-pack therapy and massage increases or reduces blood flow to the painful area, affecting stimulus reception and transmittal.

You can influence your patient's pain *perception* by giving her medication, as well as by distracting her with such activities as listening to music. Or, she can try self-hypnosis or a relaxation technique. Usually, some combination of these measures will prove most effective, rather than relying solely on medication.

However, for severe chronic pain, medication will be the foundation of the pain control program. To achieve the best results when using pain medi-

cation, keep these important points in mind.
• Be aware that the doctor may order aspirin or acetaminophen for mild pain; aspirin or acetaminophen plus codeine or oxycodone hydrochloride for moderate pain; methadone hydrochloride, morphine sulfate, or hydromorphone hydrochloride for severe pain; and morphine sulfate by continuous I.V. drip for intractable pain.
• Provide a continuous level of pain relief, to prevent awareness of pain from surfacing. That way, the medication doesn't have to overcome a present pain stimulus or the patient's memory of severe pain. When the patient becomes convinced that she'll get pain medication before she experiences pain, her anxiety will decrease. The lower her pain and anxiety levels, the lower the dosage necessary to relieve or prevent pain. *Note:* If the patient can sleep through the night without waking with severe pain, she may not require medication administered during the night. But awakening her to give medication is always preferable to her awakening in pain.
• Give medication orally rather than parenterally, if possible. You probably assume that intramuscular injections are more effective. But, they *can* be painful. And, eventually, the patient's injection sites may be exhausted. Also, intramuscular injections tend to foster the patient's psychological dependence on the person administering them.

Of course, oral dosages must be greater than parenteral doses, for equivalent results, because the medication's absorbed through the gastrointestinal tract, rather than directly into the bloodstream. But, when given in adequate dosages, oral medication can be just as effective. Although pain relief onset may be slower, around-the-clock pain-relief scheduling should make fast-acting injections unnecessary.

Keep in mind that you can

always use injections as a backup. Some patients may prefer a program of alternating oral and parenteral administration. Also, some patients *require* injections for adequate pain relief, as the patient shown here does.
• Try a nonnarcotic medication first, as ordered. If it proves inadequate to control the pain, the doctor will order a narcotic. However, the nonnarcotic shouldn't be discontinued. It can enhance the narcotic's effects on the central nervous system by providing peripheral nervous system pain relief.
• When using narcotics, try to keep side effects to a minimum. Sedation can be avoided by finding the precise effective dosage—one just high enough

to give continuous pain relief, but low enough to prevent drowsiness. Your careful assessment will help the doctor pinpoint this dosage. Avoid such side effects as constipation by administering stool softeners, as ordered, and adding fiber to the patient's diet. Giving phenothiazines will help control nausea as well as reducing anxiety, a major factor in pain intensity.
• Are you worried about your patient becoming addicted? For a terminally ill patient, physical dependency is much less important than adequate pain relief. If the patient's disease suddenly goes into remission, medication dosage can usually be reduced without ill effects.
• In helping the doctor deter-

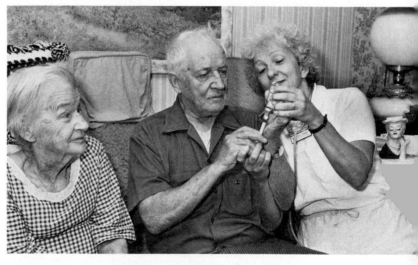

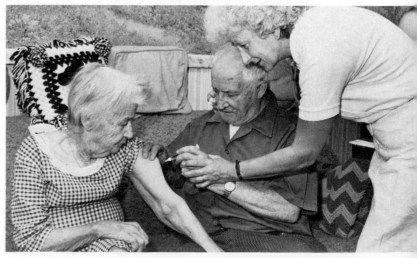

Acknowledgements

mine the correct dosage for your patient, take metabolic aging changes into consideration. Because a geriatric patient metabolizes drugs more slowly, she's more likely to experience adverse side effects.

• Keep in mind that emotional responses color pain perception. Long-term pain is almost always accompanied by anxiety and depression. Anxiety can increase muscle tension, aggravating pain. Depression often entails insomnia, which helps lower the pain threshold. Take steps to control these factors.

• Provide patient/family teaching, as necessary. Your patient may resist taking medication because she considers drug use a weakness, she fears addiction or developing a tolerance, she wants to avoid such unpleasant side effects as constipation, or she's had bad experiences with pain medication in the past. Try to build her confidence in medication use. The most effective argument will be the experience of continuous pain relief that a carefully implemented program can provide.

• If the patient's taking pain medication at home, help family members overcome any fear they may have of administering narcotics. Give the patient and family detailed information on the medication she's taking, including how it works, why she's taking it, and how to administer it. Help teach family members how to measure and administer medications correctly. Also, make them one of the charts described on pages 134 and 135 to ensure that doses are given in the right amounts—and on time.

• Remember, continuing assessment is crucial to the program's success. Medication effectiveness and side effects, as well as pain intensity, may change over time. The doctor will rely on your accurate assessment to adjust dosages, change medications, and provide other palliative measures, as necessary.

Assisting the grieving process

Grief is a normal reaction to any serious loss. The death of a family member will usually initiate a lengthy and deeply felt grieving process. This process involves immersion in and then recovery from the emotional pain associated with the patient's death. It should never be repressed or bypassed, or complete healing will probably not occur.

To successfully work through grieving, the patient and family must accomplish four major tasks. They must:
• experience grief and pain.
• accept the reality of loss (emotionally, not just intellectually).
• adjust to the idea of life without the deceased.
• emotionally disengage from the deceased after death and reinvest feelings in another person.

Important: These tasks may appear to apply solely to the family. But, the patient, if he is to be reconciled to his death, must also undertake the grieving process.

You can help the patient and family most by:
• promoting open and honest communication.
• providing emotional support.
• allowing the patient and family to express their feelings freely.
• reassuring the family that grief reactions are normal.
• making allowances for individual responses to grief as well as for differences in length of time the grieving process requires.
• reinforcing independence of family members after the patient's death.
• encouraging the bereaved to form new relationships.

We'd like to thank the following people and companies for their help with this PHOTOBOOK.

ABBEY MEDICAL
(formerly Accurate Medical Service)
Willow Grove, Pa.
Chuck Hepler
Manager

ACME UNITED CORPORATION
Medical Products Division
Bridgeport, Conn.
James F. Farrington
Senior Vice President, Marketing

AMERICAN FOUNDATION FOR
THE BLIND, INC.
New York, N.Y.
Alex H. Townsend
Consumer Resource Consultant

C.R. BARD, INC.
Bard Home Health Division
Berkeley Heights, N.J.

BELTONE ELECTRONICS CORPORATION
Chicago, Ill.
Lawrence Posen
President

BELTONE HEARING AID SERVICE
Warminster, Pa.
Robert Hirschbuhl
Director

BODY GUARD
Brigantine, N.J.
Tassy Brand
Designer

CLEO LIVING AID
Cleveland, Ohio
Shim Milder

EMERGENCY LIFE SAVING
SYSTEMS, INC.
Southampton, Pa.
Rudolph M. Wile
General Manager

FRED SAMMONS, INC.
Burr Ridge, Ill.

HEALTHDYNE, INC.
Marietta, Ga.

THE INDEPENDENCE FACTORY
Middletown, Ohio

MCNEIL PHARMACEUTICAL
A Johnson & Johnson Company
Springhouse, Pa.

MEDIC ALERT FOUNDATION
Turlock, Calif.

MEDLINE INDUSTRIES
Medcrest Division
Northbrook, Ill.
Jaimie Fankhanel
Product Manager

ROBBINS ASSOCIATES, INC.
Burnsville, Minn.

J. SKLAR MFG. CO., INC.
Long Island City, N.Y.

TEMCO HEALTHCARE INDUSTRIES, INC.
Passaic, N.J.
Alan Glatman
National Sales Manager

UNION CARBIDE CORPORATION
Moorestown, N.J.
Robert Jackson
Emergency Products

WELCH ALLYN, INC.
Skaneateles Falls, N.Y.
Douglas Hufnagle
Advertising Manager

WR MEDICAL ELECTRONICS CO.
St. Paul, Minn.

Evelina A. Bernardino, MD
St. Mary Hospital
Langhorne, Pa.

Joseph A. Bonanno, OD
The Eye Institute
Pennsylvania College of Optometry
Philadelphia, Pa.

Francis J. Connelly, Jr.
Ocularist
Philadelphia, Pa.

Also the staffs of:
BERKS VISITING NURSE HOME HEALTH
AGENCY
Supportive Care Group (hospice)
Reading, Pa.

ST. JOSEPH'S VILLA
Flourtown, Pa.
Sister St. Gregory, BS

VISITING NURSE ASSOCIATION OF
EASTERN MONTGOMERY COUNTY INC.
Abington, Pa.

Selected references

Books

Bates, Barbara. A GUIDE TO PHYSICAL EXAMINATION, 2nd ed. Philadelphia: J.B. Lippincott Co., 1979.

Birren, James E., and K. Warner Schaie. HANDBOOK OF THE PSYCHOLOGY OF AGING. New York: Van Nostrand Reinhold Co., 1977.

Bonner, Charles D. HOMBURGER AND BONNER'S MEDICAL CARE AND REHABILITATION OF THE AGED AND CHRONICALLY ILL, 3rd ed. Boston: Little, Brown, and Co., 1974.

Brocklehurst, J.C., ed. TEXTBOOK OF GERIATRIC MEDICINE AND GERONTOLOGY, 2nd ed. New York: Churchill-Livingstone, Inc., 1978.

Burnside, Irene M. NURSING AND THE AGED. New York: McGraw-Hill Book Co., 1976.

Carnevali, Doris L., and Maxine Patrick, eds. NURSING MANAGEMENT FOR THE ELDERLY. Philadelphia: J.B. Lippincott Co., 1979.

Carotenuto, Rosine, and John Bullock. PHYSICAL ASSESSMENT OF THE GERONTOLOGIC CLIENT. Philadelphia: F.A. Davis Co., 1980.

Christopherson, Victor A., et al. REHABILITATION NURSING: PERSPECTIVES AND APPLICATIONS. New York: McGraw-Hill Book Co., 1973.

COPING WITH NEUROLOGIC DISORDERS. Nursing Photobook Series. Springhouse, Pa.: Springhouse Corp., 1981.

Ebersole, Priscilla, and Patricia Hess. TOWARD HEALTHY AGING: HUMAN NEEDS AND NURSING RESPONSE. St. Louis: C.V. Mosby Co., 1981.

ELDER-ED: USING MEDICINES WISELY (DHEW Publication No. [ADM] 78-705). Washington, D.C.: U.S. Department of Health, Education, and Welfare, 1979.

Epstein, Charlotte. NURSING THE DYING PATIENT. Reston, Va.: Reston Publishing Co., Inc., 1975.

Forbes, Elizabeth Jane, and Virginia Marken Fitzsimons. THE OLDER ADULT: A PROCESS FOR WELLNESS. St. Louis: C.V. Mosby Co., 1981.

Hess, Patricia, and Candra Day. UNDERSTANDING THE AGING PATIENT. Bowie, Md.: The Robert J. Brady Co., 1977.

IMPLEMENTING UROLOGIC PROCEDURES. Nursing Photobook Series. Springhouse, Pa.: Springhouse Corp., 1981.

Kubler-Ross, Elisabeth, ed. DEATH: THE FINAL STAGE OF GROWTH. Englewood Cliffs, N.J.: Prentice-Hall, Inc., 1975.

Libow, Leslie S., and F.T. Sherman. THE CORE OF GERIATRIC MEDICINE: A GUIDE FOR STUDENTS AND PRACTITIONERS. St. Louis: C.V. Mosby Co., 1980.

Malasanos, Lois, et al. HEALTH ASSESSMENT, 2nd ed. St. Louis: C.V. Mosby Co., 1981.

NURSING DRUG HANDBOOK. Nursing84 Books. Springhouse, Pa.: Springhouse Corp., 1984.

Parad, Howard J., ed. CRISIS INTERVENTION: SELECTED READINGS. New York: Family Service Association of America, 1965.

Pegels, C. Carl. HEALTH CARE AND THE ELDERLY. Rockville, Md.: Aspen Systems Corp., 1981.

PROVIDING EARLY MOBILITY. Nursing Photobook Series. Springhouse, Pa.: Springhouse Corp., 1980.

Reichel, William. CLINICAL ASPECTS OF AGING. Baltimore: William and Wilkins Co., 1978.

Scheie, Harold G., and Daniel M. Albert. TEXTBOOK OF OPHTHALMOLOGY, 9th ed. Philadelphia: W.B. Saunders Co., 1977.

Skeist, Robert J. TO YOUR GOOD HEALTH: A PRACTICAL GUIDE FOR OLDER AMERICANS, THEIR FAMILIES AND FRIENDS. Chicago: Chicago Review Press, Inc., 1980.

Stoddard, Sandol. THE HOSPICE MOVEMENT: A BETTER WAY OF CARING FOR THE DYING. Briarcliff Manor, N.Y.: Stein and Day, 1977.

Stryker, Ruth. REHABILITATIVE ASPECTS OF ACUTE AND CHRONIC NURSING CARE, 2nd ed. Philadelphia: W.B. Saunders Co., 1977.

Yurick, Ann G., et al. THE AGED PERSON AND THE NURSING PROCESS. New York: Appleton-Century-Crofts, 1980.

Periodicals

Abdellah, F.G., et al. *PACE: An Approach to Improving the Care of the Elderly,* AMERICAN JOURNAL OF NURSING, 79:1109-1110, June 1979.

Allen, Marcia D. *Drug Therapy in the Elderly,* AMERICAN JOURNAL OF NURSING, 80:1474-1475, August 1980.

Anderson, Cheryl L. *Abuse and Neglect Among the Elderly,* JOURNAL OF GERONTOLOGICAL NURSING, 7:77-85, February 1981.

Beck, Cornelia M., and Doris Ferguson. *Aged Abuse,* JOURNAL OF GERONTOLOGICAL NURSING, 7:333-336, June 1981.

Bozian, M.W. *Symposium on on Gerontological Nursing: Nutrition for the Aged or Aged Nutrition?* NURSING CLINICS OF NORTH AMERICA, 11:169-177, March 1976.

Ellmyer, P., and N.J. Thomas. *A Guide to Your Patient's Safe Home Use of Oxygen,* NURSING82, 12:55-57, January 1982.

Falcioni, Denise. *Assessing the Abused Elderly,* JOURNAL OF GERONTOLOGICAL NURSING, 8:208-212, April 1982.

Hanan, Zachary I. *Geriatric Medication: How the Aged Are Hurt by Drugs Meant to Help, Part 1,* RN, 41:57-61, January 1978.

Heller, Barbara R., and Edward B. Gaynor. *Hearing Loss and Aural Rehabilitation of the Elderly,* TOPICS IN CLINICAL NURSING, 3:21-29, April 1981.

Holder, Lynnette. *Hearing Aids: Handle with Care,* NURSING82, 12:64-67, April 1982.

Isler, Charlotte. *Teaching the Elderly to Avoid Accidental Drug Abuse,* RN, 40:39-42, November 1977.

Jacox, A.K. *Assessing Pain,* AMERICAN JOURNAL OF NURSING, 79:895-900, May 1979.

Kavchak-Keyes, M.A. *Treating Decubitus Ulcers Using Four Proven Steps,* NURSING77, 7:44-45, October 1977.

Kroner, Kristine. *Dealing With the Confused Patient. Using Crisis Intervention Wisely,* NURSING79, 79:71-78, November 1979.

Kweskin, S. *Stroke: Early Care and Assessment,* PATIENT CARE, 13:28-29, January 30, 1979.

Kweskin, S. *Stroke: Mobilizing and Planning Therapy,* PATIENT CARE, 13:50-52, January 30, 1979.

Loomis, Jean, et al. *Discharge Planning: Good Planning Means Fewer Hospitalizations for the Chronically Ill,* NURSING81, 11:70-75, May 1981.

Meissner, J.E. *Assessing a Geriatric Patient's Need for Institutional Care: Tested Assessment Tools,* NURSING80, 10:86-87, March 1980.

O'Donnell, Lynne, and Bernice Papciak. *When All Else Fails: Continuous Morphine Infusion for Controlling Intractable Pain,* NURSING81, 11:68-72, August 1981.

Price, J.H. *Oral Health for the Geriatric Patient,* JOURNAL OF GERONTOLOGICAL NURSING, 5:25-29, March-April 1979.

Rovinski, Christine. *Hospice Nursing: Intensive Caring,* CANCER NURSING, 2:19-26, February 1979.

Sataloff, Robert T., and Lawrence A. Vassallo. *Choosing the Right Hearing Aid,* HOSPITAL PRACTICE, 16:32, May 1981.

Taylor, V.E. *Decubitus Prevention Through Early Assessment,* JOURNAL OF GERONTOLOGICAL NURSING, 6:389-391, July 1980.

Tichy, A.M., and L.J. Malasanos. *Physiological Parameters of Aging, Part 1* JOURNAL OF GERONTOLOGICAL NURSING, 5:42-46, January-February 1979.

Williams, E.J. *Food for Thought: Meeting the Nutritional Needs of the Elderly,* NURSING80, 10:60-63, September 1980.

Yen, P.K. *What is an Adequate Diet for the Older Adult?* GERIATRIC NURSING: AMERICAN JOURNAL OF CARE FOR THE AGING, 1:64, May-June 1980.

Index

Index